W9-AYX-973

CLINICIAN'S POCKET DRUG REFERENCE 2006

EDITORS

Leonard G. Gomella, MD, FACS
The Bernard W. Godwin, Jr., Professor
Chairman, Department of Urology
Jefferson Medical College
Thomas Jefferson University
Philadelphia, Pennsylvania

Steven A. Haist, MD, MS, FACP
Professor of Medicine
Division of General Medicine
Department of Internal Medicine
University of Kentucky Medical Center
Lexington, Kentucky

Aimee G. Adams, PharmD
Assistant Professor
College of Pharmacy and Department of Internal Medicine
Clinical Specialist, Primary Care
University of Kentucky Medical Center
Lexington, Kentucky

Kelly M. Smith, PharmD
Associate Professor
Department of Pharmacy Practice and Science
University of Kentucky College of Pharmacy
Clinical Specialist, Medication Use Policy
University of Kentucky Medical Center
Lexington, Kentucky

McGraw-Hill
MEDICAL PUBLISHING DIVISION

New York Chicago San Francisco Lisbon
London Madrid Mexico City Milan New Delhi
San Juan Seoul Singapore Sydney Toronto

The McGraw·Hill Companies

Clinician's Pocket Drug Reference 2006
Copyright © 2006 by Leonard G. Gomella. Published by The McGraw-Hill Companies, Inc. All rights reserved. Printed in Canada. Except as permitted under the United States Copyright Act of 1976, no part of this publication may be reproduced or distributed in any form or by any means, or stored in a data base or retrieval system, without the prior written permission of the publisher.

1 2 3 4 5 6 7 8 9 0   TRA/TRA   0 9 8 7 6 5

ISBN: 0-07-146024-1
ISSN: 1540-6725

The book was set in Times Roman by Pine Tree Composition, Inc.
The editors were Jim Shanahan and Harriet Lebowitz.
The senior production supervisor was Sherri Souffrance.
The text designer was Marsha Cohen/Parallelogram Graphics.
The indexer was Katherine Pitcoff.
Transcontinental Gagne was printer and binder.

This book is printed on acid-free paper.

CONTENTS

iii

PREFACE

We are pleased to present the fifth edition of the *Clinician's Pocket Drug Reference*. This book is based on the drug presentation style used since 1983 in the *Clinician's Pocket Reference*, popularly known as the Scut Monkey Book.

Our goal is to identify the most frequently used and clinically important medications based on input from our readers and editorial board. The book includes over 1000 generic medications and is designed to represent a cross section of those used in medical practices across the country.

The style of drug presentation includes key "must know" facts of commonly used medications, essential information for both the student and practicing physician. A unique feature is the inclusion of common uses of medications rather than just the official labeled indications. These recommendations are based on the actual uses of the medication supported by publications and community standards of care. All uses have been reviewed by our editorial board.

It is essential that students and residents in training learn more than the name and dose of the medications they prescribe. Certain common side effects and significant contraindications are associated with most prescription medications. Although health care providers should ideally be completely familiar with the entire package insert of any medication prescribed, such a requirement is unreasonable. References such as the *Physician's Desk Reference* and the drug manufacturer's Web site make package inserts readily available for many medications, but may not provide key data for generic drugs and those available over the counter.

The limitations of difficult-to-read package inserts were acknowledged by the Food and Drug Administration in early 2001, when it noted that physicians do not have time to read the many pages of small print in the typical package insert. In the future, package inserts will likely be redesigned to ensure that important drug interactions, contraindications, and common side effects are highlighted for easier practitioner reference. The editorial board has analyzed the information on both brand and generic medications and has made this key prescribing information available in this pocket-sized book. Information in this book is meant for use by health care professionals who are familiar with these commonly prescribed medications.

We are pleased about the popularity of the first four editions. This 2006 edition has been completely reviewed and updated by our editorial board. Over 30 new drugs have been added, and changes in other medications based on FDA actions have been incorporated. New to this edition is a section on commonly used and significant herbal and natural products and expanded cytochrome p450 interaction data.

We express special thanks to our spouses and families for their long-term support of this book and the entire Scut Monkey project. The contributions of the members of the editorial board are deeply appreciated. Linda Davoli, and the team at McGraw-Hill, have been supportive in our goal of creating this companion drug manual to the *Clinician's Pocket Reference*.

Your comments and suggestions are always welcome and encouraged because improvements to this and all our books would be impossible without the interest and feedback of our readers. We hope this book will help you learn some of the key elements in prescribing medications and allow you to care for your patients in the best way possible.

Leonard G. Gomella, MD, FACS
Philadelphia, PA
Leonard.Gomella@jefferson.edu

Steven A. Haist, MD, MS, FACP
Lexington, KY
sahaist@uky.edu

Aimee G. Adams, PharmD
Lexington, KY
argelh1@email.uky.edu

Kelly M. Smith, PharmD
Lexington, KY
ksmit1@email.uky.edu

MEDICATION KEY

Medications are listed by prescribing class, and the individual medications are then listed in alphabetical order by generic name. Some of the more commonly recognized trade names are listed for each medication (in parentheses after the generic name).

Generic Drug Name (Selected Common Brand Names [Controlled Substance]) **WARNING:** Summarized version of the "Black Box" precautions deemed necessary by the FDA. These are significant precautions and contraindications concerning the individual medication. **Uses:** This includes both FDA labeled indications bracketed by * and other "off label" uses of the medication. Because many medications are used to treat various conditions based on the medical literature and not listed in their package insert, we list common uses of the medication rather than the official "labeled indications" (FDA approved) based on input from our editorial board **Action:** How the drug works. This information is helpful in comparing classes of drugs and understanding side effects and contraindications. *Spectrum:* Specifies activity against selected microbes **Dose:** *Adults.* Where no specific pediatric dose is given, the implication is that this drug is not commonly used or indicated in that age group. At the end of the dosing line, important dosing modifications may be noted (ie, take with food, avoid antacids, etc) **Caution:** [pregnancy/fetal risk categories, breast-feeding (as noted above)] cautions concerning the use of the drug in specific settings **Contra:** Contraindications **Supplied:** Common dosing forms **SE:** Common or significant side effects **Notes:** Other key information about the drug.

CONTROLLED SUBSTANCE CLASSIFICATION

Medications under the control of the US Drug Enforcement Agency (Schedule I–V controlled substances) are indicated by the symbol [C]. Most medications are "uncontrolled" and do not require a DEA prescriber number on the prescription. The following is a general description of the schedules of DEA controlled substances:

Schedule (C-I) I: All nonresearch use forbidden (eg, heroin, LSD, mescaline, etc).

Schedule (C-II) II: High addictive potential; medical use accepted. No telephone call-in prescriptions; no refills. Some states require special prescription form (eg, cocaine, morphine, methadone).

Schedule (C-III) III: Low to moderate risk of physical dependence, high risk of psychologic dependence; prescription must be rewritten after 6 months or five refills (eg, acetaminophen plus codeine).

Schedule (C-IV) IV: Limited potential for dependence; prescription rules same as for schedule III (eg, benzodiazepines, propoxyphene).

Schedule (C-V) V: Very limited abuse potential; prescribing regulations often same as for uncontrolled medications; some states have additional restrictions.

FDA FETAL RISK CATEGORIES

Category A: Adequate studies in pregnant women have not demonstrated a risk to the fetus in the first trimester of pregnancy; there is no evidence of risk in the last two trimesters.

Category B: Animal studies have not demonstrated a risk to the fetus, but no adequate studies have been done in pregnant women.

or

Animal studies have shown an adverse effect, but adequate studies in pregnant women have not demonstrated a risk to the fetus during the first trimester of pregnancy and there is no evidence of risk in the last two trimesters.

Category C: Animal studies have shown an adverse effect on the fetus, but no adequate studies have been done in humans. The benefits from the use of the drug in pregnant women may be acceptable despite its potential risks.

or

No animal reproduction studies and no adequate studies in humans have been done.

Category D: There is evidence of human fetal risk, but the potential benefits from the use of the drug in pregnant women may be acceptable despite its potential risks.

Category X: Studies in animals or humans or adverse reaction reports, or both, have demonstrated fetal abnormalities. The risk of use in pregnant women clearly outweighs any possible benefit.

Category ?: No data available (not a formal FDA classification; included to provide complete data set).

BREAST-FEEDING

No formally recognized classification exists for drugs and breast-feeding. This shorthand was developed for the *Clinician's Pocket Drug Reference.*

+	Compatible with breast-feeding
M	Monitor patient or use with caution
±	Excreted, or likely excreted, with unknown effects or at unknown concentrations
?/–	Unknown excretion, but effects likely to be of concern
–	Contraindicated in breast-feeding
?	No data available

ABBREVIATIONS

Ab: antibody
ABMT: autologous bone marrow transplantation
ACE: angiotensin-converting enzyme
ACLS: advanced cardiac life support
ACS: acute coronary syndrome, American Cancer Society, American College of Surgeons
ADH: antidiuretic hormone
ADHD: attention-deficit hyperactivity disorder
ADR: adverse drug reaction
AF: atrial fibrillation
ALL: acute lymphocytic leukemia
ALT: alanine aminotransferase
AMI: acute myocardial infarction
AML: acute myelogenous leukemia
amp: ampule
ANC: absolute neutrophil count
aPTT: activated partial thromboplastin time
APAP: acetaminophen [*N*-acetyl-*p*-aminophenol]
ARB: angiotensin II receptor blocker
ARDS: adult respiratory distress syndrome
ASA: aspirin (acetylsalicylic acid)
AUC: area under the curve
AV: atrioventricular
AVM: arteriovenous malformation
BCL: B-cell lymphoma
BM: bone marrow; bowel movement

BMT: bone marrow transplantation
BOO: bladder outlet obstruction
BSA: body surface area
BUN: blood urea nitrogen
Ca: calcium
CA: cancer
CAD: coronary artery disease
CAP: cancer of the prostate
CBC: complete blood count
CCB: calcium channel blocker
CF: cystic fibrosis
CHF: congestive heart failure
CLL: chronic lymphocytic leukemia
CML: chronic myelogenous leukemia
CMV: cytomegalovirus
Contra: contraindicated
COPD: chronic obstructive pulmonary disease
CP: chest pain
CPP: central precocious puberty
CR: controlled release
CrCl: creatinine clearance
CRF: chronic renal failure
CV: cardiovascular
CVA: cerebrovascular accident, costovertebral angle
CVH: common variable hypergammaglobulinemia
D: diarrhea
D_5LR: 5% dextrose in lactated Ringer's solution
D_5NS: 5% dextrose in normal saline

D$_5$W: 5% dextrose in water
D/C: discontinue
DI: diabetes insipidus
DKA: diabetic ketoacidosis
dL: deciliter
DM: diabetes mellitus
DMARD (Dz-modifying
    antirheumatic drug)
DN: diabetic nephropathy
dppr: dropper
DVT: deep venous thrombosis
Dz: disease
EC: enteric-coated
ECC: emergency cardiac care
ECG: electrocardiogram
ED: erectile dysfunction
ELISA: enzyme-linked
    immunosorbent assay
EMIT: enzyme-multiplied
    immunoassay text
EPS: extrapyramidal symptoms
ESRD: end-stage renal disease
ET: endotracheal
EtOH: ethanol
FSH: follicle-stimulating hormone
5-FU: fluorouracil
Fxn: function
G-CSF: granulocyte colony-
    stimulating factor
gen: generation
GERD: gastroesophageal reflux
    disease
GF: growth factor
GFR: glomerular filtration rate
GI: gastrointestinal
GIST: Gastrointestinal stromal tumor
GM-CSF: granulocyte-macrophage
    colony-stimulating factor
GnRH: gonadotropin-releasing
    hormone
gt, gtt: drop, drops (*gutta*)
HA: headache

HCL: hairy cell leukemia
Hct: hematocrit
HCTZ: hydrochlorothiazide
HD: hemodialysis
Hgb: hemoglobin
HIT: heparin-induced
    thrombocytopenia
HIV: human immunodeficiency
    virus
HMG-CoA: hydroxymethylglutaryl
    coenzyme A
hs: at bedtime (*hora somni*)
HSV: herpes simplex virus
5-HT: 5-hydroxytryptamine
HTN: hypertension
Hx: history of
IBD: irritable bowel disease
IBS: irritable bowel syndrome
ICP: intracranial pressure
Ig: immunoglobulin
IM: intramuscular
Infxn: infection
Inh: inhalation
INH: isoniazid
INR: international normalized ratio
intravag: intravaginal
ISA: intrinsic sympathomimetic
    activity
IT: intrathecal
ITP: idiopathic thrombocytopenic
    purpura
IV: intravenous
K: potassium
LDL: low-density lipoprotein
LFT: liver function test
LH: luteinizing hormone
LHRH: luteinizing hormone-
    releasing hormone
LMW: low molecular weight
LVD: left ventricular dysfunction
LVSD: left ventricular systolic
    dysfunction

MAC: *Mycobacterium avium* complex

MAO/MAOI: monoamine oxidase/inhibitor

mEq: milliequivalent

MI: myocardial infarction, mitral insufficiency

mL: milliliter

MoAb: monoclonal antibody

MRSA: methicillin-resistant *Staphylococcus aureus*

MS: multiple sclerosis

MSSA: methicillin-sensitive *Staphylococcus aureus*

MTT: monotetrazolium

MTX: methotrexate

MyG: myasthenia gravis

N: nausea

NA: narrow angle

ng: nanogram

NG: nasogastric

NHL: non-Hodgkin's lymphoma

NIDDM: non-insulin-dependent diabetes mellitus

nl: normal

NPO: nothing by mouth (*nil per os*)

NRTI: nucleoside reverse transcriptase inhibitor

NS: normal saline

NSAID: nonsteroidal antiinflammatory drug

NSCLC: non-small-cell lung cancer

N/V: nausea and vomiting

N/V/D: nausea, vomiting, diarrhea

OAB: overactive bladder

OCP: oral contraceptive pill

OD: overdose

OK: recommended

OTC: over the counter

PAT: paroxysmal atrial tachycardia

pc: after eating (*post cibum*)

PCN: penicillin

PCP: *Pneumocystis jiroveci* (formerly *carinii*) pneumonia

PCWP: pulmonary capillary wedge pressure

PDGF: platelet-derived growth factor

PE: pulmonary embolus, physical examination, pleural effusion

PFT: pulmonary function test

pg: picogram

PID: pelvic inflammatory disease

plt: platelet

PMDD: premenstrual dysphoric disorder

PO: by mouth (*per os*)

PPD: purified protein derivative

PR: by rectum

PRG: pregnancy

PRN: as often as needed (*pro re nata*)

PSVT: paroxysmal supraventricular tachycardia

pt: patient

PT: prothrombin time

PTCA: percutaneous transluminal coronary angioplasty

PTH: parathyroid hormone

PTT: partial thromboplastin time

PUD: peptic ulcer disease

PVC: premature ventricular contraction

PWP: pulmonary wedge pressure

q: every (*quaque*)

q_h: every _ hours

qd: every day

qh: every hour

qhs: every hour of sleep (before bedtime)

qid: four times a day (*quater in die*)

qod: every other day

RA: rheumatoid arthritis

RCC: renal cell carcinoma

RDA: recommended dietary allowance

RDS: respiratory distress syndrome
resp: respiratory
RSV: respiratory syncytial virus
RT: reverse transcriptase
RTA: renal tubular acidosis
Rx: treatment
Rxn: reaction
SCr: serum creatinine
SIADH: syndrome of inappropriate
   antidiuretic hormone
SL: sublingual
SLE: systemic lupus erythematosus
soln: solution
SPAG: small particle aerosol
   generator
Sp: species
SQ: subcutaneous
SSRI: selective serotonin reuptake
   inhibitor
SSS: sick sinus syndrome
S/Sys: signs & symptoms
stat: immediately (*statim*)
supl: supplement
supp: suppository
SVT: supraventricular tachycardia
Sx: symptom
Sz: seizure
tab/tabs: tablet/tablets

TB: tuberculosis
TCA: tricyclic antidepressant
TTS: transdermal therapeutic system
TFT: thyroid function test
TIA: transient ischemic attack
tid: three times a day (*ter in die*)
TMP: trimethoprim
TMP—SMX: trimethoprim—
   sulfamethoxazole
tox: toxicity
TPA: tissue plasminogen activator
tri: trimester
TTP: thrombotic thrombocytopenic
   purpura
uln: upper limits of normal
URI: upper respiratory infection
UTI: urinary tract infection
VF: ventricular fibrillation
VRE: vancomycin-resistant
   Enterococcus
VT: ventricular tachycardia
WHI: Women's Health Initiative
WNL: within normal limits
WPW: Wolff—Parkinson—White
   syndrome
XR: extended release
ZE: Zollinger—Ellison (syndrome)

CLASSIFICATION (Generic and common brand names)

ALLERGY

Antihistamines

Azelastine (Astelin, Optivar)
Cetirizine (Zyrtec, Zyrtec D)
Chlorpheniramine (Chlor-Trimeton)

Clemastine Fumarate (Tavist)
Cyproheptadine (Periactin)
Desloratadine (Clarinex)
Diphenhydramine (Benadryl)

Fexofenadine (Allegra)
Hydroxyzine (Atarax, Vistaril)
Loratadine (Claritin, Alavert)

Miscellaneous Antiallergy Agents

Budesonide (Rhinocort, Pulmicort)

Cromolyn Sodium (Intal, NasalCrom, Opticrom)

Montelukast (Singulair)

ANTIDOTES

Acetylcysteine (Acetadote, Mucomyst)
Amifostine (Ethyol)
Charcoal (Superchar, Actidose, Liqui-Char Activated)

Dexrazoxane (Zinecard)
Digoxin Immune Fab (Digibind)
Flumazenil (Romazicon)
Ipecac Syrup (OTC Syrup)

Mesna (Mesnex)
Naloxone (Narcan)
Physostigmine (Antilirium)
Succimer (Chemet)

ANTIMICROBIAL AGENTS

Antibiotics

AMINOGLYCOSIDES

Amikacin (Amikin)
Gentamicin (Garamycin, G-Mycitin)

Neomycin
Streptomycin

Tobramycin (Nebcin)

CARBAPENEMS

Ertapenem (Invanz)

Imipenem–Cilastatin (Primaxin)

Meropenem (Merrem)

CEPHALOSPORINS, FIRST GENERATION

Cefadroxil (Duricef, Ultracef)

Cefazolin (Ancef, Kefzol)

Cephalexin (Keflex, Keftab)

Cephradine (Velosef)

CEPHALOSPORINS, SECOND GENERATION

Cefaclor (Ceclor)

Cefmetazole (Zefazone)

Cefonicid (Monocid)

Cefotetan (Cefotan)

Cefoxitin (Mefoxin)

Cefprozil (Cefzil)

Cefuroxime (Ceftin [oral], Zinacef [parenteral])

Loracarbef (Lorabid)

CEPHALOSPORINS, THIRD GENERATION

Cefdinir (Omnicef)

Cefditoren (Spectracef)

Cefixime (Suprax)

Cefoperazone (Cefobid)

Cefotaxime (Claforan)

Cefpodoxime (Vantin)

Ceftazidime (Fortaz, Ceptaz, Tazidime, Tazicef)

Ceftibuten (Cedax)

Ceftizoxime (Cefizox)

Ceftriaxone (Rocephin)

CEPHALOSPORINS, FOURTH GENERATION

Cefepime (Maxipime)

FLUOROQUINOLONES

Ciprofloxacin (Cipro)

Gatifloxacin (Tequin)

Gemifloxacin (Factive)

Levofloxacin (Levaquin, Quixin Ophthalmic)

Lomefloxacin (Maxaquin)

Moxifloxacin (Avelox)

Norfloxacin (Noroxin, Chibroxin Ophthalmic)

Ofloxacin (Floxin, Ocuflox Ophthalmic)

Sparfloxacin (Zagam)

Trovafloxacin (Trovan)

MACROLIDES

Azithromycin (Zithromax)

Clarithromycin (Biaxin)

Dirithromycin (Dynabac)

Erythromycin (E-Mycin, E.E.S., Ery-Tab)

Erythromycin & Sulfisoxazole (Eryzole, Pediazole)

KETOLIDE

Telithromycin (Ketek)

PENICILLINS

Amoxicillin (Amoxil, Polymox)
Amoxicillin & Clavulanic Acid (Augmentin)
Ampicillin (Amcill, Omnipen)
Ampicillin–Sulbactam (Unasyn)
Dicloxacillin (Dynapen, Dycill)

Mezlocillin (Mezlin)
Nafcillin (Nallpen)
Oxacillin (Bactocill, Prostaphlin)
Penicillin G, Aqueous (Potassium or Sodium) (Pfizerpen, Pentids)
Penicillin G Benzathine (Bicillin)

Penicillin G Procaine (Wycillin)
Penicillin V (Pen-Vee K, Veetids)
Piperacillin (Pipracil)
Piperacillin–Tazobactam (Zosyn)
Ticarcillin (Ticar)
Ticarcillin/Potassium Clavulanate (Timentin)

TETRACYCLINES

Doxycycline (Vibramycin)

Tetracycline (Achromycin V, Sumycin)

Tigecycline (Tygacil)

Miscellaneous Antibiotic Agents

Aztreonam (Azactam)
Clindamycin (Cleocin, Cleocin-T)
Fosfomycin (Monurol)
Linezolid (Zyvox)
Metronidazole (Flagyl, MetroGel)

Quinupristin–Dalfopristin (Synercid)
Rifaximin (Xifaxan)
Trimethoprim–Sulfamethoxazole [Co-Trimoxazole] (Bactrim, Septra)

Vancomycin (Vancocin, Vancoled)

Antifungals

Amphotericin B (Fungizone)
Amphotericin B Cholesteryl (Amphotec)
Amphotericin B Lipid Complex (Abelcet)
Amphotericin B Liposomal (AmBisome)

Caspofungin (Cancidas)
Clotrimazole (Lotrimin, Mycelex)
Clotrimazole & Betamethasone (Lotrisone)
Econazole (Spectazole)
Fluconazole (Diflucan)
Itraconazole (Sporanox)
Ketoconazole (Nizoral)

Miconazole (Monistat)
Nystatin (Mycostatin)
Oxiconazole (Oxistat)
Sertaconazole (Ertaczo)
Terbinafine (Lamisil)
Triamcinolone & Nystatin (Mycolog-II)
Voriconazole (VFEND)

Antimycobacterials

Clofazimine (Lamprene)
Dapsone (Avlosulfon)
Ethambutol
 (Myambutol)

Isoniazid (INH)
Pyrazinamide
Rifabutin (Mycobutin)
Rifampin (Rifadin)

Rifapentine (Priftin)
Streptomycin

Antiprotozoals

Nitazoxanide (Alinia)

Tinidazole (Tindamax)

Antiretrovirals

Abacavir (Ziagen)
Amprenavir (Agenerase)
Delavirdine (Rescriptor)
Didanosine [ddI] (Videx)
Efavirenz (Sustiva)
Fosamprenavir (Lexiva)
Indinavir (Crixivan)
Lamivudine (Epivir,
 Epivir-HBV)

Lopinavir/Ritonavir
 (Kaletra)
Nelfinavir (Viracept)
Nevirapine (Viramune)
Ritonavir (Norvir)
Saquinavir (Fortovase)
Stavudine (Zerit)
Tenofovir (Viread)

Tenofovir/Emtricitabine
 (Truvada)
Zalcitabine (Hivid)
Zidovudine (Retrovir)
Zidovudine &
 Lamivudine
 (Combivir)

Antivirals

Acyclovir (Zovirax)
Adefovir (Hepsera)
Amantadine (Symmetrel)
Atazanavir (Reyataz)
Cidofovir (Vistide)
Emtricitabine (Emtriva)
Enfuvirtide (Fuzeon)
Famciclovir (Famvir)
Foscarnet (Foscavir)

Ganciclovir (Cytovene,
 Vitrasert)
Interferon Alfa-2b &
 Ribavirin Combo
 (Rebetron)
Oseltamivir (Tamiflu)
Palivizumab (Synagis)
Peg Interferon Alfa 2a
 (Pegasys)

Penciclovir (Denavir)
Ribavirin (Virazole)
Rimantadine
 (Flumadine)
Valacyclovir (Valtrex)
Valganciclovir (Valcyte)
Zanamivir (Relenza)

Miscellaneous Antimicrobial Agents

Atovaquone (Mepron)
Atovaquone/Proguanil
 (Malarone)

Daptomycin (Cubicin)
Pentamidine (Pentam
 300, NebuPent)

Trimetrexate (Neutrexin)

ANTINEOPLASTIC AGENTS

Alkylating Agents

Altretamine (Hexalen)
Busulfan (Myleran, Busulfex)
Carboplatin (Paraplatin)

Cisplatin (Platinol)
Oxaliplatin (Eloxatin)
Procarbazine (Matulane)

Triethylenetriphosphamide (Thio-Tepa, Tespa, TSPA)

NITROGEN MUSTARDS

Chlorambucil (Leukeran)
Cyclophosphamide (Cytoxan, Neosar)

Ifosfamide (Ifex, Holoxan)
Mechlorethamine (Mustargen)

Melphalan [L-PAM] (Alkeran)

NITROSOUREAS

Carmustine [BCNU] (BiCNU, Gliadel)

Streptozocin (Zanosar)

Antibiotics

Bleomycin Sulfate (Blenoxane)
Dactinomycin (Cosmegen)

Daunorubicin (Daunomycin, Cerubidine)
Doxorubicin (Adriamycin, Rubex)

Epirubicin (Ellence)
Idarubicin (Idamycin)
Mitomycin (Mutamycin)

Antimetabolites

Clofarabine (Clolar)
Cytarabine [ARA-C] (Cytosar-U)
Cytarabine Liposome (DepoCyt)
Floxuridine (FUDR)

Fludarabine Phosphate (Flamp, Fludara)
Fluorouracil [5-FU] (Adrucil)
Gemcitabine (Gemzar)
Mercaptopurine [6-MP] (Purinethol)

Methotrexate (Folex, Rheumatrex)
Pemetrexed (Alimta)
6-Thioguanine [6-TG] (Tabloid)

Hormones

Anastrozole (Arimidex)
Bicalutamide (Casodex)
Estramustine Phosphate (Estracyt, Emcyt)
Exemestane (Aromasin)

Fluoxymesterone (Halotestin)
Flutamide (Eulexin)
Fulvestrant (Faslodex)
Goserelin (Zoladex)
Leuprolide (Lupron, Viadur, Eligard)

Levamisole (Ergamisol)
Megestrol Acetate (Megace)
Nilutamide (Nilandron)
Tamoxifen (Nolvadex)
Triptorelin (Trelstar Depot, Trelstar LA)

Mitotic Inhibitors

Etoposide [VP-16] (VePesid)

Vinblastine (Velban, Velbe)

Vincristine (Oncovin, Vincasar PFS)

Vinorelbine (Navelbine)

Monoclonal Antibodies

Cetuximab (Erbitux)

Erlotinib (Tarceva)

Trastuzumab (Herceptin)

Miscellaneous Antineoplastic Agents

Aldesleukin [Interleukin-2, IL-2] (Proleukin)
Aminoglutethimide (Cytadren)
L-Asparaginase (Elspar, Oncaspar)
BCG [Bacillus Calmette-Guérin] (TheraCys, Tice BCG)
Bevacizumab (Avastin)
Bortezomib (Velcade)
Cladribine (Leustatin)

Dacarbazine (DTIC)
Docetaxel (Taxotere)
Gefitinib (Iressa)
Gemtuzumab Ozogamicin (Mylotarg)
Hydroxyurea (Hydrea, Droxia)
Imatinib (Gleevec)
Irinotecan (Camptosar)
Letrozole (Femara)
Leucovorin (Wellcovorin)

Mitoxantrone (Novantrone)
Paclitaxel (Taxol, Abraxane)
Pemetrexed (Alimta)
Rasburicase (Elitek)
Thalidomide (Thalomid)
Topotecan (Hycamtin)
Tretinoin, Topical [Retinoic Acid] (Retin-A, Avita, Renova)

CARDIOVASCULAR (CV) AGENTS

Aldosterone Antagonist

Eplerenone (Inspra)

Alpha$_1$-Adrenergic Blockers

Doxazosin (Cardura)

Prazosin (Minipress)

Terazosin (Hytrin)

Angiotensin-Converting Enzyme (ACE) Inhibitors

Benazepril (Lotensin)
Captopril (Capoten)
Enalapril (Vasotec)
Fosinopril (Monopril)

Lisinopril (Prinivil, Zestril)
Moexipril (Univasc)
Perindopril Erbumine (Aceon)

Quinapril (Accupril)
Ramipril (Altace)
Trandolapril (Mavik)

Angiotensin II Receptor Antagonists

Candesartan (Atacand)
Eprosartan (Teveten)
Irbesartan (Avapro)
Losartan (Cozaar)
Telmisartan (Micardis)
Valsartan (Diovan)

Antiarrhythmic Agents

Adenosine (Adenocard)
Amiodarone (Cordarone, Pacerone)
Atropine
Digoxin (Lanoxin, Lanoxicaps)
Disopyramide (Norpace, NAPamide)
Dofetilide (Tikosyn)
Esmolol (Brevibloc)
Flecainide (Tambocor)
Ibutilide (Corvert)
Lidocaine (Anestacon Topical, Xylocaine)
Mexiletine (Mexitil)
Procainamide (Pronestyl, Procan)
Propafenone (Rythmol)
Quinidine (Quinidex, Quinaglute)
Sotalol (Betapace, Betapace AF)

Beta-Adrenergic Blockers

Acebutolol (Sectral)
Atenolol (Tenormin)
Atenolol & Chlorthalidone (Tenoretic)
Betaxolol (Kerlone)
Bisoprolol (Zebeta)
Carteolol (Cartrol, Ocupress Ophthalmic)
Carvedilol (Coreg)
Labetalol (Trandate, Normodyne)
Metoprolol (Lopressor, Toprol XL)
Nadolol (Corgard)
Penbutolol (Levatol)
Pindolol (Visken)
Propranolol (Inderal)
Timolol (Blocadren)

Calcium Channel Antagonists

Amlodipine (Norvasc)
Diltiazem (Cardizem, Cartia XT, Dilacor, Diltia XT, Tiamate, Tiazac)
Felodipine (Plendil)
Isradipine (DynaCirc)
Nicardipine (Cardene)
Nifedipine (Procardia, Procardia XL, Adalat, Adalat CC)
Nimodipine (Nimotop)
Nisoldipine (Sular)
Verapamil (Calan, Isoptin)

Centrally Acting Antihypertensive Agents

Clonidine (Catapres)
Methyldopa (Aldomet)

Diuretics

Acetazolamide (Diamox)
Amiloride (Midamor)
Bumetanide (Bumex)
Chlorothiazide (Diuril)
Chlorthalidone (Hygroton)
Furosemide (Lasix)
Hydrochlorothiazide (HydroDIURIL, Esidrix)
Hydrochlorothiazide & Amiloride (Moduretic)

Hydrochlorothiazide &
  Spironolactone
  (Aldactazide)
Hydrochlorothiazide &
  Triamterene (Dyazide,
  Maxzide)

Indapamide (Lozol)
Mannitol
Metolazone (Mykrox,
  Zaroxolyn)
Spironolactone
  (Aldactone)

Torsemide (Demadex)
Triamterene (Dyrenium)

Inotropic/Pressor Agents

Digoxin (Lanoxin,
  Lanoxicaps)
Dobutamine (Dobutrex)
Dopamine (Intropin)
Epinephrine (Adrenalin,
  Sus-Phrine, EpiPen)

Inamrinone (Inocor)
Isoproterenol (Isuprel)
Milrinone (Primacor)
Nesiritide (Natrecor)
Norepinephrine
  (Levophed)

Phenylephrine (Neo-
  Synephrine)

Lipid-Lowering Agents

Atorvastatin (Lipitor)
Cholestyramine
  (Questran,
  LoCHOLEST)
Colesevelam (Welchol)
Colestipol (Colestid)

Ezetimibe (Zetia)
Fenofibrate (Tricor)
Fluvastatin (Lescol)
Gemfibrozil (Lopid)
Lovastatin (Mevacor,
  Altocor)

Niacin (Niaspan)
Pravastatin (Pravachol)
Rosuvastatin (Crestor)
Simvastatin (Zocor)

Lipid-Lowering/Antihypertensive Combos

Amlodipine/Atorvastatin
  (Caduet)

Vasodilators

Alprostadil
  [Prostaglandin E_1]
  (Prostin VR)
Epoprostenol (Flolan)
Fenoldopam (Corlopam)
Hydralazine
  (Apresoline)
Iloprost (Ventavis)
Isosorbide Dinitrate
  (Isordil, Sorbitrate,
  Dilatrate-SR)

Isosorbide Mononitrate
  (Ismo, Imdur)
Minoxidil (Loniten,
  Rogaine)
Nitroglycerin (Nitrostat,
  Nitrolingual, Nitro-
  Bid Ointment, Nitro-
  Bid IV, Nitrodisc,
  Transderm-Nitro)
Nitroprusside (Nipride,
  Nitropress)

Tolazoline (Priscoline)
Treprostinil Sodium
  (Remodulin)

CENTRAL NERVOUS SYSTEM AGENTS

Antianxiety Agents

Alprazolam (Xanax)
Buspirone (BuSpar)
Chlordiazepoxide (Librium, Mitran, Libritabs)
Clorazepate (Tranxene)

Diazepam (Valium)
Doxepin (Sinequan, Adapin)
Hydroxyzine (Atarax, Vistaril)
Lorazepam (Ativan)

Meprobamate (Equanil, Miltown)
Oxazepam (Serax)

Anticonvulsants

Carbamazepine (Tegretol)
Clonazepam (Klonopin)
Diazepam (Valium)
Ethosuximide (Zarontin)
Fosphenytoin (Cerebyx)
Gabapentin (Neurontin)

Lamotrigine (Lamictal)
Levetiracetam (Keppra)
Lorazepam (Ativan)
Oxcarbazepine (Trileptal)
Pentobarbital (Nembutal)
Phenobarbital

Phenytoin (Dilantin)
Tiagabine (Gabitril)
Topiramate (Topamax)
Valproic Acid (Depakene, Depakote)
Zonisamide (Zonegran)

Antidepressants

Amitriptyline (Elavil)
Bupropion (Wellbutrin, Zyban)
Citalopram (Celexa)
Desipramine (Norpramin)
Doxepin (Sinequan, Adapin)

Duloxetine (Cymbalta)
Escitalopram (Lexapro)
Fluoxetine (Prozac, Sarafem)
Fluvoxamine (Luvox)
Imipramine (Tofranil)
Mirtazapine (Remeron)
Nefazodone (Serzone)

Nortriptyline (Aventyl, Pamelor)
Paroxetine (Paxil)
Phenelzine (Nardil)
Sertraline (Zoloft)
Trazodone (Desyrel)
Venlafaxine (Effexor)

Antiparkinson Agents

Amantadine (Symmetrel)
Apomorphine (Apokyn)
Benztropine (Cogentin)
Bromocriptine (Parlodel)

Carbidopa/Levodopa (Sinemet)
Entacapone (Comtan)
Pergolide (Permax)
Pramipexole (Mirapex)

Ropinirole (Requip)
Selegiline (Eldepryl)
Tolcapone (Tasmar)
Trihexyphenidyl (Artane)

Antipsychotics

Aripiprazole (Abilify)
Chlorpromazine (Thorazine)

Clozapine (Clozaril)
Fluphenazine (Prolixin, Permitil)

Haloperidol (Haldol)
Lithium Carbonate (Eskalith, Lithobid)

Mesoridazine (Serentil)
Molindone (Moban)
Olanzapine (Zyprexa)
Perphenazine (Trilafon)

Prochlorperazine
(Compazine)
Quetiapine (Seroquel)
Risperidone (Risperdal)
Thioridazine (Mellaril)

Thiothixene (Navane)
Trifluoperazine
(Stelazine)
Ziprasidone (Geodon)

Sedative Hypnotics

Chloral Hydrate
(Aquachloval,
Supprettes)
Diphenhydramine
(Benadryl)
Estazolam (ProSom)
Eszopiclone (Lunesta)

Flurazepam (Dalmane)
Hydroxyzine (Atarax,
Vistaril)
Midazolam (Versed)
Pentobarbital
(Nembutal)
Phenobarbital

Propofol (Diprivan)
Quazepam (Doral)
Secobarbital (Seconal)
Temazepam (Restoril)
Triazolam (Halcion)
Zaleplon (Sonata)
Zolpidem (Ambien)

Miscellaneous CNS Agents

Atomoxetine (Strattera)
Galantamine (Reminyl)
Memantine (Namenda)

Nimodipine (Nimotop)
Rivastigmine (Exelon)

Sodium Oxybate (Xyrem)
Tacrine (Cognex)

DERMATOLOGIC AGENTS

Acitretin (Soriatane)
Acyclovir (Zovirax)
Alefacept (Amevive)
Anthralin (Anthra-Derm)
Amphotericin B
(Fungizone)
Bacitracin, Topical
(Baciguent)
Bacitracin & Polymyxin
B, Topical (Polysporin)
Bacitracin, Neomycin, &
Polymyxin B, Topical
(Neosporin Ointment)
Bacitracin, Neomycin,
Polymyxin B, &
Hydrocortisone,
Topical (Cortisporin)
Bacitracin, Neomycin,
Polymyxin B, &

Lidocaine, Topical
(Clomycin)
Calcipotriene (Dovonex)
Capsaicin (Capsin,
Zostrix)
Ciclopirox (Loprox)
Ciprofloxacin (Cipro)
Clindamycin (Cleocin)
Clotrimazole &
Betamethasone
(Lotrisone)
Dibucaine (Nupercainal)
Doxepin, Topical
(Zonalon)
Econazole (Spectazole)
Efalizumab (Raptiva)
Erythromycin, Topical
(A/T/S, Eryderm,
Erycette, T-Stat)

Finasteride (Proscar,
Propecia)
Gentamicin, Topical
(Garamycin,
G-Mycitin)
Haloprogin (Halotex)
Imiquimod Cream, 5%
(Aldara)
Isotretinoin [13-*cis*
Retinoic acid]
(Accutane,
Amnesteem, Claravis,
Sotret)
Ketoconazole (Nizoral)
Lactic Acid &
Ammonium Hydroxide
[Ammonium Lactate]
(Lac-Hydrin)
Lindane (Kwell)

Metronidazole (Flagyl, MetroGel)
Miconazole (Monistat)
Minoxidil (Loniten, Rogaine)
Mupirocin (Bactroban)
Naftifine (Naftin)
Neomycin Sulfate (Myciguent)
Nystatin (Mycostatin)
Oxiconazole (Oxistat)
Penciclovir (Denavir)
Permethrin (Nix, Elimite)
Pimecrolimus (Elidel)

Podophyllin (Podocon-25, Condylox Gel 0.5%, Condylox)
Pramoxine (Anusol Ointment, Proctofoam-NS)
Pramoxine & Hydrocortisone (Enzone, Proctofoam-HC)
Selenium Sulfide (Exsel Shampoo, Selsun Blue Shampoo, Selsun Shampoo)

Silver Sulfadiazine (Silvadene)
Steroids, Topical (Table 5, page 207)
Tacrolimus (Prograf, Protopic)
Tazarotene (Tazorac)
Terbinafine (Lamisil)
Tolnaftate (Tinactin)
Tretinoin [Retinoic Acid] (Retin-A, Avita, Renova)

DIETARY SUPPLEMENTS

Calcium Acetate (Calphron, Phos-Ex, PhosLo)
Calcium Glubionate (Neo-Calglucon)
Calcium Salts [Chloride, Gluconate, Gluceptate]
Cholecalciferol [Vitamin D_3] (Delta D)
Cyanocobalamin [Vitamin B_{12}]

Ferric Gluconate Complex (Ferrlecit)
Ferrous Gluconate (Fergon)
Ferrous Sulfate
Folic Acid
Iron Dextran (DexFerrum, InFeD)
Iron Sucrose (Venofer)
Magnesium Oxide (Mag-Ox 400)
Magnesium Sulfate

Phytonadione [Vitamin K] (Aqua-MEPHYTON)
Potassium Supplements (Kaon, Kaochlor, K-Lor, Slow-K, Micro-K, Klorvess)
Pyridoxine [Vitamin B_6]
Sodium Bicarbonate [$NaHCO_3$]
Thiamine [Vitamin B_1]

EAR (OTIC) AGENTS

Acetic Acid & Aluminum Acetate (Otic Domeboro)
Benzocaine & Antipyrine (Auralgan)
Ciprofloxacin, Otic (Cipro HC Otic)
Neomycin, Colistin, & Hydrocortisone

(Cortisporin-TC Otic Drops)
Neomycin, Colistin, Hydrocortisone, & Thonzonium (Cortisporin-TC Otic Suspension)

Polymyxin B & Hydrocortisone (Otobiotic Otic)
Sulfacetamide & Prednisolone (Blephamide)
Triethanolamine (Cerumenex)

ENDOCRINE SYSTEM AGENTS

Antidiabetic Agents

Acarbose (Precose)
Chlorpropamide
 (Diabinese)
Glimepiride (Amaryl)
Glipizide (Glucotrol)
Glyburide (DiaBeta,
 Micronase, Glynase)

Glyburide/Metformin
 (Glucovance)
Insulins (Table 6, page
 210)
Metformin (Glucophage)
Miglitol (Glyset)
Nateglinide (Starlix)

Pioglitazone (Actos)
Pioglitazone/Metformin
 (ActoPlus Met)
Repaglinide (Prandin)
Rosiglitazone (Avandia)
Tolazamide (Tolinase)
Tolbutamide (Orinase)

Hormone & Synthetic Substitutes

Calcitonin (Cibacalcin,
 Miacalcin)
Calcitriol (Rocaltrol)
Cortisone Systemic,
 Topical
Desmopressin (DDAVP,
 Stimate)
Dexamethasone
 (Decadron)

Fludrocortisone Acetate
 (Florinef)
Glucagon
Hydrocortisone Topical
 & Systemic (Cortef,
 Solu-Cortef)
Methylprednisolone
 (Solu-Medrol)
Prednisolone

Prednisone
Testosterone (AndroGel,
 Androderm, Striant,
 Testim, Testoderm)
Vasopressin [Antidiuretic
 Hormone, ADH]
 (Pitressin)

Hypercalcemia/Osteoporosis Agents

Etidronate Disodium
 (Didronel)

Gallium Nitrate (Ganite)
Ibandronate (Boniva)

Pamidronate (Aredia)
Zoledronic acid (Zometa)

Obesity

Sibutramine (Meridia)

Osteoporosis Agents

Alendronate (Fosamax)
Raloxifene (Evista)

Risedronate (Actonel)
Teriparatide (Forteo)

Zoledronic Acid
 (Zometa)

Thyroid/Antithyroid

Levothyroxine
 (Synthroid, Levoxyl)
Liothyronine (Cytomel)
Methimazole (Tapazole)

Potassium iodide [Lugol
 Solution] (SSKI,
 Thyro-Block)

Propylthiouracil [PTU]

Miscellaneous Endocrine Agents

Cinacalcet (Sensipar)

Demeclocycline (Declomycin)

Diazoxide (Hyperstat, Proglycem)

EYE (OPHTHALMIC) AGENTS

Glaucoma Agents

Acetazolamide (Diamox)
Apraclonidine (Iopidine)
Betaxolol, Ophthalmic (Betopic)
Brimonidine (Alphagan)
Brinzolamide (Azopt)
Carteolol (Cartrol, Ocupress Ophthalmic)
Ciprofloxacin, Ophthalmic (Ciloxan)
Cyclosporine, Ophthalmic (Restasis)
Dipivefrin (Propine)
Dorzolamide (Trusopt)

Dorzolamide & Timolol (Cosopt)
Echothiophate Iodine (Phospholine Ophthalmic)
Epinastine (Elestat)
Gatifloxacin Ophthalmic (Zymar Ophthalmic)
Latanoprost (Xalatan)
Levobunolol (A-K Beta, Betagan)
Levocabastine (Livostin)
Levofloxacin (Levaquin, Quixin & Iquix Ophthalmic)

Lodoxamide (Alomide)
Moxifloxacin (Vigamox)
Neomycin, Polymyxin, & Hydrocortisone (Cortisporin Ophthalmic & Otic)
Norfloxin (Chibroxin)
Ofloxacin (Ocuflox Ophthalmic)
Rimexolone (Vexol Ophthalmic)
Timolol, Ophthalmic (Timoptic)

Ophthalmic Antibiotics

Bacitracin, Ophthalmic (AK-Tracin Ophthalmic)
Bacitracin & Polymyxin B, Ophthalmic (AK Poly Bac Ophthalmic, Polysporin Ophthalmic)
Bacitracin, Neomycin, & Polymyxin B (AK Spore Ophthalmic, Neosporin Ophthalmic)
Bacitracin, Neomycin, Polymyxin B, &

Hydrocortisone, Ophthalmic (AK Spore HC Ophthalmic, Cortisporin Ophthalmic)
Ciprofloxacin, Ophthalmic (Ciloxan)
Erythromycin, Ophthalmic (Ilotycin Ophthalmic)
Gentamicin, Ophthalmic (Garamycin, Genoptic, Gentacidin, Gentak)
Neomycin & Dexamethasone (AK-

Neo-Dex Ophthalmic, NeoDecadron Ophthalmic)
Neomycin, Polymyxin B, & Dexamethasone (Maxitrol)
Neomycin, Polymyxin B, & Prednisolone (Poly-Pred Ophthalmic)
Ofloxacin (Floxin, Ocuflox Ophthalmic)
Silver Nitrate (Dey-Drop)
Sulfacetamide (Bleph-10, Cetamide, Sodium Sulamyd)

Sulfacetamide & Prednisolone (Blephamide)

Tobramycin, Ophthalmic (AKTob, Tobrex)

Tobramycin & Dexamethasone (TobraDex)
Trifluridine (Viroptic)

Miscellaneous Ophthalmic Agents

Artificial Tears (Tears Naturale)
Cromolyn Sodium (Opticrom)
Cyclopentolate (Cyclogyl)
Cyclosporine Ophthalmic (Restasis)
Dexamethasone, Ophthalmic (AK-Dex

Ophthalmic, Decadron Ophthalmic)
Emedastine (Emadine)
Ketorolac, Ophthalmic (Acular)
Ketotifen (Zaditor)
Lodoxamide (Alomide)
Naphazoline & Antazoline (Albalon-A Ophthalmic)

Naphazoline & Pheniramine Acetate (Naphcon A)
Olopatadine (Patanol)
Pemirolast (Alamast)
Rimexolone (Vexol Ophthalmic)

GASTROINTESTINAL AGENTS

Antacids

Alginic Acid (Gaviscon)
Aluminum Hydroxide (Amphojel, AlternaGEL)
Aluminum Hydroxide with Magnesium Carbonate (Gaviscon)
Aluminum Hydroxide with Magnesium Hydroxide (Maalox)

Aluminum Hydroxide with Magnesium Hydroxide & Simethicone (Mylanta, Mylanta II, Maalox Plus)
Aluminum Hydroxide with Magnesium Trisilicate (Gaviscon, Gaviscon-2)

Calcium Carbonate (Tums, Alka-Mints)
Magaldrate (Riopan, Lowsium)
Simethicone (Mylicon)

Antidiarrheals

Bismuth Subsalicylate (Pepto-Bismol)
Diphenoxylate with Atropine (Lomotil)

Kaolin-Pectin (Kaodene, Kao-Spen, Kapectolin, Parepectolin)
Lactobacillus (Lactinex Granules)

Loperamide (Imodium)
Octreotide (Sandostatin, Sandostatin LAR)
Paregoric [Camphorated Tincture of Opium]

Antiemetics

Aprepitant (Emend)
Chlorpromazine
 (Thorazine)
Dimenhydrinate
 (Dramamine)
Dolasetron (Anzemet)
Dronabinol (Marinol)
Droperidol (Inapsine)

Granisetron (Kytril)
Meclizine (Antivert)
Metoclopramide (Reglan,
 Clopra, Octamide)
Ondansetron (Zofran)
Palonosetron (Aloxi)
Prochlorperazine
 (Compazine)

Promethazine
 (Phenergan)
Scopolamine (Scopace)
Thiethylperazine
 (Torecan)
Trimethobenzamide
 (Tigan)

Antiulcer Agents

Cimetidine (Tagamet)
Esomeprazole (Nexium)
Famotidine (Pepcid)
Lansoprazole (Prevacid)

Nizatidine (Axid)
Omeprazole (Prilosec,
 Zegerid)
Pantoprazole (Protonix)

Rabeprazole (Aciphex)
Ranitidine Hydrochloride
 (Zantac)
Sucralfate (Carafate)

Cathartics/Laxatives

Bisacodyl (Dulcolax)
Docusate Calcium
 (Surfak)
Docusate Potassium
 (Dialose)
Docusate Sodium (Doss,
 Colace)
Glycerin Suppository

Lactulose (Chronulac,
 Cephulac, Enulose)
Magnesium Citrate
Magnesium Hydroxide
 (Milk of Magnesia)
Mineral Oil

Polyethylene Glycol-
 Electrolyte Solution
 (GoLYTELY, CoLyte)
Psyllium (Metamucil,
 Serutan, Effer-Syllium)
Sodium Phosphate
 (Visicol)
Sorbitol

Enzymes

Pancreatin (Pancrease,
 Cotazym, Creon,
 Ultrase)

Miscellaneous GI Agents

Alosetron (Lotronex)
Balsalazide (Colazal)
Dexpanthenol (Ilopan-
 Choline Oral, Ilopan)
Dibucaine (Nupercainal)
Dicyclomine (Bentyl)

Hydrocortisone, Rectal
 (Anusol-HC
 Suppository, Cortifoam
 Rectal, Proctocort)
Hyoscyamine (Anaspaz,
 Cystospaz, Levsin)

Hyoscyamine, Atropine,
 Scopolamine, &
 Phenobarbital
 (Donnatal)
Infliximab (Remicade)

Mesalamine (Rowasa, Asacol, Pentasa)
Metoclopramide (Reglan, Clopra, Octamide)
Misoprostol (Cytotec)
Olsalazine (Dipentum)

Pramoxine (Anusol Ointment, Proctofoam-NS)
Pramoxine with Hydrocortisone (Enzone, Proctofoam-HC)

Propantheline (Pro-Banthine)
Sulfasalazine (Azulfidine)
Tegaserod Maleate (Zelnorm)
Vasopressin (Pitressin)

HEMATOLOGIC AGENTS

Anticoagulants

Ardeparin (Normiflo)
Argatroban (Acova)
Bivalirudin (Angiomax)
Dalteparin (Fragmin)

Enoxaparin (Lovenox)
Fondaparinux (Arixtra)
Heparin
Lepirudin (Refludan)

Protamine
Tinzaparin (Innohep)
Warfarin (Coumadin)

Antiplatelet Agents

Abciximab (ReoPro)
Aspirin (Bayer, Ecotrin, St. Joseph's)
Clopidogrel (Plavix)

Dipyridamole (Persantine)
Dipyridamole & Aspirin (Aggrenox)

Eptifibatide (Integrilin)
Reteplase (Retavase)
Ticlopidine (Ticlid)
Tirofiban (Aggrastat)

Antithrombotic Agents

Alteplase, Recombinant [tPA] (Activase)
Aminocaproic Acid (Amicar)
Anistreplase (Eminase)

Aprotinin (Trasylol)
Danaparoid (Orgaron)
Dextran 40 (Rheomacrodex)
Reteplase (Retavase)

Streptokinase (Streptase, Kabikinase)
Tenecteplase (TNKase)
Urokinase (Abbokinase)

Hematopoietic Stimulants

Darbepoetin Alfa (Aranesp)
Epoetin Alfa [Erythropoietin, EPO] (Epogen, Procrit)

Filgrastim [G-CSF] (Neupogen)
Oprelvekin (Neumega)
Pegfilgrastim (Neulasta)

Sargramostim [GM-CSF] (Prokine, Leukine)

Volume Expanders

Albumin (Albuminar, Buminate, Albutein)

Dextran 40 (Rheomacrodex)
Hetastarch (Hespan)

Plasma Protein Fraction (Plasmanate)

Miscellaneous Hematologic Agents

Antihemophilic Factor VIII (Monoclate)

Desmopressin (DDAVP, Stimate)

Pentoxifylline (Trental)

IMMUNE SYSTEM AGENTS

Immunomodulators

Adalimumab (Humira)
Anakinra (Kineret)
Etanercept (Enbrel)
Interferon Alfa (Roferon-A, Intron A)

Interferon Alfacon-1 (Infergen)
Interferon Beta-1b (Betaseron)
Interferon Gamma-1b (Actimmune)

Mycophenolic Acid (Myfortic)
Natalizumab (Tysabri)
Peg Interferon Alfa-2b (PEG-Intron)

Immunosuppressive Agents

Azathioprine (Imuran)
Basiliximab (Simulect)
Cyclosporine (Sandimmune, NePO)
Daclizumab (Zenapax)
Lymphocyte Immune Globulin

[Antithymocyte Globulin, ATG] (Atgam)
Muromonab-CD3 (Orthoclone OKT3)
Mycophenolate Mofetil (CellCept)

Sirolimus (Rapamune)
Steroids, Systemic (Table 4, page 206)
Tacrolimus (Prograf, Protopic)

Vaccines/Serums/Toxoids

Cytomegalovirus Immune Globulin [CMV-IG IV] (CytoGam)
Diphtheria, Tetanus Toxoids, & Acellular Pertussis Adsorbed, Hepatitis B (recombinant), & Inactivated Poliovirus Vaccine (IPV) Combined (Pediarix)
Haemophilus B Conjugate Vaccine (ActHIB, HibTITER, PedvaxHIB, Prohibit)

Hepatitis A Vaccine (Havrix, Vaqta)
Hepatitis A (Inactivated) & Hepatitis B Recombinant Vaccine (Twinrix)
Hepatitis B Immune Globulin (HyperHep, H-BIG)
Hepatitis B Vaccine (Engerix-B, Recombivax HB)
Immune Globulin, IV (Gamimune N, Sandoglobulin, Gammar IV)

Influenza Vaccine (Fluzone, FluShield, Fluvirin)
Influenza Virus Vaccine Live, Intranasal (FluMist)
Measles, Mumps, Rubella and Varicella Virus Vaccine Live (Proquad)
Meningococcal Polysaccharide Vaccine (Menomune)
Pneumococcal 7-Valent Conjugate Vaccine (Prevnar)

Pneumococcal Vaccine, Polyvalent (Pneumovax-23)

Tetanus Immune Globulin
Tetanus Toxoid

Varicella Virus Vaccine (Varivax)

MUSCULOSKELETAL AGENTS

Antigout Agents

Allopurinol (Zyloprim, Lopurin, Alloprim)

Colchicine
Probenecid (Benemid)

Sulfinpyrazone (Anturane)

Muscle Relaxants

Baclofen (Lioresal)
Carisoprodol (Soma)
Chlorzoxazone (Paraflex, Parafon Forte DSC)

Cyclobenzaprine (Flexeril)
Dantrolene (Dantrium)
Diazepam (Valium)
Metaxalone (Skelaxin)

Methocarbamol (Robaxin)
Orphenadrine (Norflex)

Neuromuscular Blockers

Atracurium (Tracrium)
Pancuronium (Pavulon)
Rocuronium (Zemuron)

Succinylcholine (Anectine, Quelicin, Sucostrin)

Vecuronium (Norcuron)

Miscellaneous Musculoskeletal Agents

Edrophonium (Tensilon)
Leflunomide (Arava)

Methotrexate (Folex, Rheumatrex)

OB/GYN AGENTS

Contraceptives

Estradiol Cypionate & Medroxyprogesterone Acetate (Lunelle)
Etonogestrel/Ethinyl Estradiol (NuvaRing)
Levonorgestrel Implant (Norplant)

Medroxyprogesterone (Provera, Depo-Provera)
Norgestrel (Ovrette)
Oral Contraceptives, Monophasic (Table 7, page 211)

Oral Contraceptives, Multiphasic (Table 7, page 213)
Oral Contraceptives, Progestin Only (Table 7, page 214)

Emergency Contraceptives

Ethinyl Estradiol, &
Levonorgestrel
(Preven)

Levonorgestrel (Plan B)

Estrogen Supplementation Agents

Esterified Estrogens
(Estratab, Menest)
Esterified Estrogens with
Methyltestosterone
(Estratest)
Estradiol (Estrace)
Estradiol, Transdermal
(Estraderm, Climara,
Vivelle)
Estrogen, Conjugated
(Premarin)

Estrogen, Conjugated-
Synthetic (Cenestin)
Estrogen, Conjugated
with Medroxypro-
gesterone (Prempro,
Premphase)
Estrogen, Conjugated
with Methylproges-
terone (Premarin with
Methylprogesterone)

Estrogen, Conjugated
with Methyltesto-
sterone (Premarin
with Methyltestoster-
one)
Ethinyl Estradiol
(Estinyl, Feminone)
Norethindrone
Acetate/Ethinyl
Estradiol (FemHRT)

Vaginal Preparations

Amino-Cerv pH 5.5
Cream

Miconazole (Monistat)
Nystatin (Mycostatin)

Terconazole (Terazol 7)
Tioconazole (Vagistat)

Miscellaneous Ob/Gyn Agents

Dinoprostone (Cervidil
Vaginal Insert,
Prepidil Vaginal Gel)
Gonadorelin
(Lutrepulse)
Leuprolide (Lupron)
Lutropin Alfa (Luveris)

Magnesium Sulfate
Medroxyprogesterone
(Provera,
Depo-Provera)
Methylergonovine
(Methergine)

Mifepristone [RU 486]
(Mifeprex)
Oxytocin (Pitocin)
Terbutaline (Brethine,
Bricanyl)

PAIN MEDICATIONS

Local Anesthetics (See Table 3, page 205)

Benzocaine &
Antipyrine (Auralgan)
Bupivacaine (Marcaine)
Capsaicin (Capsin,
Zostrix)
Cocaine

Dibucaine (Nupercainal)
Lidocaine (Anestacon
Topical, Xylocaine)
Lidocaine & Prilocaine
(EMLA, LMX)

Pramoxine (Anusol
Ointment,
Proctofoam-NS)

Migraine Headache Medications

Acetaminophen with
Butalbital w/wo
Caffeine (Fioricet,
Medigesic, Repan,
Sedapap-10 Two-
Dyne, Triapin, Axocet,
Phrenilin Forte)
Almotriptan (Axert)

Aspirin & Butalbital
Compound (Fiorinal)
Aspirin with Butalbital,
Caffeine, & Codeine
(Fiorinal with
Codeine)
Eletriptan (Relpax)
Frovatriptan (Frova)

Naratriptan (Amerge)
Serotonin 5-HT$_1$
Receptor Agonists
(See Table 11, page
218)
Sumatriptan (Imitrex)
Zolmitriptan (Zomig)

Narcotic Analgesics

Acetaminophen with
Codeine (Tylenol No.
1, 2, 3, 4)
Alfentanil (Alfenta)
Aspirin with Codeine
(Empirin No. 2, 3, 4)
Buprenorphine
(Buprenex)
Butorphanol (Stadol)
Codeine
Dezocine (Dalgan)
Fentanyl (Sublimaze)
Fentanyl, Transdermal
(Duragesic)
Fentanyl, Transmucosal
(Actiq System)
Hydrocodone &
Acetaminophen
(Lorcet, Vicodin)

Hydrocodone & Aspirin
(Lortab ASA)
Hydrocodone &
Ibuprofen
(Vicoprofen)
Hydromorphone
(Dilaudid)
Levorphanol
(Levo-Dromoran)
Meperidine (Demerol)
Methadone (Dolophine)
Morphine (Avinza XR,
Duramorph,
Infumorph, MS
Contin, Kadian SR,
Oramorph SR,
Palladone, Roxanol)
Morphine, Liposomal
(DepoDur)
Nalbuphine (Nubain)

Oxycodone (OxyContin,
OxyIR, Roxicodone)
Oxycodone &
Acetaminophen
(Percocet, Tylox)
Oxycodone & Aspirin
(Percodan, Percodan-
Demi)
Oxymorphone
(Numorphan)
Pentazocine (Talwin)
Propoxyphene (Darvon)
Propoxyphene &
Acetaminophen
(Darvocet)
Propoxyphene & Aspirin
(Darvon Compound-
65, Darvon-N with
Aspirin)

Nonnarcotic Analgesics

Acetaminophen [APAP]
(Tylenol)

Aspirin (Bayer, Ecotrin,
St. Joseph's)
Tramadol (Ultram)

Tramadol/Acetaminophen
(Ultracet)

Nonsteroidal Antiinflammatory Agents

Celecoxib (Celebrex)
Diclofenac (Cataflam, Voltaren)
Diflunisal (Dolobid)
Etodolac (Lodine)
Fenoprofen (Nalfon)
Flurbiprofen (Ansaid)
Ibuprofen (Motrin, Rufen, Advil)

Indomethacin (Indocin)
Ketoprofen (Orudis, Oruvail)
Ketorolac (Toradol)
Meloxicam (Mobic)
Nabumetone (Relafen)
Naproxen (Aleve, Naprosyn, Anaprox)
Oxaprozin (Daypro)

Piroxicam (Feldene)
Sulindac (Clinoril)
Tolmetin (Tolectin)
Valdecoxib (Bextra)

Miscellaneous Pain Medications

Amitriptyline (Elavil)
Imipramine (Tofranil)

Pregabalin (Lyrica)
Tramadol (Ultram)

Ziconotide (Prialt)

RESPIRATORY AGENTS

Antitussives, Decongestants, & Expectorants

Acetylcysteine (Acetadote, Mucomyst)
Benzonatate (Tessalon Perles)
Codeine
Dextromethorphan (Mediquell, Benylin DM, PediaCare 1)
Guaifenesin (Robitussin)
Guaifenesin & Codeine (Robitussin AC, Brontex)

Guaifenesin & Dextromethorphan
Hydrocodone & Guaifenesin (Hycotuss Expectorant)
Hydrocodone & Homatropine (Hycodan, Hydromet)
Hydrocodone & Pseudoephedrine (Detussin, Histussin-D)

Hydrocodone, Chlorpheniramine, Phenylephrine, Acetaminophen, & Caffeine (Hycomine)
Potassium Iodide (SSKI, Thyro-Block)
Pseudoephedrine (Sudafed, Novafed, Afrinol)

Bronchodilators

Albuterol (Proventil, Ventolin, Volmax)
Albuterol & Ipratropium (Combivent)
Aminophylline
Bitolterol (Tornalate)
Ephedrine

Epinephrine (Adrenalin, Sus-Phrine, EpiPen)
Formoterol (Foradil Aerolizer)
Isoproterenol (Isuprel)
Levalbuterol (Xopenex)
Metaproterenol (Alupent, Metaprel)

Pirbuterol (Maxair)
Salmeterol (Serevent)
Terbutaline (Brethine, Bricanyl)
Theophylline (Theo24, TheoChron)

Respiratory Inhalants

Acetylcysteine
(Acetadote,
Mucomyst)
Beclomethasone
(Beconase, Vancenase
Nasal Inhaler)
Beclomethasone
(QVAR)
Beractant (Survanta)
Budesonide (Rhinocort,
Pulmicort)

Calfactant (Infasurf)
Colfosceril Palmitate
(Exosurf Neonatal)
Cromolyn Sodium (Intal,
Nasalcrom, Opticrom)
Dexamethasone, Nasal
(Dexacort Phosphate
Turbinaire)
Flunisolide (AeroBid,
Nasalide)

Fluticasone, Oral, Nasal
(Flonase, Flovent)
Fluticasone Propionate
& Salmeterol
Xinafoate (Advair
Diskus)
Ipratropium (Atrovent)
Nedocromil (Tilade)
Tiotropium (Spiriva)
Triamcinolone
(Azmacort)

Miscellaneous Respiratory Agents

Alpha$_1$-Protease
Inhibitor (Prolastin)
Dornase Alfa
(Pulmozyme)

Montelukast (Singulair)
Omalizumab (Xolair)

Zafirlukast (Accolate)
Zileuton (Zyflo)

URINARY/GENITOURINARY AGENTS

Alprostadil,
Intracavernosal
(Caverject, Edex)
Alprostadil, Urethral
Suppository (Muse)
Ammonium Aluminum
Sulfate [Alum]
Belladonna & Opium
Suppositories (B & O
Supprettes)
Bethanechol
(Urecholine, Duvoid)
Darifenacin (Enablex)
Dimethyl Sulfoxide
[DMSO] (Rimso 50)
Flavoxate (Urispas)
Hyoscyamine (Anaspaz,
Cystospaz, Levsin)

Methenamine (Hiprex,
Urex)
Neomycin-Polymyxin
Bladder Irrigant
[Neosporin GU
Irrigant]
Nitrofurantoin
(Macrodantin,
Furadantin, Macrobid)
Oxybutynin (Ditropan,
Ditropan XL)
Oxybutynin Transdermal
System (Oxytrol)
Pentosan Polysulfate
(Elmiron)
Phenazopyridine
(Pyridium)

Potassium Citrate
(Urocit-K)
Potassium Citrate &
Citric Acid
(Polycitra-K)
Sildenafil (Viagra)
Solifenacin (VESIcare)
Sodium Citrate (Bicitra)
Tadalafil (Cialis)
Tolterodine (Detrol,
Detrol LA)
Trimethoprim (Trimpex,
Proloprim)
Trospium Chloride
(Sanctura)
Vardenafil (Levitra)

Benign Prostatic Hyperplasia Medications

Alfuzosin (Uroxatral)
Doxazosin (Cardura)
Dutasteride (Avodart)

Finasteride (Proscar,
Propecia)

Tamsulosin (Flomax)
Terazosin (Hytrin)

WOUND CARE

Becaplermin (Regranex
Gel)

Silver Nitrate
(Dey-Drop)

MISCELLANEOUS THERAPEUTIC AGENTS

Acamprosate (Campral)
Cilostazol (Pletal)
Drotrecogin Alfa
(Xigris)
Megestrol Acetate
(Megace)
Lanthanum Carbonate
(Fosrenol)
Naltrexone (ReVia)

Nicotine Gum
(Nicorette)
Nicotine Nasal Spray
(Nicotrol NS)
Nicotine Transdermal
(Habitrol, Nicoderm,
Nicotrol)
Orlistat (Xenical)
Palifermin (Kepivance)

Potassium Iodide [Lugol
Solution] (SSKI,
Thyro-Block)
Sevelamer (Renagel)
Sodium Polystyrene
Sulfonate
(Kayexalate)
Talc (Sterile Talc
Powder)

NATURAL AND HERBAL AGENTS

Black Cohosh
Chamomile
Cranberry (*Vaccinium
macrocarpon*)
Dong Quai (*Angelica
polymorpha, sinensis*)
Echinacea (*Echinacea
purpurea*)
Ephedra/MaHuang
Evening Primrose Oil
Garlic (*Allium sativum*)
Ginger (*Zingiber
officinale*)

Ginkgo Biloba
Ginseng
Glucosamine Sulfate
(chitosamine) &
Chondroitin Sulfate
Kava Kava (Kava Kava
Root Extract, *Piper
methysticum*)
Melatonin
Milk Thistle (*Silybum
marianum*)

Saw Palmetto (*Serenoa
repens*)
St. John's Wort
(*Hypericum
perforatum*)
Valerian (*Valeriana
officinalis*)
Yohimbine
(*Pausinystalia
yohimbe*)

GENERIC DRUG DATA

Abacavir (Ziagen) WARNING: Allergy (fever, rash, fatigue, GI, resp) reported; stop drug immediately & do not rechallenge; lactic acidosis & hepatomegaly/steatosis reported **Uses:** *HIV Infxn* **Action:** Nucleoside RT inhibitor **Dose:** *Adults.* 300 mg PO bid **Peds.** 8 mg/kg bid **Caution:** [C, –] CDC recommends HIV-infected mothers not breast-feed due to risk of infant transmission **Supplied:** Tabs 300 mg; soln 20 mg/mL **SE:** See Warning, ↑ LFTs, fat redistribution **Notes:** Numerous drug interactions

Abarelix (Plenaxis) (Withdrawn from U.S. market 2005)

Abciximab (ReoPro) **Uses:** *Prevent acute ischemic complications in PTCA,* MI **Action:** ↓ plt aggregation (glycoprotein IIb/IIIa inhibitor) **Dose:** 0.25 mg/kg bolus 10–60 min pre PTCA, then 0.125 mcg/kg/min (max = 10 mcg/min) cont inf × 12 h **Caution:** [C, ?/–] **Contra:** Active or recent (w/in 6 wk) internal hemorrhage, CVA w/in 2 y or CVA w/ significant neurologic deficit, bleeding diathesis or PO anticoagulants use w/in 7 d (unless PT 21.2 × control), thrombocytopenia (<100,000 cells/mcL), recent trauma or major surgery (w/in 6 wk), CNS tumor, AVM, aneurysm, severe uncontrolled HTN, vasculitis, use of dextran prior to or during PTCA, allergy to murine proteins **Supplied:** Inj 2 mg/mL **SE:** Allergic Rxns, bleeding, thrombocytopenia possible **Notes:** Use w/ heparin

Acamprosate (Campral) **Uses:** *Maint abstinence from EtOH* **Action:** ↓ Glutamatergic transmission; modulates neuronal hyperexcitability; related to GABA **Dose:** 666 mg PO tid; CrCl 30–50 mL/min: 333 mg PO tid **Caution:** [C; ?/–] **Contra:** CrCl < 30 mL/min **Supplied:** Tabs 333 mg **SE:** N/D, depression, anxiety **Notes:** Does not eliminate EtOH withdrawal Sx; continue even if relapse occurs

Acarbose (Precose) **Uses:** *Type 2 DM* **Action:** α-Glucosidase inhibitor; delays digestion of carbohydrates to ↓ glucose **Dose:** 25–100 mg PO tid (w/ 1st bite each meal) **Caution:** [B, ?] Avoid if CrCl <25 mL/min **Contra:** IBD, cirrhosis **Supplied:** Tabs 25, 50, 100 mg **SE:** Abdominal pain, D, flatulence, ↑ LFTs **Notes:** OK w/ sulfonylureas; can affect digoxin levels; LFTs q3mo for 1st y

Acebutolol (Sectral) **Uses:** *HTN, arrhythmias* **Action:** Competitively blocks β-adrenergic receptors, β₁, & ISA **Dose:** 200–800 mg/d, ↓ if CrCl <50 mL/min **Caution:** [B, D in 2nd & 3rd tri, +] Can exacerbate ischemic heart Dz, do not D/C abruptly **Contra:** 2nd-, 3rd-degree heart block **Supplied:** Caps 200, 400 mg **SE:** Fatigue, HA, dizziness, bradycardia

Acetaminophen [APAP, N-acetyl-p-aminophenol] (Tylenol, other generic) [OTC] **Uses:** *Mild–moderate pain, HA, fever* **Action:**

Nonnarcotic analgesic; ↓ CNS synthesis of prostaglandins & hypothalamic heat-regulating center **Dose:** *Adults.* 650 mg PO or PR q4–6h or 1000 mg PO q6h; max 4 g/24 h. *Peds. <12 y.* 10–15 mg/kg/dose PO or PR q4–6h; max 2.6 g/24 h. Quick dosing Table 1 (page 198). Administer q6h if CrCl 10–50 mL/min & q8h if CrCl <10 mL/min **Caution:** [B, +] Hepatotoxic in elderly & w/ EtOH use w/ >4 g/day; alcoholic liver Dz **Contra:** G6PD deficiency **Supplied:** Tabs 160, 325, 500, 650 mg; chew tabs 80, 160 mg; liq 100 mg/mL, 120 mg/2.5 mL, 120 mg/5 mL, 160 mg/5 mL, 167 mg/5 mL, 325 mg/5 mL, 500 mg/15 mL; gtt 48 mg/mL, 60 mg/0.6 mL; supp 80, 120, 125, 300, 325, 650 mg **SE:** OD causes hepatotox at 10-g dose; 15 g is potentially lethal Rx w/ *N*-acetylcysteine **Notes:** No antiinflammatory or plt-inhibiting action; avoid EtOH

Acetaminophen + Butalbital ± Caffeine (Fioricet, Medigesic, Repan, Sedapap-10, Two-Dyne, Triapin, Axocet, Phrenilin Forte) [C-III] **Uses:** *Tension HA,* mild pain **Action:** Nonnarcotic analgesic w/ barbiturate **Dose:** 1–2 tabs or caps PO q4/6h PRN; ↓ in renal/hepatic impair; 4 g/24 h APAP max **Caution:** [D, +] Alcoholic liver Dz **Contra:** G6PD deficiency **Supplied:** Caps *Medigesic, Repan, Two-Dyne:* butalbital 50 mg, caffeine 40 mg, + APAP 325 mg. Caps *Axocet, Phrenilin Forte:* butalbital 50 mg + APAP 650 mg; *Triapin:* butalbital 50 mg + APAP 325 mg. Tabs *Medigesic, Fioricet, Repan:* butalbital 50 mg, caffeine 40 mg, + APAP 325 mg; *Phrenilin:* butalbital 50 mg + APAP 325 mg; *Sedapap-10:* butalbital 50 mg + APAP 650 mg **SE:** Drowsiness, dizziness, "hangover" effect **Notes:** Butalbital habit-forming; avoid EtOH

Acetaminophen + Codeine (Tylenol No. 1, No. 2, No. 3, No. 4) [C-III, C-V] **Uses:** *Mild–moderate pain (No. 1, 2, 3); moderate–severe pain (No. 4)* **Action:** Combined APAP & narcotic analgesic **Dose:** *Adults.* 1–2 tabs q3–4h PRN (max dose APAP = 4 g/d). *Peds.* APAP 10–15 mg/kg/dose; codeine 0.5–1 mg/kg dose q4–6h (dosing guide: 3–6 y, 5 mL/dose; 7–12 y, 10 mL/dose); ↓ in renal/hepatic impair **Caution:** [C, +] Alcoholic liver Dz **Contra:** G6PD deficiency **Supplied:** Tabs 300 mg APAP + codeine; caps 325 mg APAP + codeine; helix, susp (C-V) APAP 120 mg + codeine 12 mg/5 mL **SE:** Drowsiness, dizziness, N/V **Notes:** Codeine in No. 1 = 7.5 mg, No. 2 = 15 mg, No. 3 = 30 mg, No. 4 = 60 mg

Acetazolamide (Diamox) **Uses:** *Diuresis, glaucoma, prevent high-altitude sickness, refractory epilepsy* **Action:** Carbonic anhydrase inhibitor; ↓ renal excretion of hydrogen & ↑ renal excretion of Na$^+$, K$^+$, HCO$_3^-$, & H$_2$O **Dose:** *Adults. Diuretic:* 250–375 mg IV or PO q24h. *Glaucoma:* 250–1000 mg PO q24h in ÷ doses. *Epilepsy:* 8–30 mg/kg/d PO in ÷ doses. *Altitude sickness:* 250 mg PO q8–12h or SR 500 mg PO q12–24h start 24–48 h before & 48 h after highest ascent. *Peds.* Epilepsy: 8–30 mg/kg/24 h PO in ÷ doses; max 1 g/d. *Diuretic:* 5 mg/kg/24 h PO or IV. *Alkalinization of urine:* 5 mg/kg/dose PO bid–tid. *Glaucoma:* 5–15 mg/kg/24 h PO in ÷ doses; max 1 g/d; adjust in renal impair; avoid if CrCl <10 mL/min **Caution:** [C, +] **Contra:** Renal/hepatic failure, sulfa allergy

Supplied: Tabs 125, 250 mg; SR caps 500 mg; inj 500 mg/vial **SE:** Malaise, metallic taste, drowsiness, photosensitivity, hyperglycemia **Notes:** Follow Na⁺ & K⁺; watch for metabolic acidosis; SR forms not for epilepsy

Acetic Acid & Aluminum Acetate (Otic Domeboro) Uses: *Otitis externa* **Action:** Antiinfective **Dose:** 4–6 gtt in ear(s) q2–3h **Caution:** [C, ?] **Contra:** Perforated tympanic membranes **Supplied:** 2% otic soln **SE:** Local irritation

Acetylcysteine (Acetadote, Mucomyst) Uses: *Mucolytic* adjuvant Rx for chronic bronchopulmonary Dzs & CF; *antidote to APAP hepatotox* **Action:** Splits disulfide linkages between mucoprotein molecular complexes; protects liver by restoring glutathione in APAP OD **Dose:** *Adults & Peds.* Nebulizer: 3–5 mL of 20% soln diluted w/ equal vol of H_2O or NS tid–qid. *Antidote:* PO or NG: 140 mg/kg load, then 70 mg/kg q4h for 17 doses. (Dilute 1:3 in carbonated beverage or orange juice) *Acetadote:* load 150 mg/kg over 15 min, then 50 mg/kg over 4h, then 100 mg/kg over 16h **Caution:** [C, ?] **Supplied:** Soln 10%, 20%; Acetadote IV soln **SE:** Bronchospasm (inhal), N/V, drowsiness; anaphylactoid rxns w/ IV **Notes:** Activated charcoal adsorbs acetylcysteine if given PO for APAP ingestion; start Rx for APAP overdose w/in 6–8 h

Acitretin (Soriatane) WARNING: Must not be used by females who are pregnant or intend to become pregnant during therapy or for up to 3 y following D/C of therapy; EtOH must not be ingested during therapy or for 2 mo following cessation of therapy; do not donate blood for 3 y following cessation Uses: *Severe psoriasis*; other keratinization disorders (lichen planus, etc) **Action:** Retinoid-like activity **Dose:** 25–50 mg/d PO, w/ main meal; ↑ if no response by 4 wk to 75 mg/d **Caution:** [X, –] Renal/hepatic impair; in women of reproductive potential **Contra:** See Warning **Supplied:** Caps 10, 25 mg **SE:** Cheilitis, skin peeling, alopecia, pruritus, rash, arthralgia, GI upset, photosensitivity, thrombocytosis, hypertriglyceridemia **Notes:** Follow LFTs; response often takes 2–3 mo; pt agreement/informed consent prior to use

Acyclovir (Zovirax) Uses: *Herpes simplex & zoster Infxns* **Action:** Interferes w/ viral DNA synthesis **Dose:** *Adults.* PO: Initial genital herpes: 200 mg PO q4h while awake, 5 caps/d × 10 d or 400 mg PO tid × 7–10 d. *Chronic suppression:* 400 mg PO bid. *Intermittent Rx:* As for initial Rx, except treat for 5 d, or 800 mg PO bid, at prodrome. *Herpes zoster:* 800 mg PO 5×/d for 7–10 d. IV: 5–10 mg/kg/dose IV q8h. *Topical: Initial herpes genitalis:* Apply q3h (6×/d) for 7 d. *Peds.* 5–10 mg/kg/dose IV or PO q8h or 750 mg/m²/24 h ÷ q8h. *Chickenpox:* 20 mg/kg/dose PO qid; ↓ for CrCl <50 mL/min **Caution:** [C, +] **Supplied:** Caps 200 mg; tabs 400, 800 mg; susp 200 mg/5 mL; inj; oint 5% **SE:** Dizziness, lethargy, confusion, rash, inflammation at IV site **Notes:** PO better than topical for herpes genitalis

Adalimumab (Humira) WARNING: Cases of TB have been observed; check TB skin test prior to use Uses: *Moderate–severe RA w/ an inadequate response to one or more DMARDs* **Action:** TNF-α inhibitor **Dose:** 40 mg SQ qowk; may ↑ 40 mg qwk if not on MTX **Caution:** [B, ?/–] Serious Infxns & sepsis reported **Supplied:** Prefilled 1 mL (40 mg) syringe **SE:** Inj site Rxns, serious Infxns, neurologic events, malignancies **Notes:** Refrigerate prefilled syringe, rotate inj sites, OK w/ other DMARDs

Adefovir (Hepsera) WARNING: Acute exacerbations of hepatitis may occur after therapy (monitor LFTs); chronic use may lead to nephrotox especially in pts w/ underlying renal impair (monitor renal Fxn); HIV resistance may emerge; lactic acidosis & severe hepatomegaly w/ steatosis reported when used alone or in combo w/ other antiretrovirals **Uses:** *Chronic active hepatitis B virus* **Action:** Nucleotide analog **Dose:** CrCl > 50 mL/min: 10 mg PO qd; CrCl 20–49 mL/min: 10 mg PO q48h; CrCl 10–19 mL/min: 10 mg PO q72h; HD: 10 mg PO q7d postdialysis; adjust w/ CrCl < 50 mL/min **Caution:** [C, –] **Supplied:** Tabs 10 mg **SE:** Asthenia, HA, abdominal pain; see Warning

Adenosine (Adenocard) **Uses:** *PSVT;* including associated w/ WPW **Action:** Class IV antiarrhythmic; slows AV node conduction **Dose:** *Adults.* 6 mg IV bolus; may repeat in 1–2 min; max 12 mg IV. *Peds.* 0.05 mg/kg IV bolus; may repeat q1–2 min to 0.25 mg/kg max **Caution:** [C, ?] **Contra:** 2nd- or 3rd-degree AV block or SSS (w/o pacemaker); recent MI or cerebral hemorrhage **Supplied:** Inj 6 mg/2 mL **SE:** Facial flushing, HA, dyspnea, chest pressure, ↓ BP **Notes:** Doses >12 mg not OK; can cause momentary asystole when administered; caffeine, theophylline antagonize effects

Albumin (Albuminar, Buminate, Albutein) **Uses:** *Plasma volume expansion for shock* (eg, burns, hemorrhage) **Action:** Maint of plasma colloid oncotic pressure **Dose:** *Adults.* Initial 25 g IV; subsequent dose based on response; 250 g/48h max. *Peds.* 0.5–1 g/kg/dose; inf at 0.05–0.1 g/min **Caution:** [C, ?] Severe anemia; cardiac, renal, or hepatic insuff due to added protein load & possible hypervolemia **Contra:** Cardiac failure **Supplied:** Soln 5%, 25% **SE:** Chills, fever, CHF, tachycardia, ↓ BP, hypervolemia **Notes:** Contains 130–160 mEq Na⁺/L; may precipitate pulmonary edema

Albuterol (Proventil, Ventolin, Volmax) **Uses:** *Asthma; prevent exercise-induced bronchospasm* **Action:** β-Adrenergic sympathomimetic bronchodilator; relaxes bronchial smooth muscle **Dose:** *Adults.* Inhaler: 2 inhal q4–6h PRN; 1 Rotacap inhaled q4–6h. *PO:* 2–4 mg PO tid–qid. *Neb:* 1.25–5 mg (0.25–1 mL of 0.5% soln in 2–3 mL of NS) tid–qid. *Peds.* Inhaler: 2 inhal q4–6h. *PO:* 0.1–0.2 mg/kg/dose PO; max 2–4 mg PO tid; *Neb:* 0.05 mg/kg (max 2.5 mg) in 2–3 mL of NS tid–qid **Caution:** [C, +] **Supplied:** Tabs 2, 4 mg; XR tabs 4, 8 mg; syrup 2 mg/5 mL; 90 mcg/dose met-dose inhaler; Rotacaps 200 mcg; soln for neb 0.083, 0.5% **SE:** Palpitations, tachycardia, nervousness, GI upset

Albuterol & Ipratropium (Combivent) **Uses:** *COPD* **Action:** Combo of β-adrenergic bronchodilator & quaternary anticholinergic **Dose:** 2 inhal qid **Caution:** [C, +] **Contra:** Allergy to peanut/soybean **Supplied:** Met-dose inhaler, 18 mcg ipratropium/103 mcg albuterol/puff **SE:** Palpitations, tachycardia, nervousness, GI upset, dizziness, blurred vision

Aldesleukin [IL-2] (Proleukin) **WARNING:** Use restricted to pts w/ nl pulmonary & cardiac Fxn **Uses:** *Metastatic RCC, melanoma* **Action:** Acts via IL-2 receptor; numerous immunomodulatory effects **Dose:** 600,000 IU/kg q8h × 14 doses (FDA-approved dose/schedule for RCC). Multiple cont inf & alternate schedules (including "high dose" using 24×10^6 IU/m^2 IV q8h on days 1–5 & 12–16) **Caution:** [C, ?/–] **Contra:** Organ allografts **Supplied:** Inj 1.1 mg/mL (22×10^6 IU) **SE:** Flu-like syndrome (malaise, fever, chills), N/V/D, ↑ bilirubin; capillary leak syndrome w/ ↓ BP, pulmonary edema, fluid retention, & weight gain; renal & mild hematologic tox (anemia, thrombocytopenia, leukopenia) & secondary eosinophilia; cardiac tox (ischemia, atrial arrhythmias); neurologic tox (CNS depression, somnolence, rarely coma, delirium). Pruritic rashes, urticaria, & erythroderma common. **Notes:** Cont inf less likely to cause severe ↓ BP & fluid retention

Alefacept (Amevive) **WARNING:** Must monitor CD4 before each dose; w/hold if <250; D/C if <250 × 1 month **Uses:** *Moderate/severe chronic plaque psoriasis* **Action:** Fusion protein inhibitor **Dose:** 7.5 mg IV or 15 mg IM once weekly × 12 wk **Caution:** [B, ?/–] PRG registry; associated w/ serious Infxn **Contra:** Lymphopenia **Supplied:** 7.5-, 15-mg vials **SE:** Pharyngitis, myalgia, inj site Rxn, malignancy **Notes:** IV or IM different formulations; may repeat course 12 wk later if CD4 OK

Alendronate (Fosamax) **Uses:** *Rx & prevention of osteoporosis, Rx of steroid-induced osteoporosis & Paget Dz* **Action:** ↓ nl & abnormal bone resorption **Dose:** *Osteoporosis: Rx:* 10 mg/d PO or 70 mg qwk. *Steroid-induced osteoporosis: Rx:* 5 mg/d PO. *Prevention:* 5 mg/d PO or 35 mg qwk. *Paget Dz:* 40 mg/d PO **Caution:** [C, ?] Not OK if CrCl <35 mL/min, w/NSAID use **Contra:** Esophageal anomalies, inability to sit/stand upright for 30 min, ↓ Ca^{2+} **Supplied:** Tabs 5, 10, 35, 40, 70 mg **SE:** GI disturbances, HA, pain, jaw osteonecrosis (w/dental procedures) **Notes:** Take 1st thing in AM w/ H_2O (8 oz) > 30 min before 1st food/beverage of the day. Do not lie down for 30 min after. Ca^{2+} & vitamin D supl necessary

Alfentanil (Alfenta) [C-II] **Uses:** *Adjunct in the maint of anesthesia; analgesia* **Action:** Short-acting narcotic analgesic **Dose:** *Adults & Peds >12 y.* 3–75 mcg/kg IV inf; total depends on duration of procedure **Caution:** [C, +/–] ↑ ICP, resp depression **Supplied:** Inj 500 mcg/mL **SE:** Bradycardia, ↓ BP arrhythmias, peripheral vasodilation, ↑ ICP, drowsiness, resp depression

Alfuzosin (Uroxatral) **WARNING:** May prolong QTc interval **Uses:** *BPH* **Action:** α-Blocker **Dose:** 10 mg PO daily immediately after the same meal **Caution:** [B, –] **Contra:** W/ CYP3A4 inhibitors; moderate–severe hepatic impair **Supplied:** Tabs 10 mg **SE:** Postural ↓ BP, dizziness, HA, fatigue **Notes:** XR tablet—do not cut or crush; fewest reports of ejaculatory disorders compared w/ other drugs in class

Alginic Acid + Aluminum Hydroxide & Magnesium Trisilicate (Gaviscon) [OTC] Uses: *Heartburn*; pain from hiatal hernia **Action:** Protective layer blocks gastric acid **Dose:** 2–4 tabs or 15–30 mL PO qid followed by H_2O; **Caution:** [B, –] Avoid in renal impair or Na^+-restricted diet **Supplied:** Tabs, susp **SE:** D, constipation

Allopurinol (Zyloprim, Lopurin, Aloprim) Uses: *Gout, hyperuricemia of malignancy, uric acid urolithiasis* **Action:** Xanthine oxidase inhibitor; ↓ uric acid production **Dose:** *Adults. PO:* Initial 100 mg/d; usual 300 mg/d; max 800 mg/d. *IV:* 200–400 mg/m²/d (max 600 mg/24 h); (take after meal w/ plenty of fluid). *Peds.* Only for hyperuricemia of malignancy if <10 y: 10 mg/kg/24 h PO or 200 mg/m²/d IV ÷ q6–8h (max 600 mg/24 h); ↓ in renal impair **Caution:** [C, M] **Supplied:** Tabs 100, 300 mg; inj 500 mg/30 mL (Aloprim) **SE:** Skin rash, N/V, renal impair, angioedema **Notes:** Aggravates acute gout; begin after acute attack resolves; IV dose of 6 mg/mL final conc as single daily inf or ÷ 6-, 8-, or 12-h intervals

Almotriptan (Axert) See Table 11 (page 218)

Alosetron (Lotronex) WARNING: Serious GI side effects, some fatal, including ischemic colitis reported. May be prescribed only through participation in the prescribing program for Lotronex Uses: *Severe diarrhea-predominant IBS in women who fail conventional therapy* **Action:** Selective 5-HT₃ receptor antagonist **Dose:** *Adults.* 1 mg PO qd × 4 wk; titrate to 1 mg bid max; D/C after 4 wk at max dose if Sxs not controlled **Caution:** [B, ?/–] **Contra:** Hx chronic/severe constipation, GI obstruction, strictures, toxic megacolon, GI perforation, adhesions, ischemic colitis, Crohn Dz, ulcerative colitis, diverticulitis, thrombophlebitis, or hypercoagulable state. **Supplied:** Tabs 1 mg **SE:** Constipation, abdominal pain, nausea **Notes:** D/C immediately if constipation or Sxs of ischemic colitis develop; pt must sign informed consent prior to use

Alpha₁-Protease Inhibitor (Prolastin) Uses: *α₁-Antitrypsin deficiency*; panacinar emphysema **Action:** Replace human α₁-protease inhibitor **Dose:** 60 mg/kg IV once/wk **Caution:** [C, ?] **Contra:** Selective IgA deficiencies w/ known IgA antibodies **Supplied:** Inj 500 mg/20 mL, 1000 mg/40 mL **SE:** Fever, dizziness, flu-like Sxs, allergic Rxns

Alprazolam (Xanax) [C-IV] Uses: *Anxiety & panic disorders,* anxiety w/ depression **Action:** Benzodiazepine; antianxiety agent **Dose:** *Anxiety:* Initial, 0.25–0.5 mg tid; ↑ to a max of 4 mg/d in ÷ doses. *Panic:* Initial, 0.5 mg tid; may gradually ↑ to response; ↓ in elderly, debilitated, & hepatic impair **Caution:** [D, –] **Contra:** NA glaucoma, concomitant itra-/ketoconazole **Supplied:** Tabs 0.25, 0.5, 1, 2 mg; soln 1 mg/mL **SE:** Drowsiness, fatigue, memory impair, sexual dysfunction **Notes:** Avoid abrupt D/C after prolonged use

Alprostadil [Prostaglandin E₁] (Prostin VR) Uses: *Conditions where blood flow must be maintained in ductus arteriosus* sustain pulmonary/systemic circulation until surgery (eg, pulmonary atresia/stenosis, tricuspid atresia, transposition, severe tetralogy of Fallot) **Action:** Vasodilator, plt inhibitor; ductus arteriosus smooth muscle is especially sensitive **Dose:** 0.05 mcg/kg/min IV; ↓ to lowest that maintains response **Caution:** [X, –] **Contra:** Neonatal resp distress syndrome **Supplied:** Injectable forms **SE:** Cutaneous vasodilation, Sz-like activity, jitteriness, ↑ temp, ↓ Ca^{2+}, apnea, thrombocytopenia, ↓ BP; may cause apnea **Notes:** Keep intubation kit at bedside if pt is not intubated

Alprostadil, Intracavernosal (Caverject, Edex) Uses: *Erectile dysfunction* **Action:** Relaxes smooth muscles, dilates cavernosal arteries, ↑ lacunar spaces and blood entrapment by compressing venules against tunica **Dose:** 2.5–60 mcg intracavernosal; titrate at physician's office **Caution:** [X, –] **Contra:** Predisposition to priapism (eg, sickle cell); penile deformities/implants; men in whom sexual activity is inadvisable **Supplied:** *Caverject:* 6–10 or 6–20 mcg vials ± diluent syringes. *Caverject Impulse:* Self-contained syringe (29 gauge) 10 & 20 mcg. *Edex:* 5, 10, 20, 40 mcg vials + syringes **SE:** Local pain w/ injection **Notes:** Counsel about priapism, penile fibrosis, & hematoma risks, titrate w/Obs

Alprostadil, Urethral Suppository (Muse) Uses: *Erectile dysfunction* **Action:** Urethral mucosal absorption; vasodilator, smooth muscle relaxant of corpus cavernosa **Dose:** 125–1000 mcg system 5–10 min prior to sexual activity; titrate at physician's office **Caution:** [X, –] **Contra:** Predisposition to priapism (eg, sickle cell) penile deformities/implants; men in whom sexual activity is inadvisable **Supplied:** 125, 250, 500, 1000 mcg w/ a transurethral delivery system **SE:** ↓ BP, dizziness, syncope, penile/testicular pain, urethral burning/bleeding, priapism **Notes:** Supervision, titrate w/Obs

Alteplase, Recombinant [tPA] (Activase) Uses: *AMI, PE, acute ischemic stroke, & CV cath occlusion* **Action:** Thrombolytic; binds to fibrin in the thrombus, initiates local fibrinolysis **Dose:** *AMI & PE:* 100 mg IV over 3 h (10 mg over 2 min, then 50 mg over 1 h, then 40 mg over 2 h). *Stroke:* 0.9 mg/kg (max 90 mg) inf over 60 min. *Cath occlusion:* 10–29 kg 1 mg/mL, ≥30 kg 2 mg/mL **Caution:** [C, ?] **Contra:** Active internal bleeding; uncontrolled HTN (systolic BP = > 185 mm Hg/diastolic = > 110 mm Hg); recent (w/in 3 mo) CVA, GI bleed, trauma, surgery, prolonged external cardiac massage; intracranial neoplasm, suspected aortic dissection, AVM/aneurysm/subarachnoid hemorrhage, bleeding/hemostatic defects, Sz at the time of stroke **Supplied:** Powder for inj 50, 100 mg **SE:** Bleeding, bruising (eg, venipuncture sites), ↓ BP **Notes:** Give heparin to prevent reocclusion; in AMI, doses of >150 mg associated w/ intracranial bleeding

Altretamine (Hexalen) Uses: *Epithelial ovarian CA* **Action:** Unknown; cytotoxic agent, unknown alkylating agent; ↓ nucleotide incorporation into DNA/RNA **Dose:** 260 mg/m^2/d in 4 ÷ doses for 14–21 d of a 28-d Rx cycle; dose ↑ to 150 mg/m^2/d for 14 d in multiagent regimens (Per protocols) **Caution:** [D, ?/–]. **Contra:** Preexisting BM depression or neurologic tox **Supplied:** Caps 50, 100 mg **SE:** V/D, cramps; neurologic (peripheral neuropathy, CNS depression); minimally myelosuppressive

Aluminum Hydroxide (Amphojel, AlternaGEL) [OTC] Uses: *Relief of heartburn, upset or sour stomach, or acid indigestion*; supl to Rx of hyperphosphatemia **Action:** Neutralizes gastric acid; binds PO_4^{-2} **Dose:** *Adults.* 10–30 mL or 2 tabs PO q4–6h. *Peds.* 5–15 mL PO q4–6h or 50–150 mg/kg/24 h PO ÷ q4–6h (hyperphosphatemia) **Caution:** [C, ?] **Supplied:** Tabs 300, 600 mg; chew tabs 500 mg; susp 320, 600 mg/5 mL **SE:** constipation **Notes:** OK in renal failure

Aluminum Hydroxide + Magnesium Carbonate (Gaviscon) [OTC] Uses: *Relief of heartburn, acid indigestion* **Action:** Neutralizes gastric acid **Dose:** *Adults.* 15–30 mL PO qid or PRN; avoid in renal impair **Caution:** [C, ?] **Supplied:** Liq w/ aluminum hydroxide 95 mg + magnesium carbonate 358 mg/15 mL **SE:** May cause ↑ Mg^{2+} (w/ renal insuff), constipation, D **Notes:** Doses qid are best given pc & hs; may affect absorption of some drugs

Aluminum Hydroxide + Magnesium Hydroxide (Maalox) [OTC] Uses: *Hyperacidity* (peptic ulcer, hiatal hernia, etc) **Action:** Neutralizes gastric acid **Dose:** *Adults.* 10–60 mL or 2–4 tabs PO qid or PRN. *Peds.* 5–15 mL PO qid or PRN **Caution:** [C, ?] **Supplied:** Tabs, susp **SE:** May cause ↑ Mg^{2+} in renal insuff, constipation, D **Notes:** Doses qid best given pc & hs

Aluminum Hydroxide + Magnesium Hydroxide & Simethicone (Mylanta, Mylanta II, Maalox Plus) [OTC] Uses: *Hyperacidity w/ bloating* **Action:** Neutralizes gastric acid & defoaming **Dose:** *Adults.* 10–60 mL or 2–4 tabs PO qid or PRN. *Peds.* 5–15 mL PO qid or PRN; avoid in renal impair **Caution:** [C, ?] **Supplied:** Tabs, susp **SE:** ↑ Mg^{2+} in renal insuff, D, constipation **Notes:** Mylanta II contains 2X aluminum & magnesium hydroxide of Mylanta; may affect absorption of some drugs

Aluminum Hydroxide + Magnesium Trisilicate (Gaviscon, Gaviscon-2) [OTC] Uses: *Relief of heartburn, upset or sour stomach, or acid indigestion* **Action:** Neutralizes gastric acid **Dose:** Chew 2–4 tabs qid; avoid in renal impair **Caution:** [C, ?] **Contra:** Mg^{2+}, sensitivity **Supplied:** *Gaviscon:* Aluminum hydroxide 80 mg & magnesium trisilicate 20 mg; *Gaviscon-2:* Aluminum hydroxide 160 mg & magnesium trisilicate 40 mg **SE:** ↑ Mg^{2+} in renal insuff, constipation, D **Notes:** May affect absorption of some drugs

Amantadine (Symmetrel) Uses: *Rx or prophylaxis influenza A viral Infxns, parkinsonism, & drug-induced EPS* **Action:** Prevents release of infectious viral nucleic acid into host cell; releases dopamine from intact dopaminergic terminals **Dose:** *Adults. Influenza A:* 200 mg/d PO or 100 mg PO bid. *Parkinsonism:* 100 mg PO qd–bid. *Peds. 1–9 y:* 4.4–8.8 mg/kg/24 h to 150 mg/24 h max ÷ doses daily–bid. *10–12 y:* 100–200 mg/d in 1–2 ÷ doses; ↓ in renal impair **Caution:** [C, M] **Supplied:** Caps 100 mg; tabs 100 mg; soln 50 mg/5 mL **SE:** Orthostatic ↓ BP, edema, insomnia, depression, irritability, hallucinations, dream abnormalities

Amifostine (Ethyol) Uses: *Xerostomia prophylaxis during RT (head, neck, ovarian, non-small-cell lung CA). ↓ renal tox associated w/ repeated administration of cisplatin* Action: Prodrug, dephosphorylated by alkaline phosphatase to active thiol metabolite Dose: 910 mg/m²/d 15-min IV inf 30 min prior to chemo Caution: [C, +/−] Supplied: 500-mg vials lyophilized w/ 500 mg of mannitol, reconstitute in sterile NS SE: Transient ↓ BP (>60%), N/V, flushing w/ hot or cold chills, dizziness, ↓ Ca²⁺, somnolence, sneezing Notes: Does not reduce the effectiveness of cyclophosphamide plus cisplatin chemo

Amikacin (Amikin) Uses: *Serious gram(−) bacterial Infxns * & mycobacteria Action: Aminoglycoside; ↓ protein synthesis Spectrum: Good gram(−) bacterial coverage: *Pseudomonas* sp; *Mycobacterium* sp Dose: *Adults & Peds.* 5–7.5 mg/kg/dose ÷ q8–24h based on renal Fxn. *Neonates <1200 g, 0–4 wk:* 7.5 mg/kg/dose q12h–18h. *Postnatal age <7 d, 1200–2000 g:* 7.5 mg/kg/dose q12h; *>2000 g:* 10 mg/kg/dose q12h. *Postnatal age >7 d, 1200–2000 g:* 7.5 mg/kg/dose q8h; *>2000 g:* 7.5–10 mg/kg/dose q8h Caution: [C, +/−] Supplied: Inj 100, 500 mg/2 mL SE: Nephro/oto/neurotox; avoid use w/ diuretics Notes: May be effective in gram(−) bacteria resistant to gentamicin & tobramycin; monitor renal Fxn for dosage adjustments; monitor levels (Table 2, page 200)

Amiloride (Midamor) Uses: *HTN, CHF, & thiazide-induced ↓ K⁺* Action: K⁺-sparing diuretic; interferes w/ K⁺/Na⁺ exchange in distal tubule Dose: *Adults.* 5–10 mg PO daily. *Peds.* 0.625 mg/kg/d; ↓ in renal impair Caution: [B, ?] Contra: ↑ K⁺, SCr > 1.5, BUN > 30 Supplied: Tabs 5 mg SE: ↑ K⁺ possible; monitor K⁺; HA, dizziness, dehydration, impotence

Aminocaproic Acid (Amicar) Uses: *Excessive bleeding from systemic hyperfibrinolysis & urinary fibrinolysis* Action: ↓ fibrinolysis via inhibition of TPA substances Dose: *Adults.* 5 g IV or PO (1st h) followed by 1–1.25 g/h IV or PO (max dose/d: 30 g) *Peds.* 100 mg/kg IV (1st h) then 1 g/m²/h; max 18 g/m²/d; ↓ in renal failure Caution: [C, ?] Upper urinary tract bleeding Contra: DIC Supplied: Tabs 500 mg; syrup 250 mg/mL; inj 250 mg/mL SE: ↓ BP, bradycardia, dizziness, HA, fatigue, rash, GI disturbance, ↓ plt Fxn Notes: Administer for 8 h or until bleeding controlled; not for upper urinary tract bleeding

Amino-Cerv pH 5.5 Cream Uses: *Mild cervicitis,* postpartum cervicitis/cervical tears, postcauterization, postcryosurgery, & postconization Action: Hydrating agent; removes excess keratin in hyperkeratotic conditions Dose: 1 Applicatorful intravag hs for 2–4 wk Caution: [C, ?] Use in viral skin Infxn Supplied: Vaginal cream SE: Transient stinging, local irritation Notes: AKA carbamide or urea; contains 8.34% urea, 0.5% sodium propionate, 0.83% methionine, 0.35% cystine, 0.83% inositol, & benzalkonium chloride

Aminoglutethimide (Cytadren) Uses: Adrenocortical carcinoma, *Cushing syndrome,* breast CA & CAP Action: ↓ adrenal steroidogenesis & conversion of androgens to estrogens Dose: 750–1500 mg/d in divided doses plus hydrocortisone 20–40 mg/d; ↓ in renal insuff **Caution:** [D, ?] **Supplied:** Tabs 250 mg **SE:** Adrenal insuff ("medical adrenalectomy"), hypothyroidism, masculinization, ↓ BP, vomiting, rare hepatotox, rash, myalgia, fever

Aminophylline **Uses:** *Asthma, COPD* & bronchospasm **Action:** Relaxes smooth muscle (bronchi, pulmonary vessels); stimulates diaphragm **Dose:** *Adults.* *Acute asthma:* Load 6 mg/kg IV, then 0.4–0.9 mg/kg/h IV cont inf. *Chronic asthma:* 24 mg/kg/24 h PO or PR ÷ q6h. *Peds.* Load 6 mg/kg IV, then 1 mg/kg/h IV cont inf; ↓ in hepatic insuff & w/ certain drugs (macrolide & quinolone antibiotics, cimetidine, & propranolol) **Caution:** [C, +] Uncontrolled arrhythmias/Sz disorder, hyperthyroidism, peptic ulcers **Supplied:** Tabs 100, 200 mg; soln 105 mg/5 mL; supp 250, 500 mg; inj 25 mg/mL **SE:** N/V, irritability, tachycardia, ventricular arrhythmias, Szs **Notes:** Individualize dosage; follow levels (as theophylline, Table 2, page 200); aminophylline ≅85% theophylline; erratic rectal absorption

Amiodarone (Cordarone, Pacerone) **Uses:** *Recurrent VF or hemodynamically unstable VT,* supraventricular arrhythmias, AF **Action:** Class III antiarrhythmic (Table 12, page 219) **Dose:** *Adults.* Ventricular arrhythmias: *IV:* 15 mg/min for 10 min, then 1 mg/min for 6 h, then maint 0.5 mg/min cont. inf *or PO:* Load: 800–1600 mg/d PO for 1–3 wk. Maint: 600–800 mg/d PO for 1 mo, then 200–400 mg/d. *Supraventricular arrhythmias: IV:* 300 mg IV over 1 h, then 20 mg/kg for 24 h, then 600 mg PO qd for 1 wk, then maint 100–400 mg qd *or PO:* Load: 600–800 mg/d PO for 1–4 wk. Maint: Gradually ↓ to 100–400 mg q day. *Peds.* 10–15 mg/kg/24 h ÷ q12h PO for 7–10 d, then 5 mg/kg/24 h ÷ q12h or daily (infants/neonates require higher loading); ↓ in liver insuff **Caution:** [D, –] **Contra:** Sinus node dysfunction, 2nd- or 3rd-degree AV block, sinus bradycardia (w/o pacemaker) **Supplied:** Tabs 200 mg; inj 50 mg/mL **SE:** Pulmonary fibrosis, exacerbation of arrhythmias, prolongs QT interval; CHF, hypohyperthyroidism, ↑ LFTs, liver failure, corneal microdeposits, optic neuropathy/neuritis, peripheral neuropathy, photosensitivity **Notes:** Half-life 53 d; IV conc of >0.2 mg/mL via a central catheter; may require ↓ digoxin and warfarin dose

Amitriptyline (Elavil) **WARNING:** antidepressants may ↑ risk of suicidality; consider risks and benefits of use. Monitor patients closely **Uses:** *Depression,* peripheral neuropathy, chronic pain, tension HAs **Action:** TCA; ↓ reuptake of serotonin & norepinephrine by presynaptic neurons **Dose:** *Adults.* Initial, 30–50 mg PO hs; may ↑ to 300 mg hs. *Peds.* Not OK <12 y unless for chronic pain; initial 0.1 mg/kg PO hs, ↑ over 2–3 wk to 0.5–2 mg/kg PO hs; taper when D/C **Caution:** [D, +/–] NA glaucoma, hepatic impair **Contra:** W/ MAOIs, during acute MI recovery **Supplied:** Tabs 10, 25, 50, 75, 100, 150 mg; inj 10 mg/mL **SE:** Strong anticholinergic SEs; OD may be fatal; urine retention, sedation, ECG changes, photosensitivity

Amlodipine (Norvasc) **Uses:** *HTN, stable or unstable angina* **Action:** CCB; relaxes coronary vascular smooth muscle **Dose:** 2.5–10 mg/d PO **Caution:** [C, ?] **Supplied:** Tabs 2.5, 5, 10 mg **SE:** Peripheral edema, HA, palpitations, flushing **Notes:** Take w/o regard to meals

Amlodipine/Atorvastatin (Caduet) Uses: * HTN, chronic stable/vasospastic angina, control cholesterol & triglycerides* Action: CCB & HMG-CoA reductase inhibitor Dose: Amlodipine 2.5–10 mg PO qd/ Atorvastatin 10–80 mg PO qd Caution: [X, –] Contra: Active liver Dz, ↑ serum transaminases Supplied: Tabs amlodipine/atorvastatin: 2.5/10, 2.5/20, 2.5/40, 5/10, 5/20, 5/40, 5/80, 10/10, 10/20, 10/40, 10/80 mg SE: Peripheral edema, HA, palpitations, flushing, myopathy, arthralgia, myalgia, GI upset Notes: Monitor LFTs

Ammonium Aluminum Sulfate [Alum] [OTC] Uses: *Hemorrhagic cystitis when saline bladder irrigation fails* Action: Astringent Dose: 1–2% soln w/ constant NS bladder irrigation Caution: [+/–] Supplied: Powder for reconstitution SE: Encephalopathy possible; obtain aluminum levels, especially in renal insuff; can precipitate & occlude catheters Notes: Safe to use w/o anesthesia & w/ vesicoureteral reflux

Amoxicillin (Amoxil, Polymox) Uses: *Ear, nose, & throat, lower resp, skin, urinary tract Infxns resulting from susceptible gram(+) bacteria* endocarditis prophylaxis Action: β-Lactam antibiotic; ↓ cell wall synthesis Spectrum: Gram(+) (Strep sp, Enterococcus sp); some gram(–) (H. influenzae, E. coli, N. gonorrhoeae, H. pylori & P. mirabilis) Dose: Adults. 250–500 mg PO tid or 500–875 mg bid. Peds. 25–100 mg/kg/24 h PO ÷ q8h. 200–400 mg PO bid (equivalent to 125–250 mg tid); ↓ in renal impair Caution: [B, +] Supplied: Caps 250, 500 mg; chew tabs 125, 200, 250, 400 mg; susp 50 mg/mL, 125, 200, 250 & 400 mg/5 mL; tabs 500, 875 mg SE: D; skin rash common Notes: Cross hypersensitivity PCN; many strains of E. coli-resistant

Amoxicillin & Clavulanic Acid (Augmentin, Augmentin 600 ES, Augmentin XR) Uses: *Ear, lower resp, sinus, urinary tract, skin Infxns caused by β-lactamase-producing H. influenzae, S. aureus, & E. coli* Action: Combo β-lactam antibiotic & β-lactamase inhibitor. Spectrum: Gram(+) same as amox alone, MSSA; gram(–) as w/ amox alone, β-lactamase-producing H. influenzae, Klebsiella sp, M. catarrhalis Dose: Adults. 250–500 mg PO q8h or 875 mg q12h; XR 2000 mg PO Q12H. Peds. 20–40 mg/kg/d as amoxicillin PO ÷ q8h or 45 mg/kg/d ÷ q12h; ↓ in renal impair; take w/ food Caution: [B, ?] Supplied (as amoxicillin/clavulanic acid): Tabs 250/125, 500/125, 875/125 mg; chew tabs 125/31.25, 200/28.5, 250/62.5, 400/57 mg; susp 125/31.25, 250/62.5, 200/28.5, 400/57 mg/5 mL; 600-ES 600/42.9 mg tab; XR tab 1000/62.5 mg SE: Abdominal discomfort, N/V/D, allergic Rxn, vaginitis Notes: Do not substitute two 250-mg tabs for one 500-mg tab (OD of clavulanic acid)

Amphotericin B (Fungizone) Uses: *Severe, systemic fungal Infxns; oral & cutaneous candidiasis* Action: Binds ergosterol in the fungal membrane to alter permeability Dose: Adults & Peds. Test dose: 1 mg IV adults or 0.1 mg/kg to 1 mg IV in children; then 0.25–1.5 mg/kg/24 h IV over 2–6 h (range 25–50 mg/d or qod). Total dose varies w/ indication. PO: 1 mL qid. Topical: Apply bid–qid for 1–4 wk depending on Infxn; ↓ in renal impair Caution: [B, ?] Supplied: Powder for inj 50 mg/vial; PO susp 100 mg/mL; cream, lotion, oint 3% **SE:** ↓ K⁺/Mg²⁺ from renal wasting; anaphylaxis reported, HA, fever, chills, nephrotoxicity, ↓ BP, anemia **Notes:** Monitor renal Fxn/LFTs; pretreatment w/ APAP & antihistamines (Benadryl) minimizes adverse IV effects (eg, fever, chills,)

Amphotericin B Cholesteryl (Amphotec) **Uses:** *Aspergillosis in pts intolerant or refractory to conventional amphotericin B,* systemic candidiasis **Action:** Binds sterols in the cell membrane, alters permeability **Dose:** *Adults* & *Peds.* Test dose 1.6–8.3 mg, over 15–20 min, then 3–4 mg/kg/d; 1 mg/kg/h inf; ↓ in renal insuff **Caution:** [B, ?] **Supplied:** Powder for inj 50 mg, 100 mg/vial (final = 0.6 mg/mL) **SE:** Anaphylaxis reported; fever, chills, HA, ↓ K⁺, ↓ Mg²⁺, nephrotox, ↓ BP, anemia **Notes:** Do not use in-line filter; monitor LFT & electrolytes

Amphotericin B Lipid Complex (Abelcet) **Uses:** *Refractory invasive fungal Infxn in pts intolerant to conventional amphotericin B* **Action:** Binds sterols in cell membrane, alters permeability **Dose:** *Adults* & *Peds.* 5 mg/kg/d IV single daily dose; 2.5 mg/kg/h inf **Caution:** [B, ?] **Supplied:** Inj 5 mg/mL **SE:** Anaphylaxis: fever, chills, HA, ↓ K⁺, ↓ Mg²⁺, nephrotox, ↓ BP, anemia **Notes:** Filter soln w/5-mcm filter needle; do not mix in electrolyte-containing solns; if inf >2 h, manually mix bag

Amphotericin B Liposomal (AmBisome) **Uses:** *Refractory invasive fungal Infxn in pts intolerant to conventional amphotericin B, cryptococcal meningitis in HIV, empiric Rx for febrile neutropenia, visceral leishmaniasis* **Action:** Binds to sterols in cell membrane, changes membrane permeability **Dose:** *Adults* & *Peds.* 3–5 mg/kg/d, inf 60–120 min; ↓ in renal insuff **Caution:** [B, ?] **Supplied:** Powder for inj 50 mg **SE:** Anaphylaxis reported; fever, chills, HA, ↓ K⁺, ↓ Mg²⁺ nephrotox, ↓ BP, anemia **Notes:** Filter w/ no less than 1-mcm filter

Ampicillin (Amcill, Omnipen) **Uses:** *Resp, GU, or GI tract Infxns, meningitis due to gram(−) & gram(+) bacteria; endocarditis prophylaxis* **Action:** β-Lactam antibiotic; ↓ cell wall synthesis. *Spectrum:* Gram(+) (*Streptococcus* sp, *Staphylococcus* sp, *Listeria*); gram(−) (*Klebsiella* sp, *E. coli, H. influenzae, P. mirabilis, Shigella* sp, *Salmonella* sp) **Dose:** *Adults.* 500 mg–2 g IM or IV q6h or 250–500 mg PO q6h. *Peds. Neonates* <7 d: 50–100 mg/kg/24 h IV ÷ q8h. *Term infants:* 75–150 mg/kg/24 h ÷ q6–8h IV or PO. *Children >1 mo:* 100–200 mg/kg/24 h ÷ q4–6h IM or IV; 50–100 mg/kg/24 h ÷ q6h PO up to 250 mg/dose. *Meningitis:* 200–400 mg/kg/24 h ÷ q4–6h IV; ↓ in renal impair; take on empty stomach **Caution:** [B, M] Cross hypersensitivity w/ PCN **Supplied:** Caps 250, 500 mg; susp 100 mg/mL (reconstituted as drops), 125 mg/5 mL, 250 mg/5 mL, 500 mg/5 mL; powder for inj 125 mg, 250 mg, 500 mg. 1 g, 2 g, 10 g/vial **SE:** D, skin rash, allergic Rxn **Notes:** Many strains of *E. coli*-resistant

Ampicillin–Sulbactam (Unasyn) **Uses:** *Gynecologic, intraabdominal, skin Infxns caused by β-lactamase-producing strains of S. aureus, Enterococcus, H. influenzae, P. mirabilis, & Bacteroides sp* **Action:** Combo β-lactam antibiotic & a β-lactamase inhibitor. *Spectrum:* Gram(+) & gram(−) as for amp alone; also

Enterobacter, Acinetobacter, Bacteroides **Dose:** *Adults.* 1.5–3 g IM or IV q6h. **Peds.** 100–200 mg ampicillin/kg/d (150–300 mg Unasyn) q6h; ↓ in renal failure **Caution:** [B, M] **Supplied:** Powder for inj 1.5, 3.0 g/vial **SE:** Allergy Rxns, rash, D, pain at injection site **Notes:** A 2:1 ratio ampicillin:sulbactam

Amprenavir (Agenerase) **WARNING:** PO soln contra in children <4 y (potential tox from large volume of polypropylene glycol in formulation) **Uses:** *HIV Infxn* **Action:** Protease inhibitor; prevents the maturation of the virion to mature virus **Dose:** *Adults.* 1200 mg bid. **Peds.** 20 mg/kg bid or 15 mg/kg tid up to 2400 mg/d **Caution:** [C, ?] CDC recommends HIV-infected mothers not breast-feed (risk of HIV transmission); Hx sulfonamides allergy **Contra:** CYP450 3A4 substrates (ergot derivatives, midazolam, triazolam, etc); soln < 4 y, PRG, hepatic or renal failure, disulfram, or metronidazole **Supplied:** Caps 50, 150 mg; soln 15 mg/mL **SE:** Life-threatening rash, hyperglycemia, hypertriglyceridemia, fat re-distribution, N/V/D, depression **Notes:** Caps & soln contain vitamin E exceeding RDA ; avoid high-fat meals; many drug interactions

Anakinra (Kineret) **WARNING:** Associated w/ ↑ incidence of serious Infxn; D/C w/ serious Infxn **Uses:** *Reduce signs & Sxs of moderate/severe active RA, failed 1 or more DMARD* **Action:** Human IL-1 receptor antagonist **Dose:** 100 mg SQ qd **Caution:** [B, ?] **Contra:** Allergy to *E. coli*-derived proteins, active Infxn, <18 y **Supplied:** 100-mg prefilled syringes **SE:** Neutropenia especially when used w/ TNF-blocking agents, inj site Rxn, Infxn

Anastrozole (Arimidex) **Uses:** *Breast CA: postmenopausal w/ metasta-tic breast CA, adjuvant Rx of postmenopausal w/ early hormone-receptor(+) breast CA* **Action:** Selective nonsteroidal aromatase inhibitor, ↓ circ estradiol **Dose:** 1 mg/d **Caution:** [C, ?] **Contra:** PRG **Supplied:** Tabs 1 mg **SE:** May ↑ choles-terol; D, HTN, flushing, ↑ bone & tumor pain, HA, somnolence **Notes:** No effect on adrenal corticosteroids or aldosterone

Anistreplase (Eminase) **Uses:** *AMI* **Action:** Thrombolytic; activates conversion of plasminogen to plasmin, ↑ thrombolysis **Dose:** 30 units IV over 2–5 min **Caution:** [C, ?] **Contra:** Active internal bleeding, Hx CVA, recent (<2 mo) in-tracranial or intraspinal surgery/trauma, intracranial neoplasm, AVM, aneurysm, bleeding diathesis, severe uncontrolled HTN **Supplied:** Vials w/30 units **SE:** Bleeding, ↓ BP, hematoma **Notes:** Ineffective if readministered >5 d after the pre-vious dose of anistreplase or streptokinase, or streptococcal Infxn (production of antistreptokinase Ab)

Anthralin (Anthra-Derm) **Uses:** *Psoriasis* **Action:** Keratolytic **Dose:** Apply qd **Caution:** [C, ?] **Contra:** Acutely inflamed psoriatic eruptions, erythro-derma **Supplied:** Cream, oint 0.1, 0.2, 0.25, 0.4, 0.5, 1% **SE:** Irritation; hair/finger-nails/skin discoloration

Antihemophilic Factor [AHF, Factor VIII] (Monoclate) **Uses:** *Classic hemophilia A, von Willebrand Dz* **Action:** Provides factor VIII needed to convert prothrombin to thrombin **Dose:** *Adults & Peds.* 1 AHF unit/kg ↑ factor

VIII level ≅2%. Units required = (kg) (desired factor VIII ↑ as % nl) × (0.5). Prevent spontaneous hemorrhage = 5% nl. Hemostasis after trauma/surgery = 30% nl. Head injuries, major surgery, or bleeding = 80–100% nl. Determine pt's % of nl factor VIII before dosing **Caution:** [C, ?] **Supplied:** Check each vial for units contained **SE:** Rash, fever, HA, chills, N/V

Antithymocyte Globulin. See Lymphocyte Immune Globulin, page 123

Apomorphine (Apokyn) WARNING: Do not administer IV **Uses:** *Acute, intermittent hypomobility ("off") episodes of Parkinson Dz* **Action:** Dopamine agonist **Dose:** *Adults.* 0.2-mL SQ test dose under medical supervision; if BP OK, initial 0.2 mL SQ during "off" periods; only 1 dose per "off" period; requires careful titration; 0.6 mL max single doses; requires concomitant antiemetic; ↓ in renal impair **Caution:** [C, +/–] Avoid EtOH; antihypertensives, vasodilators, cardio or cerebrovascular Dz, hepatic impair **Contra:** 5HT3 antagonists, sulfite allergy **Supplied:** Inj 10 mg/mL, 3-mL prefilled pen cartridges; 2-mL amp **SE:** Emesis, syncope, QT prolongation, orthostatic ↓ BP, somnolence, ischemia, injection site Rxn, abuse potential, dyskinesia, fibrotic conditions, priapism **Notes:** Potential for daytime somnolence may limit activities; trimethobenzamide 300 mg tid PO or other non-5HT3 antagonist antiemetic given 3 d prior to & up to 2 mo following initiation

Apraclonidine (Iopidine) **Uses:** *Glaucoma, postop intraocular HTN* **Action:** α₂-Adrenergic agonist **Dose:** 1–2 gtt of 0.5% tid **Caution:** [C, ?] **Contra:** MAOI use **Supplied:** 0.5, 1% soln **SE:** Ocular irritation, lethargy, xerostomia

Aprepitant (Emend) **Uses:** *N/V assoc w/ emetogenic CA chemo (eg, cisplatin) (use in combo w/ other antiemetics)* **Action:** Substance P/neurokinin 1(NK₁) receptor antagonist **Dose:** 125 mg PO day 1, 1 h before chemo, then 80 mg PO q AM on days 2 & 3 **Caution:** [B, ?/–]; substrate & moderate inhibitor of CYP3A4; inducer of CYP2C9 **Contra:** Use w/ pimozide **Supplied:** Caps 80, 125 mg **SE:** Fatigue, asthenia, hiccups **Notes:** ↓ Effectiveness of PO contraceptives; ↓ effect of warfarin

Aprotinin (Trasylol) **Uses:** *↓/Prevents blood loss during CABG* **Action:** Protease inhibitor, antifibrinolytic **Dose:** 1-mL IV test dose. *High dose:* 2 million KIU load, 2 million KIU to prime pump, then 500,000 KIU/h until surgery ends. *Low dose:* 1 million KIU load, 1 million KIU to prime pump, then 250,000 KIU/h until surgery ends; 7 million KIU max total **Caution:** [B, ?] Thromboembolic Dz requiring anticoagulants or blood factor administration **Supplied:** Inj 1.4 mg/mL (10,000 KIU/mL) **SE:** AF, MI, heart failure, dyspnea, postop renal dysfunction **Notes:** 1000/KIU = 0.14 mg of aprotinin

Ardeparin (Normiflo) **Uses:** *Prevents DVT/PE following knee replacement* **Action:** LMW heparin **Dose:** 35–50 units/kg SQ q12h. Begin day of surgery, continue up to 14 d **Caution:** [C, ?] ↓ renal Fxn **Contra:** Active hemorrhage; allergy to pork products **Supplied:** Inj 5000, 10,000 IU/0.5 mL **SE:** Bleeding, bruising, thrombocytopenia, pain at inj site, ↑ serum transaminases **Notes:** Lab monitoring usually not necessary

Argatroban (Acova) Uses: *Prophylaxis or Rx of thrombosis in HIT, PCI in pts w/ risk of HIT* **Action:** Anticoagulant, direct thrombin inhibitor **Dose:** 2 mcg/kg/min IV; adjust until aPTT 1.5–3× baseline not to exceed 100 s; 10 mcg/kg/min max; ↓ in hepatic impair **Caution:** [B, ?] Avoid PO anticoagulants, ↑ bleeding risk; avoid concomitant use of thrombolytics **Contra:** Overt major bleed **Supplied:** Inj 100 mg/ml **SE:** AF, cardiac arrest, cerebrovascular disorder, ↓ BP, VT, N/V/D, sepsis, cough, renal tox, ↓ Hgb **Note:** steady state in 1–3h

Aripiprazole (Abilify) WARNING: Increased mortality in elderly with dementia-related psychosis **Uses:** *Schizophrenia* **Action:** Dopamine & serotonin antagonist **Dose:** *Adults.* 10–15 mg PO qd; ↓ when used w/ potent CYP3A4 or CYP2D6 inhibitors (page 220); ↑ when used w/ inducer of CYP3A4 **Caution:** [C, –] **Supplied:** Tabs 5, 10, 15, 20, 30 mg; soln 1 mg/ml **SE:** Neuroleptic malignant syndrome, tardive dyskinesia, orthostatic ↓ BP, cognitive & motor impair, hyperglycemia

Artificial Tears (Tears Naturale) [OTC] Uses: *Dry eyes* **Action:** Ocular lubricant **Dose:** 1–2 gtt tid–qid **Supplied:** OTC soln

L-Asparaginase (Elspar, Oncaspar) Uses: *ALL* (in combo w/ other agents) **Action:** Protein synthesis inhibitor **Dose:** 500–20,000 IU/m²/d for 1–14 d (Per protocols) **Caution:** [C, ?] **Contra:** Active/Hx pancreatitis **Supplied:** Inj 10,000 IU **SE:** Allergy 20–35% (from urticaria to anaphylaxis test dose recommended); rare GI tox (mild nausea/anorexia, pancreatitis)

Aspirin (Bayer, Ecotrin, St. Joseph's) [OTC] Uses: *Angina, CABG, PTCA, carotid endarterectomy, ischemic stroke, TIA, MI, arthritis, pain,* HA, *fever,* inflammation, Kawasaki Dz **Action:** Prostaglandin inhibitor **Dose:** *Adults.* Pain, fever: 325–650 mg q4–6h PO or PR. *RA:* 3–6 g/d PO in ÷ doses. *Plt inhibitor:* 81–325 mg PO qd. *Prevent MI:* 81–325 mg PO qd. **Peds.** *Antipyretic:* 10–15 mg/kg/dose PO or PR q4h up to 80 mg/kg/24 h. *RA:* 60–100 mg/kg/24 h PO ÷ q4–6h (keep levels between 15 & 30 mg/dL); avoid w/ CrCl <10 mL/min, in severe liver Dz **Caution:** [C, M] Use linked to Reye syndrome; avoid w/ viral illness in children **Contra:** Allergy to ASA, chickenpox/flu Sxs, syndrome of nasal polyps, asthma, rhinitis **Supplied:** Tabs 325, 500 mg; chew tabs 81 mg; EC tabs 165, 325, 500, 650, 975 mg; SR tabs 650, 800 mg; effervescent tabs 325, 500 mg; supp 120, 200, 300, 600 mg **SE:** GI upset & erosion **Notes:** D/C 1 wk prior to surgery to ↓ bleeding; avoid/limit EtOH

Aspirin & Butalbital Compound (Fiorinal) [C-III] Uses: *Tension HA,* pain **Action:** Combo barbiturate & analgesic **Dose:** 1–2 PO q4h PRN, max 6 tabs/d; avoid w/ CrCl <10 mL/min & severe liver Dz **Caution:** [C (D if prolonged use or high doses at term), ?] **Contra:** ASA allergy, GI ulceration, bleeding disorder, porphyria, syndrome of nasal polyps, angioedema, & bronchospasm to NSAIDs **Supplied:** Caps (Fiorgen PF, Fiorinal) Tabs (Fiorinal, Lanorinal) ASA 325 mg/butalbital 50 mg/caffeine 40 mg **SE:** Drowsiness, dizziness, GI upset, ulceration, bleeding **Notes:** Butalbital habit-forming; avoid or limit EtOH intake

Aspirin + Butalbital, Caffeine, & Codeine (Fiorinal + Codeine) [C-III] Uses: Mild *pain*, HA, especially when associated w/ stress Action: Sedative analgesic, narcotic analgesic Dose: 1–2 tabs (caps) PO q4–6h PRN Caution: [D, ?] Contra: Allergy to ASA Supplied: Cap/tab contains 325 mg ASA, 40 mg caffeine, 50 mg of butalbital, 30 mg of codeine SE: Drowsiness, dizziness, GI upset, ulceration, bleeding

Aspirin + Codeine (Empirin No. 2, No. 3, No. 4) [C-III] Uses: Mild to *moderate pain* Action: Combined effects of ASA & codeine Dose: Adults. 1–2 tabs PO q4–6h PRN. Peds. ASA 10 mg/kg/dose; codeine 0.5–1 mg/kg/dose q4h Caution: [D, M] Contra: Allergy to ASA/codeine, PUD, bleeding, anticoagulant Rx, children w/ chickenpox or flu Sxs Supplied: Tabs 325 mg of ASA & codeine (Codeine in No. 2 = 15 mg, No. 3 = 30 mg, No. 4 = 60 mg) SE: Drowsiness, dizziness, GI upset, ulceration, bleeding

Atazanavir (Reyataz) WARNING: Hyperbilirubinemia may require drug D/C Uses: *HIV-1 Infxn* Action: Protease inhibitor Dose: 400 mg PO qd w/ food; when given w/ efavirenz 600 mg, administer atazanavir 300 mg + ritonavir 100 mg once/d; separate doses from buffered didanosine administration; ↓ in hepatic impair Caution: [B, –]; ↑ levels of statins, sildenafil, antiarrhythmics, warfarin, cyclosporine, TCAs; atazanavir ↓ by St. John's wort Contra: Use w/midazolam, triazolam, ergots, cisapride, pimozide Supplied: Caps 100, 150, 200 mg SE: HA, N/V/D, rash, abdominal pain, DM, photosensitivity, ↑ PR interval Notes: May have less adverse effect on cholesterol

Atenolol (Tenormin) Uses: *HTN, angina, MI* Action: Competitively blocks β-adrenergic receptors, β₁ Dose: HTN & angina: 50–100 mg/d PO. AMI: 5 mg IV ×2 over 10 min, then 50 mg PO bid if tolerated; ↓ in renal impair Caution: [D, M] DM, bronchospasm; abrupt D/C can exacerbate angina & ↑ MI risk Contra: Bradycardia, cardiogenic shock, cardiac failure, 2nd- or 3rd- degree AV block Supplied: Tabs 25, 50, 100 mg; inj 5 mg/10 mL SE: Bradycardia, ↓ BP, 2nd- or 3rd-degree AV block, dizziness, fatigue

Atenolol & Chlorthalidone (Tenoretic) Uses: *HTN* Action: β-Adrenergic blockade w/ diuretic Dose: 50–100 mg/d PO; ↓ in renal impair Caution: [D, M] DM, bronchospasm Contra: Use atenolol; anuria Supplied: Tenoretic 50: Atenolol 50 mg/chlorthalidone 25 mg; Tenoretic 100: Atenolol 100 mg/chlorthalidone 25 mg SE: Bradycardia, ↓ BP, 2nd- or 3rd-degree AV block, dizziness, fatigue, ↓ K⁺, photosensitivity

Atomoxetine (Strattera) WARNING: Severe liver injury may occur in rare cases. DK w/jaundice or ↑ LFT Uses: * ADHD* Action: Selective norepinephrine reuptake inhibitor Dose: Adults & children >70 kg. 40 mg × 3 days, ↑ to 80–100 mg + daily–bid. Peds < 70 kg. 0.5 mg/kg × 3 d, then ↑ 1.2 mg/kg max daily or bid Caution: [C, ? /–] Contra: NA glaucoma, use w/ or w/in 2 wk of D/C an MAOI Supplied: Caps 10, 18, 25, 40, 60 mg SE: ↑ BP, tachycardia, weight loss, sexual dysfunction Notes: ↓ dose w/ hepatic insuff, ↓ in combo w/ inhibitors of CYP2D6 (p. 220)

Atorvastatin (Lipitor) Uses: *↑ cholesterol & triglycerides* Action: HMG-CoA reductase inhibitor Dose: Initial 10 mg/d, may ↑ to 80 mg/d Caution: [X, –] Contra: Active liver Dz, unexplained ↑ of transaminases Supplied: Tabs 10, 20, 40, 80 mg SE: Myopathy, HA, arthralgia, myalgia, GI upset Notes: monitor LFTs

Atovaquone (Mepron) Uses: *Rx & prevention PCP* Action: ↓ nucleic acid & ATP synthesis Dose: Rx: 750 mg PO bid for 21 d. Prevention: 1500 mg PO once/d (w/ meals) Caution: [C, ?] Supplied: Suspension 750 mg/5 mL SE: Fever, HA, anxiety, insomnia, rash, N/V

Atovaquone/Proguanil (Malarone) Uses: *Prevention or Rx P. falciparum malaria* Action: Antimalarial Dose: Adults: Prevention: 1 tab PO 2 d before, during, & 7 d after leaving endemic region; Rx: 4 tabs PO single dose qd ×3 d. Peds. See insert Caution: [C, ?] Contra: CrCl < 30 mL/min Supplied: Tab atovaquone 250 mg/proguanil 100 mg; peds 62.5/25 mg SE: HA, fever, myalgia

Atracurium (Tracrium) Uses: *Anesthesia adjunct to facilitate ET intubation* Action: Nondepolarizing neuromuscular blocker Dose: Adults & Peds. 0.4–0.5 mg/kg IV bolus, then 0.08–0.1 mg/kg q20–45 min PRN Caution: [C, ?] Supplied: Inj 10 mg/mL SE: Flushing Notes: Pt must be intubated & on controlled ventilation; use adequate amounts of sedation & analgesia

Atropine Uses: *Preanesthetic; symptomatic bradycardia & asystole* Action: Antimuscarinic agent; blocks acetylcholine at parasympathetic sites Dose: Adults. ECC: 0.5–1 mg IV q3–5min. Preanesthetic: 0.3–0.6 mg IM. Peds. ECC: 0.01–0.03 mg/kg IV q2–5min, max 1 mg, min dose 0.1 mg. Preanesthetic: 0.01 mg/kg/dose SC/IV (max 0.4 mg) Caution: [C, +] Contra: Glaucoma Supplied: Tabs 0.3, 0.4, 0.6 mg; inj 0.05, 0.1, 0.3, 0.4, 0.5, 0.8, 1 mg/mL; ophth 0.5, 1, 2% SE: Blurred vision, urinary retention, constipation, dried mucous membranes

Azathioprine (Imuran) Uses: *Adjunct to prevent renal transplant rejection, RA,* SLE Action: Immunosuppressive; antagonizes purine metabolism Dose: Adults & Peds. 1–3 mg/kg/d IV or PO (↓ in renal failure) Caution: [D, ?] Contra: PRG Supplied: Tabs 50 mg; inj 100 mg/20 mL SE: GI intolerance, fever, chills, leukopenia, thrombocytopenia; chronic use may ↑ neoplasia Notes: Handle inj w/ cytotoxic precautions; interaction w/ allopurinol; do not administer live vaccines to a pt taking azathioprine

Azelastine (Astelin, Optivar) Uses: *Allergic rhinitis (rhinorrhea, sneezing, nasal pruritus); allergic conjunctivitis* Action: Histamine H₁-receptor antagonist Dose: Nasal: 2 sprays/nostril bid. Ophth: 1 gtt into each affected eye bid Caution: [C, ?/–] Contra: Component sensitivity Supplied: Nasal 137 mcg/spray; ophth soln 0.05% SE: Somnolence, bitter taste

Azithromycin (Zithromax) Uses: *Community-acquired pneumonia, pharyngitis, otitis media, skin Infxns, nongonococcal urethritis, & PID; Rx & prevention of MAC in HIV* Action: Macrolide antibiotic; ↓ protein synthesis. Spectrum: Chlamydia, H. ducreyi, H. influenzae, Legionella, M. catarrhalis, M. pneumoniae, M.

hominis, N. gonorrhoeae, S. aureus, S. agalactiae, S. pneumoniae, S. pyogenes **Dose: Adults. PO:** *Resp tract Infxns:* 500 mg day 1, then 250 mg/d PO ×4 d; 500 mg/d PO × 3 days; or 2g PO × 1. *Nongonococcal urethritis:* 1 g PO single dose. *Prevention of MAC:* 1200 mg PO once/wk. *IV:* 500 mg ×2 d, then 500 mg PO ×7–10 d. **Peds.** *Otitis media:* 10 mg/kg PO day 1, then 5 mg/kg/d days 2–5. *Pharyngitis:* 12 mg/kg PO ×5 d (take susp on an empty stomach; tabs may be taken w/wo food) **Caution:** [B, +] **Supplied:** Tabs 250, 600 mg; Z-Pack (5-day); Tri-Pak (500-mg tabs × 3); susp 1-g; single-dose packet Zmax (2 gm); susp 100, 200 mg/5 mL; inj 500 mg **SE:** GI upset

Aztreonam (Azactam) **Uses:** *Aerobic gram(–) UTIs, lower resp, intraabdominal, skin, gynecologic Infxns & septicemia* **Action:** Monobactam; ↓ Cell wall synthesis. **Spectrum:** Gram(–) (*Pseudomonas, E. coli, Klebsiella, H. influenzae, Serratia, Proteus, Enterobacter, Citrobacter*) **Dose: Adults.** 1–2 g IV/IM q6–12h. **Peds.** *Premature:* 30 mg/kg/dose IV q12h. *Term & children:* 30 mg/kg/dose q6–8h; ↓ in renal impair **Caution:** [B, +] **Supplied:** Inj 500 mg, 1 g, 2 g **SE:** N/V/D, rash, pain at injection site **Notes:** No gram(+) or anaerobic activity; OK in PCN-allergic pts

Bacitracin, Ophthalmic (AK-Tracin Ophthalmic); Bacitracin & Polymyxin B, Ophthalmic (AK Poly Bac Ophthalmic, Polysporin Ophthalmic); Bacitracin, Neomycin, & Polymyxin B, Ophthalmic (AK Spore Ophthalmic, Neosporin Ophthalmic); Bacitracin, Neomycin, Polymyxin B, & Hydrocortisone, Ophthalmic (AK Spore HC Ophthalmic, Cortisporin Ophthalmic) **Uses:** *Steroid-responsive inflammatory ocular conditions* **Action:** Topical antibiotic w/antiinflammatory **Dose:** Apply q3–4h into conjunctival sac **Caution:** [C, ?] **Contra:** Viral, mycobacterial, fungal eye Infxn **Supplied:** See Bacitracin, Topical equivalents, below

Bacitracin, Topical (Baciguent); Bacitracin & Polymyxin B, Topical (Polysporin); Bacitracin, Neomycin, & Polymyxin B, Topical (Neosporin Ointment); Bacitracin, Neomycin, Polymyxin B, & Hydrocortisone, Topical (Cortisporin); Bacitracin, Neomycin, Polymyxin B, & Lidocaine, Topical (Clomycin) **Uses:** Prevent/Rx of *minor skin Infxns* **Action:** Topical antibiotic w/ added components (antiinflammatory & analgesic) **Dose:** Apply sparingly bid–qid **Caution:** [C, ?] **Supplied:** Bacitracin 500 U/g oint; Bacitracin 500 U/polymyxin B sulfate 10,000 U/g oint & powder; Bacitracin 400 U/neomycin 3.5 mg/polymyxin B 5000 U/g oint (Neosporin Cream, see page 136); Bacitracin 400 U/neomycin 3.5 mg/polymyxin B/10,000 U/hydrocortisone 10 mg/g oint; Bacitracin 500 U/neomycin 3.5 g/ polymyxin B 5000 U/lidocaine 40 mg/g oint **Notes:** Systemic & irrigation forms available, but not generally used due to potential tox

Baclofen (Lioresal) **Uses:** *Spasticity due to severe chronic disorders (eg, MS, ALS, or spinal cord lesions),* trigeminal neuralgia, hiccups **Action:** Centrally acting skeletal muscle relaxant; ↓ transmission of both monosynaptic & polysynaptic cord reflexes **Dose:** *Adults.* Initial, 5 mg PO tid; ↑ q3d to effect; max 80 mg/d. *Intrathecal:* via implantable pump *Peds.* 2–7 y: 10–15 mg/d ÷ q8h; titrate, max 40 mg/d. *>8 y:* Max 60 mg/d. *IT:* via implantable pump; in renal impair; w/ food or milk **Caution:** [C, +] Epilepsy, neuropsychiatric disturbances; withdrawal may occur w/ abrupt D/C **Supplied:** Tabs 10, 20 mg; IT inj 10 mg/20 mL, 10 mg/5 mL **SE:** Dizziness, drowsiness, insomnia, ataxia, weakness, ↓ BP

Balsalazide (Colazal) **Uses:** *Ulcerative colitis* **Action:** 5-ASA derivative, antiinflammatory, ↓ leukotriene synthesis **Dose:** 2.25 g (3 caps) tid ×8–12 wk **Caution:** [B, ?] Severe renal/hepatic failure **Contra:** Mesalamine or salicylate hypersensitivity **Supplied:** Caps 750 mg **SE:** Dizziness, HA, nausea, agranulocytosis, pancytopenia, renal impair, allergic Rxns **Notes:** Daily dose of 6.75 g = to 2.4 g mesalamine

Basiliximab (Simulect) **Uses:** *Prevent acute organ transplant rejection* **Action:** IL-2 receptor antagonists **Dose:** *Adults.* 20 mg IV 2 h before transplant, then 20 mg IV 4 d posttransplant. *Peds.* 12 mg/m² ↑ to max of 20 mg 2 h prior to transplant; the same dose IV 4 d posttransplant **Caution:** [B, ?/–] **Contra:** Hypersensitivity to Murine proteins **Supplied:** Inj 20 mg **SE:** Edema, HTN, HA, dizziness, fever, pain, Infxn, GI effects, electrolyte disturbances **Notes:** Murine/human MoAb

BCG [Bacillus Calmette-Guérin] (TheraCys, Tice BCG) **Uses:** *Bladder carcinoma (superficial),* *TB prophylaxis* **Action:** Immunomodulator **Dose:** Bladder CA, 1 vial prepared & instilled in bladder for 2 h. Repeat once/wk for 6 wk; then maint 3/wk at 3, 6, 12, 18, & 24 mo after initial therapy **Caution:** [C, ?] Asthma, do not administer w/traumatic catheterization or UTI **Contra:** Immunosuppression, UTI, steroid use, acute illness, fever of unknown origin **Supplied:** Inj 81 mg (10.5 ± 8.7 × 10⁸ CFU vial) (TheraCys), 1–8 × 10⁸ CFU/vial (Tice BCG) **SE:** *Intravesical:* Hematuria, urinary frequency, dysuria, bacterial UTI, rare BCG sepsis **Notes:** Routine US adult BCG immunization not OK; occasionally used in high-risk children who are PPD(–) & cannot take INH

Becaplermin (Regranex Gel) **Uses:** Adjunct to local wound care w/*diabetic foot ulcers* **Action:** Recombinant PDGF, enhances granulation tissue **Dose:** Based on lesion; 1⅓-in. ribbon from 2-g tube, ⅔-in. ribbon from 7.5- or 15-g tube/in.² of ulcer; apply & cover w/moist gauze; rinse after 12h; do not reapply; repeat in 12 h **Caution:** [C, ?] **Contra:** Neoplasm/or active site Infxn **Supplied:** 0.01% gel in 2-, 7.5-, 15-g tubes **SE:** Erythema, local pain **Notes:** Use w/ good wound care; wound must be vascularized

Beclomethasone (Beconase, Vancenase Nasal Inhaler) **Uses:** *Allergic rhinitis* refractory to antihistamines & decongestants; *nasal polyps* **Action:** Inhaled steroid **Dose:** *Adults.* 1 spray intranasal bid–qid. *Aqueous inhal:* 1–2 sprays/nostril daily. *Peds 6–12 y.* 1 spray intranasal tid **Caution:** [C, ?] **Supplied:** Nasal met-dose inhaler **SE:** Local irritation, burning, epistaxis **Notes:** Nasal spray delivers 42 mcg/dose & 84 mcg/dose

Beclomethasone (QVAR) Uses: Chronic *asthma* Action: Inhaled corticosteroid Dose: *Adults & Peds.* 1–4 inhal bid (Rinse mouth/throat after) Caution: [C, ?] Contra: Acute asthma Supplied: PO met-dose inhaler; 40, 80 mcg/inhal SE: HA, cough, hoarseness, oral candidiasis Notes: Not effective for acute asthma

Belladonna & Opium Suppositories (B & O Supprettes) [C-II] Uses: *Bladder spasms; moderate/severe pain* Action: Antispasmodic, analgesic Dose: 1 supp PR q6h PRN; 15A = 30 mg powdered opium/16.2 mg belladonna extract; 16A = 60 mg powdered opium/16.2 mg belladonna extract Caution: [C, ?] Supplied: Supp 15A, 16A SE: Anticholinergic (sedation, urinary retention, constipation)

Benazepril (Lotensin) Uses: *HTN,* DN, CHF Action: ACE inhibitor Dose: 10–40 mg/d PO Caution: [C (1st tri), D (2nd & 3rd tri), +] Contra: Angioedema, Hx edema Supplied: Tabs 5, 10, 20, 40 mg SE: Symptomatic ↓ BP w/ diuretics; dizziness, HA, ↓ K⁺, nonproductive cough

Benzocaine & Antipyrine (Auralgan) Uses: *Analgesia in severe otitis media* Action: Anesthetic w/ local decongestant Dose: Fill ear & insert a moist cotton plug; repeat 1–2 h PRN Caution: [C, ?] Contra: w/ perforated eardrum Supplied: Soln SE: Local irritation

Benzonatate (Tessalon Perles) Uses: Symptomatic relief of *cough* Action: Anesthetizes the stretch receptors in the resp passages Dose: *Adults & Peds >10 y.* 100 mg PO tid Caution: [C, ?] Supplied: Caps 100 mg SE: Sedation, dizziness, GI upset Notes: Do not chew or puncture the caps

Benztropine (Cogentin) Uses: *Parkinsonism & drug-induced extrapyramidal disorders* Action: Partially blocks striatal cholinergic receptors Dose: *Adults.* 0.5–6 mg PO, IM, or IV in ÷ doses/d. *Peds >3 y.* 0.02–0.05 mg/kg/dose 1–2/d Caution: [C, ?] Contra: < 3 y Supplied: Tabs 0.5, 1, 2 mg; inj 1 mg/mL SE: Anticholinergic side effects Notes: Physostigmine 1–2 mg SC/IV to reverse severe Sxs

Beractant (Survanta) Uses: *Prevention & Rx of RDS in premature infants* Action: Replaces pulmonary surfactant Dose: 100 mg/kg via ET tube; may repeat 3× q6h; max 4 doses/48 h Supplied: Susp 25 mg of phospholipid/mL SE: Transient bradycardia, desaturation, apnea Notes: Administer via 4-quadrant method

Betaxolol (Kerlone) Uses: *HTN* Action: Competitively blocks β-adrenergic receptors, β₁ Caution: [C (1st tri), D (2nd or 3rd tri), +/–] Contra: Sinus bradycardia, AV conduction abnormalities, cardiac failure Dose: 10–20 mg/d Supplied: Tabs 10, 20 mg SE: Dizziness, HA, bradycardia, edema, CHF

Betaxolol, Ophthalmic (Betoptic) Uses: Glaucoma Action: Competitively blocks β-adrenergic receptors, β₁ Dose: 1 gt bid Caution: [C (1st tri), D (2nd or 3rd tri), ?/–] Supplied: Soln 0.5%; susp 0.25% SE: Local irritation, photophobia

Bethanechol (Urecholine, Duvoid, others) Uses: *Neurogenic bladder atony w/ retention,* acute *postop* & postpartum functional *(nonobstructive) urinary retention* **Action:** Stimulates cholinergic smooth muscle receptors in bladder & GI tract **Dose:** *Adults.* 10–50 mg PO tid–qid or 2.5–5 mg SQ tid–qid & PRN. *Peds.* 0.6 mg/kg/24 h PO ÷ tid–qid or 0.15–2 mg/kg/d SQ ÷ 3–4× (take on empty stomach) **Caution:** [C, ?/–] **Contra:** BOO, PUD, epilepsy, hyperthyroidism, bradycardia, COPD, AV conduction defects, parkinsonism, ↓ BP, vasomotor instability **Supplied:** Tabs 5, 10, 25, 50 mg; inj 5 mg/mL **SE:** Abdominal cramps, D, salivation, ↓ BP **Notes:** Do not use IM/IV

Bevacizumab (Avastin) **WARNING:** Associated w/ GI perforation, wound dehiscence, & fatal hemoptysis **Uses:** *Colorectal metastatic carcinoma, w/ 5-FU* Nonsquamous NSCLC w/ paclitaxel and carboplatin **Action:** Vascular endothelial GF inhibitor **Dose:** *Adults.* 5 mg/kg IV q14d; 1st dose over 90 min; 2nd over 60 min, 3rd over 30 min if tolerated **Caution:** [C, –] Do not use w/in 28 d of surgery if time for separation of drug & anticipated surgical procedures is unknown; D/C w/ serious adverse events **Supplied:** 100 mg/4 mL, 400 mg/16 mL vials **SE:** Wound dehiscence, GI perforation, hemoptysis, hemorrhage, HTN, proteinuria, CHF, inf Rxns, D, leucopenia, thromboembolism **Notes:** Monitor for ↑ BP & proteinuria

Bicalutamide (Casodex) Uses: *Advanced CAP (metastatic)* (w/ GnRH agonists [eg, leuprolide, goserelin]) **Action:** Nonsteroidal antiandrogen **Dose:** 50 mg/d **Caution:** [X, ?] **Contra:** Women **Supplied:** Caps 50 mg **SE:** Hot flashes, loss of libido, impotence, D/N/V, gynecomastia, & LFT elevation

Bicarbonate (See Sodium Bicarbonate, page 167)

Bisacodyl (Dulcolax) [OTC] Uses: *Constipation; preop bowel prep* **Action:** Stimulates peristalsis **Dose:** *Adults.* 5–15 mg PO or 10 mg PR PRN. *Peds.* <2 y: 5 mg PR PRN. >2 y: 5 mg PO or 10 mg PR PRN (do not chew tabs or give w/in 1 h of antacids or milk) **Caution:** [B, ?] **Contra:** Acute abdomen or bowel obstruction, appendicitis, gastroenteritis **Supplied:** EC tabs 5 mg; supp 10 mg **SE:** Abdominal cramps, proctitis, & inflammation w/ suppositories

Bismuth Subsalicylate (Pepto-Bismol) [OTC] Uses: Indigestion, nausea, & *D;* combo for Rx of *H. pylori* Infxn* **Action:** Antisecretory & antiinflammatory effects **Dose:** *Adults.* 2 tabs or 30 mL PO PRN (max 8 doses/24 h). *Peds. 3–6 y:* ⅓ tab or 5 mL PO PRN (max 8 doses/24 h). *6–9 y:* ⅔ tab or 10 mL PO PRN (max 8 doses/24 h). *9–12 y:* 1 tab or 15 mL PO PRN (max 8 doses/24 h) **Caution:** [C, D (3rd tri), –] Avoid in renal failure **Contra:** Influenza or chickenpox (↑ risk of Reye syndrome), ASA allergy **Supplied:** Chew tabs 262 mg; liq 262, 524 mg/15 mL **SE:** May turn tongue & stools black

Bisoprolol (Zebeta) Uses: *HTN* **Action:** Competitively blocks β₁-adrenergic receptors **Dose:** 5–10 mg/d (max dose 20 mg/d); ↓ in renal impair **Caution:** [C (D 2nd & 3rd tri), +/–] **Contra:** Sinus bradycardia, AV conduction abnormalities, cardiac failure **Supplied:** Tabs 5, 10 mg **SE:** Fatigue, lethargy, HA, bradycardia, edema, CHF **Notes:** Not dialyzed

Bitolterol (Tornalate) Uses: Prophylaxis & Rx of *asthma* & reversible bronchospasm Action: Sympathomimetic bronchodilator; stimulates pulmonary β₂-adrenergic receptors Dose: *Adults & Peds >12 y.* 2 inhal q8h Caution: [C, ?] Supplied: Aerosol 0.8% SE: Dizziness, nervousness, trembling, HTN, palpitations

Bivalirudin (Angiomax) Uses: *Anticoagulant w/ ASA in unstable angina undergoing PTCA* Action: Anticoagulant, thrombin inhibitor Dose: 1 mg/kg IV bolus, then 2.5 mg/kg/h over 4 h; PRN, use 0.2 mg/kg/h for up to 20 h (give w/ aspirin 300–325 mg/d); start pre-PTCA) Caution: [B, ?] Contra: Major bleeding Supplied: Powder for inj SE: Bleeding, back pain, nausea, HA

Bleomycin Sulfate (Blenoxane) Uses: *Testis CA; Hodgkin Dz & NHLs; cutaneous lymphomas; & squamous cell CA (head & neck, larynx, cervix, skin, penis); sclerosing agent for malignant pleural effusion* Action: Induces breakage (scission) of DNA Dose: 10–20 mg (units)/m² 1–2/wk (Per protocols); ↓ in renal impair Caution: [D, ?] Severe pulmonary Dz Supplied: Inj 15 mg (15 U) SE: Hyperpigmentation (skin staining) & allergy (rash to anaphylaxis); fever in 50%; lung tox (idiosyncratic & dose related); pneumonitis may progress to fibrosis; Raynaud phenomenon, N/V Notes: Test dose 1 mg (U) OK, especially in lymphoma pts; lung tox w/ total dose >400 mg (U)

Bortezomib (Velcade) **WARNING:** May worsen preexisting neuropathy Uses: *Progression of multiple myeloma despite two previous Rxs* Action: Proteasome inhibitor Dose: 1.3 mg/m² bolus IV 2×/wk × 2 wk, w/ 10-day rest period (= 1 cycle); ↓ dose w/hematologic tox, neuropathy Caution: [D, ?/–] Supplied: 3.5-mg vial SE: Asthenia, GI upset, anorexia, dyspnea, HA, orthostatic ↓ BP, edema, insomnia, dizziness, rash, pyrexia, arthralgia, neuropathy Notes: May interact w/ drugs metabolized via CYP450

Brimonidine (Alphagan) Uses: *Open-angle glaucoma, ocular HTN* Action: α₂-Adrenergic agonist Dose: 1 gt in eye(s) tid (wait 15 min to insert contacts) Caution: [B, ?] Contra: MAOI therapy Supplied: 0.2% soln SE: Local irritation, HA, fatigue

Brinzolamide (Azopt) Uses: *Open-angle glaucoma, ocular HTN* Action: Carbonic anhydrase inhibitor Dose: 1 gt in eye(s) tid Caution: [C, ?] Supplied: 1% susp SE: Blurred vision, dry eye, blepharitis, taste disturbance

Bromocriptine (Parlodel) Uses: *Parkinson Dz, hyperprolactinemia, acromegaly, pituitary tumors* Action: Direct-acting on the striatal dopamine receptors; ↓ prolactin secretion Dose: Initial, 1.25 mg PO bid; titrate to effect Caution: [C, ?] Contra: Severe ischemic heart Dz or PVD Supplied: Tabs 2.5 mg; caps 5 mg SE: ↓ BP, Raynaud phenomenon, dizziness, nausea, hallucinations

Budesonide (Rhinocort, Pulmicort) Uses: *Allergic & nonallergic rhinitis, asthma* Action: Steroid Dose: *Intranasal:* 2 sprays/nostril bid or 4 sprays/nostril/d. *Aqueous:* 1 spray/nostril/d. *PO inhaled:* 1–4 inhal bid. *Peds.* 1–2 inhal bid (Rinse mouth after PO use) Caution: [C, ?/–] Supplied: Met-dose Turbuhaler, nasal inhaler, & aqueous spray SE: HA, cough, hoarseness, *Candida* Infxn, epistaxis

Bumetanide (Bumex) Uses: *Edema from CHF, hepatic cirrhosis, & renal Dz* **Action:** Loop diuretic; ↓ reabsorption of Na^+ & Cl^-, in the ascending loop of Henle & the distal tubule **Dose:** *Adults.* 0.5–2 mg/d PO; 0.5–1 mg IV q8–24h (max 10 mg/d). *Peds.* 0.015–0.1 mg/kg/d PO, IV, or IM ÷ q6–24h **Caution:** [D, ?] **Contra:** Anuria, hepatic coma, severe electrolyte depletion **Supplied:** Tabs 0.5, 1, 2 mg; inj 0.25 mg/mL **SE:** ↓ K^+, ↓ Na^+, ↑ creatinine, ↑ uric acid, dizziness, ototox **Notes:** Monitor fluid & electrolytes

Bupivacaine (Marcaine) Uses: *Local, regional, & spinal anesthesia, local & regional analgesia* **Action:** Local anesthetic **Dose:** *Adults & Peds.* Dose-dependent on procedure (ie, tissue vascularity, depth of anesthesia, etc) (Table 3, page 205) **Caution:** [C, ?] **Contra:** Severe bleeding, ↓ BP, shock & arrhythmias, local Infxns at anesthesia site, septicemia **Supplied:** Inj 0.25, 0.5, 0.75% **SE:** ↓ BP, bradycardia, dizziness, anxiety

Buprenorphine (Buprenex) [C-V] Uses: *Moderate/severe pain* **Action:** Opiate agonist–antagonist **Dose:** 0.3–0.6 mg IM or slow IV push q6h PRN **Caution:** [C, ?/–] **Supplied:** Inj 0.324 mg/mL (= 0.3 mg of buprenorphine) **SE:** Sedation, ↓ BP, resp depression **Notes:** withdrawal if opioid-dependent

Bupropion (Wellbutrin, Wellbutrin SR, Wellbutrin XL, Zyban) WARNING: Closely monitor for worsening depression or emergence of suicidality Uses: *Depression, adjunct to smoking cessation* **Action:** Weak inhibitor of neuronal uptake of serotonin & norepinephrine; ↓ neuronal dopamine reuptake **Dose:** *Depression:* 100–450 mg/d ÷ bid–tid; SR 100–200 mg bid; XL 150–300 mg qd. *Smoking cessation:* 150 mg/d × 3 d, then 150 mg bid ×8–12 wk; ↓ in renal/hepatic impair **Caution:** [B, ?/–] **Contra:** Sz disorder, Hx anorexia nervosa or bulimia, MAOI, abrupt D/C of EtOH or sedatives **Supplied:** Tabs 75, 100 mg; SR tabs 100, 150, 200 mg; XL tabs 150, 300 mg **SE:** Associated w/ Szs; agitation, insomnia, HA, tachycardia **Notes:** Avoid EtOH & other CNS depressants

Buspirone (BuSpar) WARNING: Closely monitor for worsening depression or emergence of suicidality Uses: Short-term relief of *anxiety* **Action:** Antianxiety; antagonizes CNS serotonin receptors **Dose:** 5–10 mg PO tid; ↑ to effect; usual 20–30 mg/d; max 60 mg/d; ↓ in severe hepatic insuff **Caution:** [B, ?/–] **Supplied:** Tabs 5, 10, 15, 30 mg dividose **SE:** Drowsiness, dizziness; HA, N **Notes:** No abuse potential or physical/psychologic dependence

Busulfan (Myleran, Busulfex) Uses: *CML,* preparative regimens for allogeneic & ABMT in high doses **Action:** Alkylating agent **Dose:** 4–12 mg/d for several wks; 16 mg/kg once or 4 mg/kg/d for 4 d w/ another agent in BMT. (Per protocol) **Caution:** [D, ?] **Supplied:** Tabs 2 mg, inj 60 mg/10 mL **SE:** Myelosuppression, pulmonary fibrosis, nausea (high-dose therapy), gynecomastia, adrenal insuff, & skin hyperpigmentation

Butorphanol (Stadol) [C-IV] Uses: *Anesthesia adjunct, pain* & migraine HA **Action:** Opiate agonist–antagonist w/ central analgesic actions **Dose:** 1–4 mg IM or IV q3–4h PRN. *HA:* 1 spray in 1 nostril; may repeat ×1 if pain not relieved in 60–90 min; ↓ in renal impair **Caution:** [C (D if high doses or prolonged periods at term), +] **Supplied:** Inj 1, 2 mg/mL; nasal spray 10 mg/ mL **SE:** Drowsiness, dizziness, nasal congestion **Notes:** May induce withdrawal in opioid dependency

Calcipotriene (Dovonex) Uses: *Plaque psoriasis* Action: Keratolytic **Dose:** Apply bid **Caution:** [C, ?] **Contra:** ↑ Ca²⁺; vitamin D tox; do not apply to face **Supplied:** Cream; oint; soln 0.005% **SE:** Skin irritation, dermatitis

Calcitonin (Cibacalcin, Miacalcin) Uses: *Paget Dz of bone, ↑ Ca²⁺,* osteogenesis imperfecta, *postmenopausal osteoporosis* Action: Polypeptide hormone **Dose:** *Paget Dz salmon form:* 100 units/d IM/SC initial, 50 units/d or 50–100 units q1–3d maint. *Paget Dz human form:* 0.5 mg/d initial; maint 0.5 mg 2–3 ×/wk or 0.25 mg/d, max 0.5 mg bid. ↑ *Ca²⁺ salmon calcitonin:* 4 units/kg IM/SC q12h; ↑ to 8 units/kg q12h, max q6h. *Osteoporosis salmon calcitonin:* 100 units/d IM/SQ; intranasal 200 units = 1 nasal spray/d **Caution:** [C, ?] **Supplied:** Spray, nasal 200 units/activation; inj, human (Cibacalcin) 0.5 mg/vial, salmon 200 units/mL (2 mL) **SE:** Facial flushing, nausea, injection site edema, nasal irritation, polyuria **Notes:** Human (Cibacalcin) & salmon forms; human only approved for Paget bone Dz

Calcitriol (Rocaltrol) Uses: *Reduction of ↑ PTH levels, ↓ Ca²⁺ on dialysis* Action: 1,25-Dihydroxycholecalciferol (vitamin D analog) **Dose:** *Adults.* Renal failure: 0.25 mcg/d PO, ↑ 0.25 mcg/d q4–6wk PRN; ↑ 0.5 mcg 3×/wk IV, ↑ PRN. *Hyperparathyroidism:* 0.5–2 mcg/d. *Peds.* Renal failure: 15 ng/kg/d, ↑ PRN; maint 30–60 ng/kg/d. *Hyperparathyroidism:* <5 y, 0.25–0.75 mcg/d. >6 y, 0.5–2 mcg/d **Caution:** [C, ?] **Contra:** ↑ Ca²⁺; vitamin D tox **Supplied:** Inj 1, 2 mcg/mL (in 1-mL); caps 0.25, 0.5 mcg **SE:** ↑ Ca²⁺ possible **Notes:** Monitor to keep Ca²⁺ WNL

Calcium Acetate (Calphron, Phos-Ex, PhosLo) Uses: *ESRD-associated hyperphosphatemia* Action: Ca²⁺ supl w/o aluminum to ↓ PO₄⁻² **Dose:** 2–4 tabs PO w/ meals **Caution:** [C, ?] **Contra:** ↑ Ca²⁺ **Supplied:** Caps Phos-Ex 500 mg (125 mg Ca); tabs Calphron & PhosLo 667 mg (169 mg Ca) **SE:** Can ↑ Ca²⁺, hypophosphatemia, constipation **Notes:** Monitor Ca²⁺

Calcium Carbonate (Tums, Alka-Mints) [OTC] Uses: *Hyperacidity associated w/ peptic ulcer Dz, hiatal hernia,* etc **Action:** Neutralizes gastric acid **Dose:** 500 mg–2 g PO PRN; ↓ in renal impair **Caution:** [C, ?] **Supplied:** Chew tabs 350, 420, 500, 550, 750, 850 mg; susp **SE:** ↑ Ca²⁺, hypophosphatemia, constipation

Calcium Glubionate (Neo-Calglucon) [OTC] Uses: *Rx & prevent calcium deficiency* Action: Ca²⁺ supl **Dose:** *Adults.* 6–18 g/d ÷ doses. *Peds.* 600–2000 mg/kg/d ÷ qid (9 g/d max); ↓ in renal impair **Caution:** [C, ?] **Contra:** ↑ Ca²⁺ **Supplied:** OTC syrup 1.8 g/5 mL = Ca 115 mg/5 mL **SE:** ↑ Ca²⁺, hypophosphatemia, constipation

Calcium Salts (Chloride, Gluconate, Gluceptate) Uses: *Ca²⁺ replacement,* VF, Ca²⁺ blocker tox, Mg²⁺ intox, tetany, *hyperphosphatemia in*

ESRD* Action: Ca^{2+} supl/replacement Dose: *Adults. Replacement:* 1–2 g/d PO. *Cardiac emergencies:* CaCl 0.5–1 g IV q 10 min or Ca gluconate 1–2 g IV q 10 min. *Tetany:* 1 g CaCl over 10–30 min; repeat in 6 h PRN. **Peds.** *Replacement:* 200–500 mg/kg/24 h PO or IV ÷ qid. *Cardiac emergency:* 100 mg/kg/dose IV gluconate salt q 10 min. *Tetany:* 10 mg/kg CaCl over 5–10 min; repeat in 6 h or use inf (200 mg/kg/d max). **Adult & Peds.** ↓ Ca^{2+} due to citrated blood inf: 0.45 mEq Ca/100 mL citrated blood inf (↓ in renal impair) **Caution:** [C, ?] **Contra:** ↑ Ca^{2+} **Supplied:** CaCl inj 10% = 100 mg/mL = Ca 27.2 mg/mL = 10-mL amp; Ca gluconate inj 10% = 100 mg/mL = Ca 9 mg/mL; tabs 500 mg = 45 mg Ca, 650 mg = 58.5 mg Ca, 975 mg = 87.75 mg Ca, 1 g = 90 mg Ca; Ca gluceptate inj 220 mg/mL = 18 mg/mL Ca **SE:** Bradycardia, cardiac arrhythmias, ↑ Ca^{2+} **Notes:** CaCl 270 mg (13.6 mEq) elemental Ca/g, & calcium gluconate 90 mg (4.5 mEq) Ca/g. *RDA for Ca:* Adults = 800 mg/d; Peds = <6 mo 360 mg/d, 6 mo–1 y 540 mg/d, 1–10 y 800 mg/d, 10–18 y 1200 mg/d

Calfactant (Infasurf) Uses: *Prevention & Rx of RSD in infants* Action: Exogenous pulmonary surfactant Dose: 3 mL/kg instilled into lungs. Can retreat for a total of 3 doses given 12 h apart Caution: [?, ?] Supplied: Intratracheal susp 35 mg/mL SE: Monitor for cyanosis, airway obstruction, bradycardia during administration

Candesartan (Atacand) Uses: *HTN,* DN, CHF Action: Angiotensin II receptor antagonist Dose: 2–32 mg/d (usual 16 mg/d) Caution: [X, –] Contra: Primary hyperaldosteronism; bilateral renal artery stenosis Supplied: Tabs 4, 8, 16, 32 mg SE: Dizziness, HA, flushing, angioedema

Capsaicin (Capsin, Zostrix, others) [OTC] Uses: Pain due to *postherpetic neuralgia,* chronic neuralgia, *arthritis, diabetic neuropathy,* postop pain, psoriasis, intractable pruritus Action: Topical analgesic Dose: Apply tid–qid Caution: [?, ?] Supplied: OTC creams; gel; lotions; roll-ons SE: Local irritation, neurotox, cough

Captopril (Capoten, others) Uses: *HTN, CHF, MI,* LVD, DN Action: ACE inhibitor Dose: *Adults. HTN:* Initial, 25 mg PO bid–tid; ↑ to maint q1–2wk by 25-mg increments/dose (max 450 mg/d) to effect. *CHF:* Initial, 6.25–12.5 mg PO tid; titrate PRN *LVD:* 50 mg PO tid. *DN:* 25 mg PO tid. **Peds.** *Infants <2 mo:* 0.05–0.5 mg/kg/dose PO q8–24h. *Children:* Initial, 0.3–0.5 mg/kg/dose PO; ↑ to 6 mg/kg/d max (1 h before meals) Caution: [C (1st tri); D (2nd & 3rd tri); unknown effects in renal impair +] Contra: Hx angioedema Supplied: Tabs 12.5, 25, 50, 100 mg SE: Rash, proteinuria, cough, ↑ K^+

Carbamazepine (Tegretol) WARNING: Aplastic anemia & agranulocytosis have been reported w/ carbamazepine Uses: *Epilepsy, trigeminal neuralgia,* EtOH withdrawal Action: Anticonvulsant Dose: *Adults.* Initial, 200 mg PO bid; ↑ by 200 mg/d; usual 800–1200 mg/d ÷ doses. **Peds.** *<6 y:* 5 mg/kg/d, ↑ to 10–20 mg/kg/d ÷ in 2–4 doses. *6–12 y:* Initial, 100 mg PO bid or 10 mg/kg/24 h PO ÷ qd–bid; ↑ to maint 20–30 mg/kg/24 h ÷ tid–qid; ↓ in renal impair (take w/

food) **Caution:** [D, +] **Contra:** MAOI use, Hx BM suppression **Supplied:** Tabs 200 mg; chew tabs 100 mg; XR tabs 100, 200, 400 mg; susp 100 mg/5 mL **SE:** Drowsiness, dizziness, blurred vision, N/V, rash, ↓ Na^+, leukopenia, agranulocytosis **Notes:** Monitor CBC & serum levels (Table 2, page 200), generic products not interchangeable

Carbidopa/Levodopa (Sinemet) Uses: *Parkinson Dz* Action: ↑ CNS dopamine levels **Dose:** 25/100 mg bid–qid; ↑ as needed (max 200/2000 mg/d) **Caution:** [C, ?] **Contra:** NA glaucoma, suspicious skin lesion (may activate melanoma),melanoma, MAOI use **Supplied:** Tabs (mg carbidopa/mg levodopa) 10/100, 25/100, 25/250; tabs SR (mg carbidopa/mg levodopa) 25/100, 50/200 **SE:** Psychiatric disturbances, orthostatic ↓ BP, dyskinesias, cardiac arrhythmias

Carboplatin (Paraplatin) Uses: *Ovarian, lung, head & neck, testicular, urothelial,* & brain *CA, NHL,* & allogeneic & ABMT in high doses **Action:** DNA cross-linker; forms DNA-platinum adducts **Dose:** 360 mg/m² (ovarian carcinoma); AUC dosing 4–7 mg/mL (Culvert formula: mg = AUC × [25 + calculated GFR]); adjust based on pretreatment plt count, CrCl, & BSA (Egorin formula); up to 1500 mg/m² used in ABMT setting (Per protocols) **Caution:** [D, ?] **Contra:** Severe BM suppression, excessive bleeding **Supplied:** Inj 50, 150, 450 mg **SE:** Myelosuppression, N/V/D, nephrotox, hematuria, neurotox, ↑ LFTs **Notes:** Physiologic dosing based on either Culvert or Egorin formula allows ↑ doses w/↓ tox

Carisoprodol (Soma) Uses: *Adjunct to sleep & physical therapy to relieve painful musculoskeletal conditions* **Action:** Centrally acting muscle relaxant **Dose:** 350 mg PO tid–qid **Caution:** [C, M] Tolerance may result; w/ renal/hepatic impair **Contra:** Allergy to meprobamate; acute intermittent porphyria **Supplied:** Tabs 350 mg **SE:** CNS depression, drowsiness, dizziness, tachycardia **Notes:** Avoid EtOH & other CNS depressants; available in combo w/ ASA or codeine.

Carmustine [BCNU] (BiCNU, Gliadel) Uses: *Primary brain tumors, melanoma, Hodgkin lymphoma & NHLs, multiple myeloma, & induction for allogeneic & ABMT in high doses; adjunct to surgery in pts w/ recurrent glioblastoma* **Action:** Alkylating agent; nitrosourea forms DNA cross-links **Dose:** 150–200 mg/m² q6–8wk single or ÷ dose qd inj over 2 d; 20–65 mg/m² q4–6wk; 300–900 mg/m² in BMT (Per protocols); ↓ in hepatic impair **Caution:** [D, ?] ↓ WBC, RBC, plt counts, renal/hepatic impair **Contra:** Myelosuppression, PRG **Supplied:** Inj 100 mg/vial; wafer: 7.7 mg **SE:** ↓ BP, N/V, myelosuppression (WBC & plt), phlebitis, facial flushing, hepatic/renal dysfunction, pulmonary fibrosis, optic neuroretinitis; hematologic tox may persist 4–6 wk after dose **Notes:** Do not give course more frequently than q6wk (cumulative tox); baseline PFTs OK

Carteolol (Cartrol, Ocupress Ophthalmic) Uses: *HTN,* ↑ intraocular pressure, chronic open-angle glaucoma* **Action:** Blocks β-adrenergic receptors (β₁, β₂), mild ISA **Dose:** PO 2.5–5 mg/d; ophth 1 gt in eye(s) bid; ↓ in renal impair **Caution:** [C (1st tri); D (2nd & 3rd tri), ?/–] Cardiac failure, asthma

Contra: Sinus bradycardia; heart block >1st degree; bronchospasm **Supplied:** Tabs 2.5, 5 mg; ophth soln 1% **SE:** Drowsiness, sexual dysfunction, bradycardia, edema, CHF; *ocular:* conjunctival hyperemia, anisocoria, keratitis, eye pain **Notes:** No value in CHF

Carvedilol (Coreg)
Uses: *HTN, CHF, MI* **Action:** Blocks adrenergic receptors, β_1, β_2, α **Dose:** *HTN:* 6.25–12.5 mg bid. *CHF:* 3.125–25 mg bid; w/ food to minimize ↓ BP **Caution:** [C (1st tri); D (2nd & 3rd tri), ?/–] Bradycardia, asthma, diabetes **Contra:** Decompensated cardiac failure, 2nd-/3rd-degree heart block, SSS, severe hepatic impair **Supplied:** Tabs 3.125, 6.25, 12.5, 25 mg **SE:** Dizziness, fatigue, hyperglycemia, bradycardia, edema, hypercholesterolemia **Notes:** Do not D/C abruptly; ↑ digoxin levels

Caspofungin (Cancidas)
Uses: *Invasive aspergillosis refractory/intolerant to standard therapy, esophageal candidiasis* **Action:** An echinocandin; ↓ fungal cell wall synthesis; highest activity in regions of active cell growth **Dose:** 70 mg IV load day 1, 50 mg/d IV; slow inf; ↓ in hepatic impair **Caution:** [C, ?/–] Do not use w/ cyclosporine; not studied as initial therapy **Contra:** Allergy to any component **Supplied:** IV inf **SE:** Fever, HA, N/V, thrombophlebitis at site, ↑ LFTs **Notes:** Monitor during inf; limited experience beyond 2 wk of therapy

Cefaclor (Ceclor)
Uses: * Bacterial Infxns of the upper & lower resp tract, skin, bone, urinary tract, abdomen, gynecologic system* **Action:** 2nd-gen cephalosporin; ↓ cell wall synthesis. **Spectrum:** More gram(–) activity than 1st-gen cephalosporins; effective against gram(+) (*S. aureus*); good gram(–) coverage against *Haemophilus influenzae* **Dose:** *Adults.* 250–500 mg PO tid; XR 375–500 mg bid. *Peds.* 20–40 mg/kg/d PO ÷ 8–12h; ↓ renal impair **Caution:** [B, +] **Contra:** Cephalosporin allergy **Supplied:** Caps 250, 500 mg; XR tabs 375, 500 mg; susp 125, 187, 250, 375 mg/5 mL **SE:** D, rash, eosinophilia, ↑ transaminases

Cefadroxil (Duricef, Ultracef)
Uses: *Infxns of skin, bone, upper & lower resp tract, urinary tract* **Action:** 1st-gen cephalosporin; ↓ cell wall synthesis. **Spectrum:** Good gram(+) coverage (group A β-hemolytic *Strep, Staph); gram(–) (E. coli, Proteus, Klebsiella)* **Dose:** *Adults.* 1–2 g/d PO, 2 ÷ doses *Peds.* 30 mg/kg/d ÷ bid; ↓ in renal impair **Caution:** [B, +] **Contra:** Cephalosporin allergy **Supplied:** Caps 500 mg; tabs 1 g; susp 125, 250, 500 mg/5 mL **SE:** N/V/D, rash, eosinophilia, ↑ transaminases

Cefazolin (Ancef, Kefzol)
Uses: * Infxns of skin, bone, upper & lower resp tract, urinary tract* **Action:** 1st-gen cephalosporin; ↓ cell wall synthesis. **Spectrum:** Good coverage gram(+) bacilli & cocci, (*Strep, Staph* (except *Enterococcus*); some gram(–) (*E. coli, Proteus, Klebsiella*) **Dose:** *Adults.* 1–2 g IV q8h *Peds.* 25–100 mg/kg/d IV ÷ q6–8h; ↓ in renal impair **Caution:** [B, +] **Contra:** Cephalosporin allergy **Supplied:** Inj SE: D, rash, eosinophilia, elevated transaminases, pain at inj site **Notes:** Widely used for surgical prophylaxis

Cefdinir (Omnicef)
Uses: *Infxns of the resp tract, skin, bone, & urinary tract* **Action:** 3rd-gen cephalosporin; ↓ cell wall synthesis **Spectrum:** Active

against wide range of gram(+) & gram(−) organisms; more active than cefaclor & cephalexin against *Streptococcus, Staphylococcus;* active against some anaerobes **Dose: *Adults.*** 300 mg PO bid or 600 mg/d PO. ***Peds.*** 7 mg/kg PO bid or 14 mg/kg/d PO; ↓ in renal impair **Caution:** [B, +] In PCN-sensitive pts, serum sickness-like Rxns reported **Contra:** Hypersentivity to cephalosporins **Supplied:** Caps 300 mg; susp 125 mg/5 mL **SE:** Anaphylaxis, D, rare pseudomembranous colitis

Cefditoren (Spectracef)
Uses: *Acute exacerbations of chronic bronchitis, pharyngitis, tonsillitis; skin Infxns* **Action:** 3rd-gen cephalosporin; ↓ cell wall synthesis. *Spectrum:* Good gram(+) (*Strep* & *Staph*); gram(−) (*Haemophilus influenzae* & *Moraxella catarrhalis*) **Dose: *Adults & Peds >12 y. Skin:* 200 mg PO bid × 10 days. *Chronic bronchitis, pharyngitis, tonsillitis:* 400 mg PO bid × 10 days; avoid antacids w/in 2 h; take w/ meals; ↓ in renal impair **Caution:** [B, ?] Renal/hepatic impair **Contra:** Cephalosporin/PCN allergy, milk protein, or carnitine deficiency **Supplied:** 200-mg tabs **SE:** HA, N/V/D, colitis, nephrotox, hepatic dysfunction, Stevens–Johnson syndrome, toxic epidermal necrolysis, allergy Rxns **Notes:** Causes renal excretion of carnitine; tablets contain milk protein

Cefepime (Maxipime)
Uses: *UTI, pneumonia, febrile neutropenia, skin/soft tissue Infxns* **Action:** 4th-gen cephalosporin; ↓ cell wall synthesis. *Spectrum:* gram(+) *S. pneumoniae, S. aureus,* gram(−) *K. pneumoniae, E. coli, P. aeruginosa,* & *Enterobacter* sp **Dose: *Adults.*** 1–2 g IV q12h. ***Peds.*** 50 mg/kg q8h for febrile neutropenia; 50 mg/kg bid for skin/soft tissue Infxns; ↓ in renal impair **Caution:** [B, +] **Contra:** Cephalosporin allergy **Supplied:** Inj 500 mg, 1, 2 g **SE:** Rash, pruritus, N/V/D, fever, HA, (+) Coombs' test w/o hemolysis **Notes:** Administered as IM or IV

Cefixime (Suprax)
Uses: *Infxns of the resp tract, skin, bone, & urinary tract* **Action:** 3rd-gen cephalosporin; ↓ cell wall synthesis. *Spectrum: S. pneumoniae, S. pyogenes, H. influenzae,* & enterobacteria. **Dose: *Adults.*** 400 mg PO qd–bid. ***Peds.*** 8 mg/kg PO qd bid PO ÷ qd–bid; ↓ in renal impair **Caution:** [B, +] **Contra:** Cephalosporin allergy **Supplied:** Tabs 200, 400 mg; susp 100 mg/5 mL **SE:** N/V/D, flatulence, & abdominal pain **Notes:** Monitor renal & hepatic Fxn; use susp for otitis media

Cefmetazole (Zefazone)
Uses: *Rx Infxns of the upper & lower resp tract, skin, bone, urinary tract, abdomen, & gynecologic system* **Action:** 2nd-gen cephalosporin; ↓ cell wall synthesis. *Spectrum:* Gram(+) against *S. aureus;* gram(−) activity & some anaerobic activity; use in mixed aerobic–anaerobic Infxns where *Bacteroides fragilis* likely **Dose: *Adults.*** 2 g IV q6–12h; ↓ in renal impair **Caution:** [B, +] **Contra:** Cephalosporin allergy **Supplied:** Inj 1, 2 g **SE:** Eosinophilia, leukopenia, N/V/D, ↑ LFTs, bleeding risk, rash, pseudomembranous colitis, disulfram Rxn **Notes:** Avoid EtOH; safety not established in children

Cefonicid (Monocid)
Uses: *Rx bacterial Infxns (resp tract, skin, bone & joint, urinary tract, gynecologic, sepsis)* **Action:** 2nd-gen cephalosporin; ↓ bacterial cell wall synthesis. *Spectrum:* Gram(+) including MSSA & many streptococci:

gram(–) bacilli including *E. coli, Klebsiella, P. mirabilis, H. influenzae,* & *Moraxella* **Dose:** 0.5–2 g/24 h IM/IV; ↓ in renal impair **Caution:** [B, +] **Contra:** Cephalosporin allergy **Supplied:** Powder for inj 500 mg, 1 g, 10 g **SE:** D, rash, ↑ plts, eosinophilia, ↑ transaminases

Cefoperazone (Cefobid) **Uses:** *Rx Infxns of the resp, skin, urinary tract, sepsis* **Action:** 3rd-gen cephalosporin; ↓ bacterial cell wall synthesis. *Spectrum:* **Adults.** (eg, *E. coli, Klebsiella*); variable against *Streptococcus* & *Staphylococcus* sp; active *P. aeruginosa* but < ceftazidime **Dose:** **Adults.** 2–4 g/d IM/IV ÷ q 8–12h (12 g/d max). **Peds.** (not approved) 100–150 mg/kg/d IM/IV ÷ bid–tid (12 g/d max); ↓ in renal/hepatic impair **Caution:**[B, +] May ↑ risk of bleeding **Contra:** Cephalosporin allergy **Supplied:** Powder for inj 1, 2 g **SE:** D, rash, eosinophilia, ↑ LFTs, hypoprothrombinemia, & bleeding (due to MTT side chain) **Notes:** May interfere w/ warfarin

Cefotaxime (Claforan) **Uses:** *Rx Infxns of resp tract, skin, bone, urinary tract, meningitis, sepsis* **Action:** 3rd-gen cephalosporin; ↓ cell wall synthesis. *Spectrum:* Most gram(–) (not *Pseudomonas*), some gram(+) cocci (not *Enterococcus*); many PCN-resistant pneumococci **Dose:** **Adults.** 1–2 g IV q4–12h. **Peds.** 50–200 mg/kg/d IV ÷ q 4–12h; ↓ dose renal/hepatic impair **Caution:** [B, +] Arrhythmia associated w/ rapid inj; caution in colitis **Contra:** Cephalosporin allergy **Supplied:** Powder for inj 500 mg, 1, 2, 10 g **SE:** D, rash, pruritus, colitis, eosinophilia, ↑ transaminases

Cefotetan (Cefotan) **Uses:** *Rx Infxns of the upper & lower resp tract, skin, bone, urinary tract, abdomen, & gynecologic system* **Action:** 2nd-gen cephalosporin; ↓ cell wall synthesis. *Spectrum:* Less active against gram(+); anaerobes including *B. fragilis;* gram(–), including *E. coli, Klebsiella,* & *Proteus* **Dose:** **Adults.** 1–2 g IV q12h. **Peds.** 20–40 mg/kg/d IV ÷ q12h; ↓ in renal impair **Caution:** [B, +] May ↑ bleeding risk; in those Hx of PCN allergies **Contra:** Cephalosporin allergy **Supplied:** Powder for inj 1, 2, 10 g **SE:** D, rash, eosinophilia, ↑ transaminases, hypoprothrombinemia, & bleeding (due to MTT side chain) **Notes:** Caution w/ other nephrotoxic drugs; may interfere w/ warfarin

Cefoxitin (Mefoxin) **Uses:** *Rx Infxns of the upper & lower resp tract, skin, bone, urinary tract, abdomen, & gynecologic system* **Action:** 2nd-gen cephalosporin; ↓ cell wall synthesis. *Spectrum:* Good gram(–) against enteric bacilli (ie, *E. coli, Klebsiella,* & *Proteus*); anaerobic activity against *B. fragilis* **Dose:** **Adults.** 1–2 g IV q6–8h. **Peds.** 80–160 mg/kg/d ÷ q4–6h; ↓ in renal impair **Caution:** [B, +] **Contra:** Cephalosporin allergy **Supplied:** Powder for inj 1, 2, 10 g **SE:** D, rash, eosinophilia, ↑ transaminases

Cefpodoxime (Vantin) **Uses:** *Rx resp, skin, & urinary tract Infxns* **Action:** 3rd-gen cephalosporin; ↓ cell wall synthesis. *Spectrum:* *S. pneumoniae* or non-β-lactamase-producing *H. influenzae;* acute uncomplicated *N. gonorrhoeae;* some uncomplicated gram(–)(*E. coli, Klebsiella, Proteus*) **Dose:** **Adults.** 200–400 mg PO q12h. **Peds.** 10 mg/kg/d PO ÷ bid; ↓ in renal impair, take w/ food **Caution:**

[B, +] **Contra:** Cephalosporin allergy **Supplied:** Tabs 100, 200 mg; susp 50, 100 mg/5 mL **SE:** D, rash, HA, eosinophilia, elevated transaminases **Notes:** Drug interactions w/ agents that ↑ gastric pH

Cefprozil (Cefzil) Uses: *Rx resp tract, skin, & urinary tract Infxns* **Action:** 2nd-gen cephalosporin; ↓ cell wall synthesis. *Spectrum:* Active against MSSA, strep, & gram(−) bacilli (*E. coli, Klebsiella, P. mirabilis, H. influenzae, Moraxella*) **Dose:** *Adults.* 250–500 mg PO daily–bid. *Peds.* 7.5–15 mg/kg/d PO ÷ bid; ↓ in renal impair **Caution:** [B, +] **Contra:** Cephalosporin allergy **Supplied:** Tabs 250, 500 mg; susp 125, 250 mg/5 mL **SE:** D, dizziness, rash, eosinophilia, ↑ transaminases **Notes:** Use higher doses for otitis & pneumonia

Ceftazidime (Fortaz, Ceptaz, Tazidime, Tazicef) Uses: *Rx resp tract, skin, bone, urinary tract Infxns, meningitis, & septicemia* **Action:** 3rd-gen cephalosporin; ↓ cell wall synthesis. *Spectrum: P. aeruginosa* sp, good gram(−) activity **Dose:** *Adults.* 500–2 g IV q8–12h. *Peds.* 30–50 mg/kg/dose IV q8h; ↓ in renal impair **Caution:** [B, +] **Contra:** Cephalosporin allergy **Supplied:** Powder for inj 1, 2, 10 g **SE:** D, rash, eosinophilia, ↑ transaminases

Ceftibuten (Cedax) Uses: *Rx resp tract, skin, urinary tract Infxns & otitis media* **Action:** 3rd-gen cephalosporin; ↓ cell wall synthesis. *Spectrum: H. influenzae* & *M. catarrhalis;* weak against *S. pneumoniae* **Dose:** *Adults.* 400 mg/d PO. *Peds.* 9 mg/kg/d PO; ↓ in renal impair; take on empty stomach **Caution:** [B, +] **Contra:** Cephalosporin allergy **Supplied:** Caps 400 mg; susp 90, 180 mg/5 mL **SE:** D, rash, eosinophilia, ↑ transaminases

Ceftizoxime (Cefizox) Uses: *Rx resp tract, skin, bone, & urinary tract Infxns, meningitis, septicemia* **Action:** 3rd-gen cephalosporin; ↓ cell wall synthesis. *Spectrum:* Good gram(−) bacilli (not *Pseudomonas*), some gram(+) cocci (not *Enterococcus*), & some anaerobes **Dose:** *Adults.* 1–2 g IV q8–12h. *Peds.* 150–200 mg/kg/d IV ÷ q6–8h; ↓ in renal impair **Caution:** [B, +] **Contra:** Cephalosporin allergy **Supplied:** Inj 500 mg, 1, 2, 10 g **SE:** D, fever, rash, eosinophilia, thrombocytosis, ↑ transaminases

Ceftriaxone (Rocephin) Uses: *Resp tract (pneumonia), skin, bone, urinary tract Infxns, meningitis, & septicemia;* * **Action:** 3rd-gen cephalosporin; ↓ cell wall synthesis. *Spectrum:* Moderate gram(+); excellent against β-lactamase producers **Dose:** *Adults.* 1–2 g IV q12–24h. *Peds.* 50–100 mg/kg/d IV ÷ q12–24h; ↓ in renal impair **Caution:** [B, +] **Contra:** Cephalosporin allergy; hyperbilirubinemic neonates (displaces bilirubin from binding sites) **Supplied:** Powder for inj 250 mg, 500 mg, 1, 2 g **SE:** D, rash, leukopenia, thrombocytosis, eosinophilia, ↑ transaminases

Cefuroxime (Ceftin [PO], Zinacef [parenteral]) Uses: *Upper & lower resp tract, skin, bone, urinary tract, abdomen, gynecologic Infxns* **Action:** 2nd-gen cephalosporin; ↓ cell wall synthesis *Spectrum:* Staphylococci, group B streptococci, *H. influenzae, E. coli, Enterobacter, Salmonella,* & *Klebsiella* **Dose:** *Adults.* 750 mg–1.5 g IV q8h or 250–500 mg PO bid. *Peds.* 100–150 mg/kg/d IV ÷

q8h or 20–30 mg/kg/d PO ÷ bid; ↓ in renal impair; take w/ food **Caution:** [B, +] **Contra:** Cephalosporin allergy **Supplied:** Tabs 125, 250, 500 mg; susp 125, 250 mg/5 mL; powder for inj 750 mg, 1.5, 7.5 g **SE:** D, rash, eosinophilia, ↑ LFTs **Notes:** Cefuroxime film-coated tablets & PO susp not bioequivalent; do not substitute on a mg/mg basis; IV crosses blood–brain barrier

Celecoxib (Celebrex) **WARNING:** ↑ Risk of serious CV thrombotic events, MI & stroke, which can be fatal; ↑ risk of serious GI adverse events including bleeding, ulceration, & perforation of the stomach or intestines, which can be fatal. **Uses:** *Osteoarthritis & RA, anklylosing spondylitis*; acute pain, primary dysmenorrhea; preventive in familial adenomatous polyposis **Action:** NSAID; ↓ the COX-2 pathway **Dose:** 100–200 mg/d or bid; ↓ in hepatic impair; take w/ food/milk **Caution:** [C/D (3rd tri), ?] Caution in renal impair **Contra:** Allergy to sulfonamides, periop CABG **Supplied:** Caps 100, 200 mg **SE:** see Warning; GI upset, HTN, edema, renal failure, HA **Notes:** Watch for Sxs of GI bleeding; no effect on plt/bleeding time; can affect drugs metabolized by P-450 pathway

Cephalexin (Keflex, Keftab) **Uses:** *Skin, bone, upper/lower resp tract, urinary tract Infxns* **Action:** 1st-gen cephalosporin; ↓ cell wall synthesis. *Spectrum:* Strep, Staph, E. coli, Proteus, Klebsiella **Dose:** *Adults.* 250–500 mg PO qid. *Peds.* 25–100 mg/kg/d PO ÷ qid; ↓ in renal impair; (on empty stomach) **Caution:** [B, +] **Contra:** Cephalosporin allergy **Supplied:** Caps 250, 500 mg; tabs 250, 500, 1000 mg; susp 125, 250 mg/5 mL **SE:** D, rash, eosinophilia, ↑ LFTs

Cephradine (Velosef) **Uses:** *Respiratory, GU, GI, skin, soft tissue, bone, & joint Infxns* **Action:** 1st-gen cephalosporin; ↓ cell wall synthesis. *Spectrum:* Gram(+) bacilli & cocci (not *Enterococcus*); some gram(−) bacilli (*E. coli, Proteus, & Klebsiella*) **Dose:** *Adults.* 250–500 mg q6–12h (8 g/d max). *Peds >9 mo.* 25–100 mg/kg/d ÷ bid–qid (4 g/d max); ↓ in renal impair **Caution:** [B, +] **Contra:** Cephalosporin allergy **Supplied:** Caps: 250, 500 mg; powder for susp 125, 250 mg/5 mL, etc **SE:** Rash, eosinophilia, ↑ LFTs, N/V/D

Cetirizine (Zyrtec, Zyrtec D) **Uses:** *Allergic rhinitis & other allergic Sxs including urticaria* **Action:** Nonsedating antihistamine **Dose:** *Adults & Children >6 y.* 5–10 mg/d. Zyrtec D 5/120 mg PO bid whole **Peds.** *6–11 mo:* 2.5 mg qd. *12–23 mo:* 2.5 mg qd–bid; ↓ in renal/hepatic impair **Caution:** [B, ?/–] Elderly & nursing mothers; >10 mg/d may cause drowsiness **Contra:** Allergy to cetirizine, hydroxyzine **Supplied:** Tabs 5, 10 mg; syrup 5 mg/5 mL **SE:** HA, drowsiness, xerostomia **Notes:** Can cause sedation Zyrtec D: Taber 5/120 mg (cetirizine/pseudoephedrine)

Cetuximab (Erbitux) **WARNING:** Severe inf Rxns including rapid onset of airway obstruction (bronchospasm, stridor, hoarseness), urticaria, & hypotension. Permanent D/C is required. **Uses:** *EGFR-expressing metastatic colorectal CA w/wo irinotecan* **Action:** Human/mouse recombinant MoAb; binds EGFR, ↓ tumor cell growth **Dose:** Per protocol; load 400 mg/m² IV over 2 h; 250 mg/m² given over 1 h × 1 wk **Caution:** [C, −] **Supplied:** Inj 100 mg/ 50 mL **SE:** Acneform rash, asthenia/malaise, N/V/D, abdominal pain, alopecia, inf Rxn, dermatologic tox, interstitial lung disease, fever, sepsis, dehydration, kidney failure, PE **Notes:** Assess tumor for EGFR before Rx; pretreat w/ diphenhydramine; w/ mild SE ↓ inf rate by 50%; limit sun exposure

Charcoal, Activated (Superchar, Actidose, Liqui-Char) **Uses:** *Emergency Rx in poisoning by most drugs & chemicals* **Action:** Adsorbent detoxicant **Dose:** Give w/ 70% sorbitol (2 mL/kg); repeated use of sorbitol not OK **Adults.** *Acute intox:* 30–100 g/dose. *GI dialysis:* 20–50 g q6h for 1–2 d. *Peds 1–12 y.* *Acute intox:* 1–2 g/kg/dose. *GI dialysis:* 5–10 g/dose q4–8h **Caution:** [C, ?] May cause vomiting (hazardous in petroleum distillate & caustic ingestions); do not mix w/ milk, ice cream, or sherbet **Contra:** Not effective for cyanide, mineral acids, caustic alkalis, organic solvents, iron, EtOH, methanol poisoning, Li; do not use sorbitol in pts w/ fructose intolerance **Supplied:** Powder, liq, caps **SE:** Some liq dosage forms in sorbitol base (a cathartic); V/D, black stools, constipation **Notes:** Charcoal w/ sorbitol not OK in children < 1 y; monitor for ↓ K^+ & Mg^{2+}; protect airway in lethargic or comatose pts

Chloral Hydrate (Aquachloral, Supprettes) [C-IV] **Uses:** *Short-term nocturnal & preop sedation* **Action:** Sedative hypnotic; active metabolite trichloroethanol **Dose:** *Adults. Hypnotic:* 500 mg–1 g PO or PR 30 min hs or before procedure. *Sedative:* 250 mg PO or PR tid. *Peds. Hypnotic:* 20–50 mg/kg/24 h PO or PR 30 min hs or before procedure. *Sedative:* 5–15 mg/kg/dose q8h; avoid w/ CrCl <50 mL/min or severe hepatic impair **Caution:** [C, +] Porphyria & neonates **Contra:** Allergy to components; severe renal, hepatic or cardiac Dz **Supplied:** Caps 500 mg; syrup 250, 500 mg/5 mL; supp 324, 500, 648 mg **SE:** GI irritation, drowsiness, ataxia, dizziness, nightmares, rash **Notes:** May accumulate; tolerance may develop >2 wk; taper dose; mix syrup in H_2O or fruit juice; avoid EtOH & CNS depressants

Chlorambucil (Leukeran) **Uses:** *CLL, Hodgkin Dz, Waldenström's macroglobulinemia* **Action:** Alkylating agent **Dose:** 0.1–0.2 mg/kg/d for 3–6 wk or 0.4 mg/kg/dose q2wk (Per protocol) **Caution:** [D, ?] Sz disorder & BM suppression; affects human fertility **Contra:** Previous resistance; alkylating agent allergy **Supplied:** Tabs 2 mg **SE:** Myelosuppression, N/V, drug fever, skin rash, chromosomal damage can cause secondary leukemias, alveolar dysplasia, pulmonary fibrosis, hepatotox **Notes:** Monitor LFTs, CBC, leukocyte counts, plts, serum uric acid; ↓ initial dosage if pt has received radiation therapy

Chlordiazepoxide (Librium, Mitran, Libritabs) [C-IV] **Uses:** *Anxiety, tension, EtOH withdrawal,* & preop apprehension **Action:** Benzodiazepine; antianxiety agent **Dose:** *Adults. Mild anxiety:* 5–10 mg PO tid–qid or PRN. *Severe anxiety:* 25–50 mg IM, IV, or PO q6–8h or PRN. *EtOH withdrawal:* 50–100 mg IM or IV; repeat in 2–4 h if needed, up to 300 mg in 24 h; gradually taper daily dose. *Peds >6 y.* 0.5 mg/kg/24 h PO or IM ÷ q6–8h; ↓ in renal impair, elderly **Caution:**[D, ?] Resp depression, CNS impair, Hx of drug dependence; avoid in hepatic impair **Contra:** Preexisting CNS depression **Supplied:** Caps 5,

10, 25 mg; tabs 10, 25 mg; inj 100 mg **SE:** Drowsiness, CP, rash, fatigue, memory impair, xerostomia, weight gain **Notes:** Erratic IM absorption

Chlorothiazide (Diuril) **Uses:** *HTN, edema* **Action:** Thiazide diuretic **Dose:** *Adults.* 500 mg–1 g PO daily–bid; 100–500 mg/d IV (for edema only). *Peds >6 mo.* 20–30 mg/kg/24 h PO ÷ bid; 4 mg/kg/d IV **Caution:** [D, +] Do not administer inj IM or SQ **Contra:** Cross-sensitivity to thiazides/sulfonamides, anuria **Supplied:** Tabs 250, 500 mg; susp 250 mg/5 mL; inj 500 mg/vial **SE:** ↓ K⁺, Na⁺, dizziness, hyperglycemia, hyperuricemia, hyperlipidemia, photosensitivity **Notes:** May be taken w/ food/milk; take early in the day to avoid nocturia; use sunblock; monitor electrolytes

Chlorpheniramine (Chlor-Trimeton, others [OTC]) **Uses:** *Allergic Rxns; common cold* **Action:** Antihistamine **Dose:** *Adults.* 4 mg PO q4–6h or 8–12 mg PO bid of SR *Peds.* 0.35 mg/kg/24 h PO ÷ q4–6h or 0.2 mg/kg/24 h SR **Caution:** [C, ?/–] BOO; NA glaucoma; hepatic insuff **Contra:** Allergy **Supplied:** Tabs 4 mg; chew tabs 2 mg; SR tabs 8, 12 mg; syrup 2 mg/5 mL; inj 10, 100 mg/mL **SE:** Anticholinergic SE & sedation common, postural ↓ BP, QT changes, extrapyramidal Rxns, photosensitivity

Chlorpromazine (Thorazine) **Uses:** *Psychotic disorders, N/V,* apprehension, intractable hiccups **Action:** Phenothiazine antipsychotic; antiemetic **Dose:** *Adults.* *Psychosis:* 10–25 mg PO or PR bid–tid (usual 30–800 mg/d in ÷ doses). *Severe Sxs:* 25 mg IM/IV initial; may repeat in 1–4 h; then 25–50 mg PO or PR tid. *Hiccups:* 25–50 mg PO bid–tid. *Children >6 mo. Psychosis & N/V:* 0.5–1 mg/kg/dose PO q4–6h or IM/IV q6–8h; avoid in severe hepatic impair **Caution:** [C, ?/–] Safety in children <6 mo not established; Szs, BM suppression **Contra:** Cross-sensitivity w/ phenothiazines; NA glaucoma **Supplied:** Tabs 10, 25, 50, 100, 200 mg; SR caps 30, 75, 150 mg; syrup 10 mg/5 mL; conc 30, 100 mg/mL; supp 25, 100 mg; inj 25 mg/mL **SE:** Extrapyramidal SE & sedation; α-adrenergic blocking properties; ↓ BP; prolongs QT interval **Notes:** Do not D/C abruptly; dilute PO conc in 2–4 oz of liq

Chlorpropamide (Diabinese) **Uses:** *Type 2 DM* **Action:** Sulfonylurea; ↑ pancreatic insulin release; ↑ peripheral insulin sensitivity; ↓ hepatic glucose output **Dose:** 100–500 mg/d; w/ food **Caution:** [C, ?/–] CrCl < 50 mL/min; ↓ in hepatic impair **Contra:** Cross-sensitivity w/ sulfonamides **Supplied:** Tabs 100, 250 mg **SE:** HA, dizziness, rash, photosensitivity, hypoglycemia, SIADH **Notes:** Avoid EtOH (disulfiram-like Rxn)

Chlorthalidone (Hygroton, others) **Uses:** *HTN* **Action:** Thiazide diuretic **Dose:** *Adults.* 50–100 mg PO daily. *Peds.* (Not approved) 2 mg/kg/dose PO 3×/wk or 1–2 mg/kg/d PO; ↓ in renal impair **Caution:** [D, +] **Contra:** Cross-sensitivity w/ thiazides or sulfonamides; anuria **Supplied:** Tabs 15, 25, 50, 100 mg **SE:** ↓ K⁺, dizziness, photosensitivity, hyperglycemia, hyperuricemia, sexual dysfunction **Notes:** May take w/ food/milk

Chlorzoxazone (Paraflex, Parafon Forte DSC, others) **Uses:** *Adjunct to rest & physical therapy to relieve discomfort associated w/ acute, painful musculoskeletal conditions* **Action:** Centrally acting skeletal muscle relaxant **Dose:** *Adults.* 250–500 mg PO tid-qid. *Peds.* 20 mg/kg/d in 3–4 ÷ doses **Caution:** [C, ?] EtOH & CNS depressants **Contra:** Severe liver Dz **Supplied:** Tabs 250; caps 250, 500 mg **SE:** Drowsiness, tachycardia, dizziness, hepatotox, angioedema

Cholecalciferol [Vitamin D₃] (Delta D)   Uses: Dietary supl to Rx vitamin D deficiency **Action:** Enhances intestinal Ca^{2+} absorption **Dose:** 400–1000 IU/d PO **Caution:** [A (D doses above the RDA), +] **Contra:** $\uparrow Ca^{2+}$, hypervitaminosis, allergy **Supplied:** Tabs 400, 1000 IU **SE:** Vitamin D tox (renal failure, HTN, psychosis) **Notes:** 1 mg cholecalciferol = 40,000 IU Vitamin D activity

Cholestyramine (Questran, LoCHOLEST)   Uses: *Hypercholesterolemia; Rx pruritus associated w/ partial biliary obstruction; diarrhea associated w/ excess fecal bile acids* **Action:** Binds intestinal bile acids, forms insoluble complexes **Dose:** *Adults.* Individualize: 4 g/d–bid ($\uparrow$ to max 24 g/d & 6 doses/d). *Peds.* 240 mg/kg/d in 3 ÷ doses **Caution:** [C, ?] Constipation, phenylketonuria **Contra:** Complete biliary obstruction; hypolipoproteinemia types III, IV, V **Supplied:** 4 g of cholestyramine resin/9 g powder; w/ aspartame: 4 g resin/5 g powder **SE:** Constipation, abdominal pain, bloating, HA, rash **Notes:** OD may result in GI obstruction; mix 4 gm in 2–6 oz of noncarbonated beverage; take other meds 1–2 h before or 6 h after

Ciclopirox (Loprox)   Uses: *Tinea pedis, tinea cruris, tinea corporis, cutaneous candidiasis, tinea versicolor* **Action:** Antifungal antibiotic in vitro cellular depletion of essential substrates &/or ions **Dose:** *Adults & Peds >10 y.* Massage into affected area bid **Caution:** [B, ?] **Contra:** Component sensitivity **Supplied:** Cream, gel, lotion 1% **SE:** Pruritus, local irritation, burning **Notes:** D/C if irritation occurs; avoid dressings; gel best for athletes foot

Cidofovir (Vistide)   WARNING: Renal impair is the major tox. Follow administration instructions **Uses:** *CMV retinitis in pts w/ HIV* **Action:** Selective inhibition of viral DNA synthesis **Dose:** *Rx:* 5 mg/kg IV over 1 h once/wk for 2 wk w/ probenecid. *Maint:* 5 mg/kg IV once/2 wk w/ probenecid. *Probenecid:* 2 g PO 3 h prior to cidofovir, then 1 g PO at 2 h & 8 h after cidofovir; $\downarrow$ in renal impair **Caution:** [C, –] SCr >1.5 mg/dL or CrCl = 55 mL/min or urine protein >100 mg/dL; w/ other nephrotoxic drugs **Contra:** Probenecid or sulfa allergy **Supplied:** Inj 75 mg/mL **SE:** Renal tox, chills, fever, HA, N/V/D, thrombocytopenia, neutropenia **Notes:** Hydrate w/ NS prior to each inf

Cilostazol (Pletal)   Uses: *Reduce Sxs of intermittent claudication* **Action:** Phosphodiesterase III inhibitor; $\uparrow$s cAMP in plts & blood vessels, vasodilation & inhibit plt aggregation **Dose:** 100 mg PO bid, ½ h before or 2 h after breakfast & dinner **Caution:** [C, +/–] $\downarrow$ dose when used w/ other drugs that inhibit CYP3A4 & CYP2C19 **Contra:** CHF **Supplied:** Tabs 50, 100 mg **SE:** HA, palpitation, D

Cimetidine (Tagamet, Tagamet HB) [OTC]   Uses: *Duodenal ulcer; ulcer prophylaxis in hypersecretory states, (eg, trauma, burns); & GERD* **Action:**

H_2 receptor antagonist **Dose:** *Adults. Active ulcer:* 2400 mg/d IV cont inf or 300 mg IV q6h; 400 mg PO bid or 800 mg hs. *Maint:* 400 mg PO hs. *GERD:* 300–600 mg PO q6h; maint 800 mg PO hs. **Peds.** *Infants:* 10–20 mg/kg/24 h PO or IV ÷ q6–12h. *Children:* 20–40 mg/kg/24 h PO or IV ÷ q6h; ↑ interval w/ renal insuff; ↓ dose in the elderly **Caution:** [B, +] Many drug interactions (P-450 system) **Contra:** Component sensitivity **Supplied:** Tabs 200, 300, 400, 800 mg; liq 300 mg/5 mL; inj 300 mg/2 mL **SE:** Dizziness, HA, agitation, thrombocytopenia, gynecomastia **Notes:** Take 1 h before or 2 h after antacids; avoid EtOH

Cinacalcet (Sensipar) Uses: *Secondary hyperparathyroidism in CRF; ↑ Ca^{2+} in parathyroid carcinoma* **Action:** ↓ PTH by ↑ calcium-sensing receptor sensitivity **Dose:** *Secondary hyperparathyroidism:* 30 mg PO daily. *Parathyroid carcinoma:* 30 mg PO bid; titrate q2–4wk based on calcium & PTH levels; swallow whole; take w/ food **Caution:** [C, ?/–] Dose adjust w/ addition/deletion of CYP3A4 inhibitors **Supplied:** Tabs 30, 60, 90 mg **SE:** N/V/D, myalgia, dizziness, ↓ Ca^{2+} **Notes:** Monitor Ca^{2+}, PO_4^{-2}, PTH

Ciprofloxacin (Cipro) Uses: *Rx lower resp tract, sinuses, skin & skin structure, bone/joints, & UT Infxns including prostatitis* **Action:** Quinolone antibiotic; ↓ DNA gyrase. *Spectrum:* Broad-spectrum gram(+) & gram(–) aerobics; little against *Strep;* good *Pseudomonas, E. coli, B. fragilis, P. mirabilis, K. pneumoniae, Campylobacter jejuni,* or *Shigella* **Dose:** *Adults.* 250–750 mg PO q12h; XR 500–1000 mg PO q24h; or 200–400 mg IV q12h; ↓ in renal impair **Caution:** [C, ?/–] Children <18 yr **Contra:** Component sensitivity **Supplied:** Tabs 100, 250, 500, 750 mg; Tabs XR 500, 1000 mg; susp 5 g/100 mL, 10 g/100 mL; inj 200, 400 mg **SE:** Restlessness, N/V/D, rash, ruptured tendons, ↑ LFTs **Notes:** Avoid antacids; reduce/restrict caffeine intake; interactions w/ theophylline, caffeine, sucralfate, warfarin, antacids

Ciprofloxacin, Ophthalmic (Ciloxan) Uses: *Rx & prevention of ocular Infxns (conjunctivitis, blepharitis, corneal abrasions)* **Action:** Quinolone antibiotic; ↓ DNA gyrase **Dose:** 1–2 gtt in eye(s) q2h while awake for 2 d, then 1–2 gtt q4h while awake for 5 d **Caution:** [C, ?/–] **Contra:** Component sensitivity **Supplied:** Soln 3.5 mg/mL **SE:** Local irritation

Ciprofloxacin, Otic (Cipro HC Otic) Uses: *Otitis externa* **Action:** Quinolone antibiotic; ↓ DNA gyrase **Dose:** *Adult & Peds >1 mo.* 1–2 gtt in ear(s) bid for 7 d **Caution:** [C, ?/–] **Contra:** Perforated tympanic membrane, viral Infxns of the external canal **Supplied:** Susp ciprofloxacin 0.2% & hydrocortisone 1% **SE:** HA, pruritus

Cisplatin (Platinol, Platinol AQ) Uses: *Testicular, small-cell & non-small-cell lung, bladder, ovarian, breast, head & neck, & penile CAs; osteosarcoma; ped brain tumors* **Action:** DNA-binding; denatures double helix; intrastrand cross-linking; formation of DNA adducts **Dose:** 10–20 mg/m²/d for 5 d q3wk; 50–120 mg/m² q3–4wk; (Per protocols); ↓ in renal impair **Caution:** [D, –] Cumulative renal tox may be severe; monitor Mg^{2+}, electrolytes before & w/in 48 h after cisplantin **Contra:** Allergy to platinum-containing compounds; preexisting renal insuff, myelosuppression, hearing impair **Supplied:** Inj 1 mg/mL **SE:** Allergic Rxns, N/V, nephrotox (worse w/administration of other nephrotoxic drugs; minimize by NS inf & mannitol diuresis); high-frequency hearing loss in 30%, peripheral "stocking glove"-type neuropathy, cardiotox (ST-, T-wave changes), ↓ Mg²⁺, mild myelosuppression, hepatotox; renal impair dose-related & cumulative **Notes:** Give taxanes before platinum derivatives

Citalopram (Celexa) **WARNING:** Closely monitor for worsening depression or emergence of suicidality, particularly in ped pts **Uses:** *Depression* **Action:** SSRI **Dose:** Initial 20 mg/d, may ↑ to 40 mg/d; ↓ in elderly & hepatic/renal insuff **Caution:** [C, +/−] Hx of mania, Szs & pts at risk for suicide **Contra:** MOAI or w/in 14 d of MAOI use **Supplied:** Tabs 10, 20, 40 mg; Soln 10 mg/5 mL **SE:** Somnolence, insomnia, anxiety, xerostomia, diaphoresis, sexual dysfunction **Notes:** May cause ↓ Na⁺/SIADH

Cladribine (Leustatin) **Uses:** *HCL, CLL, NHLs, progressive MS* **Action:** Induces DNA strand breakage; interferes w/ DNA repair/synthesis; purine nucleoside analog **Dose:** 0.09–0.1 mg/kg/d cont IV inf for 1–7 d (Per protocols) **Caution:** [D, ?/−] Causes neutropenia & Infxn **Contra:** Component sensitivity **Supplied:** Inj 1 mg/mL **SE:** Myelosuppression, T-lymphocyte suppression may be prolonged (26–34 wk), fever in 46% (May cause tumor lysis), Infxns (especially lung & IV sites), rash (50%), HA, fatigue **Notes:** Consider prophylactic allopurinol; monitor CBC

Clarithromycin (Biaxin, Biaxin XL) **Uses:** *Upper/lower resp tract, skin/skin structure Infxns, H. pylori Infxns, & Infxns caused by nontuberculosis (atypical) Mycobacterium; prevention of MAC Infxns in HIV-Infxn* **Action:** Macrolide antibiotic, ↓ protein synthesis. *Spectrum: H. influenzae, M. catarrhalis, S. pneumoniae, Mycoplasma pneumoniae, H. pylori* **Dose: Adults.** 250–500 mg PO bid or 1000 mg (2 × 500 mg XR tab)/d. *Mycobacterium:* 500–1000 mg PO bid. *Peds >9 mo.* 7.5 mg/kg/dose PO bid; ↓ in renal/hepatic impair **Caution:** [C, ?] Antibiotic-associated colitis; rare QT prolongation & ventricular arrhythmias, including torsades de pointes **Contra:** Allergy to macrolides; combo w/ ranitidine in pts w/ Hx of porphyria or CrCl < 25 mL/min **Supplied:** Tabs 250, 500 mg; susp 125, 250 mg/5 mL; 500 mg XR tab **SE:** Prolongs QT interval, causes metallic taste, N/D, abdominal pain, HA, rash **Notes:** Multiple drug interactions, ↑ theophylline & carbamazepine levels; do not refrigerate suspension

Clemastine Fumarate (Tavist, Tavist-1) [OTC] **Uses:** *Allergic rhinitis & Sxs of urticaria* **Action:** Antihistamine **Dose: Adults & Peds >12 y.** 1.34 mg bid–2.68 mg tid; max 8.04 mg/d *<12 y:* 0.4 mg PO bid **Caution:** [C, M] BOO **Contra:** NA glaucoma **Supplied:** Tabs 1.34, 2.68 mg; syrup 0.67 mg/5 mL **SE:** Drowsiness, dyscoordination, epigastric distress, urinary retention **Notes:** Avoid EtOH

Clindamycin (Cleocin, Cleocin-T) **Uses:** * Rx aerobic & anaerobic Infxns; topical for severe acne & vaginal Infxns* **Action:** Bacteriostatic; interferes w/ protein synthesis. *Spectrum:* Streptococci, pneumococci, staphylococci, & gram(+) & gram(–) anaerobes; no activity against gram(–) aerobes & bacterial vaginosis **Dose:** *Adults.* **PO:** 150–450 mg PO q6–8h. **IV:** 300–600 mg IV q6h or 900 mg IV q8h. *Vaginal:* 1 applicator hs for 7 d. **Topical:** Apply 1% gel, lotion, or soln bid. **Peds.** *Neonates:* (Avoid use; contains benzyl alcohol) 10–15 mg/kg/24 h ÷ q8–12h. *Children >1 mo:* 10–30 mg/kg/24 h ÷ q6–8h, to a max of 1.8 g/d PO or 4.8 g/d IV. *Topical:* Apply 1%, gel, lotion, or soln bid; ↓ in severe hepatic impair **Caution:** [B, +] Can cause fatal colitis **Contra:** Hx pseudomembranous colitis **Supplied:** Caps 75, 150, 300 mg; susp 75 mg/5 mL; inj 300 mg/2 mL; vaginal cream 2% **SE:** Diarrhea may be pseudomembranous colitis caused by *C. difficile*, rash, ↑ LFTs **Notes:** D/C drug if significant diarrhea, evaluate for *C. difficile*

Clofarabine (Clolar) **Uses:** Rx relapsed/refractory ALL after at least 2 regimens in children 1–21 y **Action:** Antimetabolite; ↓ ribonucleotide reductase w/ false nucleotide base-inhibiting DNA synthesis **Dose:** 52 mg/m² IV over 2 h qd × 5 d (repeat q2–6wk); Per protocol **Caution:** [D, –] **Supplied:** Inj 20 mg/20 mL **SE:** N/V/D, anemia, leukopenia, thrombocytopenia, neutropenia, Infxn, ↑ AST/ALT **Notes:** Monitor for tumor lysis syndrome & systemic inflammatory response syndrome (SIRS)/capillary leak syndrome

Clofazimine (Lamprene) **Uses:** *Leprosy & combo therapy for MAC in AIDS* **Action:** Bactericidal; ↓ DNA synthesis. *Spectrum:* Multibacillary dapsone-sensitive leprosy; erythema nodosum leprosum; *Mycobacterium avium-intracellulare* **Dose:** *Adults.* 100–300 mg PO qd. **Peds.** 1 mg/kg/d in combo w/ dapsone & rifampin; take w/ meals **Caution:** [C, +/–] w/ GI problems; use dosages >100 mg/d for as short a duration as possible **Contra:** Component hypersensitivity **Supplied:** Caps 50 mg **SE:** Pink/brownish-black discoloration of the skin & conjunctiva, dry skin, GI intolerance **Notes:** Orphan drug for the Rx of dapsone-resistant leprosy; monitor for GI complaints

Clonazepam (Klonopin) [C-IV] **Uses:** *Lennox–Gastaut syndrome, akinetic & myoclonic Szs, absence Szs, panic attacks,* restless legs syndrome, neuralgia, parkinsonian dysarthria, bipolar disorder **Action:** Benzodiazepine; anticonvulsant **Dose:** *Adults.* 1.5 mg/d PO in 3 ÷ doses; ↑ by 0.5–1 mg/d q3d PRN up to 20 mg/d. **Peds.** 0.01–0.03 mg/kg/24 h PO ÷ tid; ↑ to 0.1–0.2 mg/kg/24 h ÷ tid; avoid abrupt withdrawal **Caution:** [D, M] Elderly pts, resp Dz, CNS depression, severe hepatic impair, NA glaucoma **Contra:** Severe liver Dz, acute NA glaucoma **Supplied:** Tabs 0.5, 1, 2 mg **SE:** CNS side effects, including drowsiness, dizziness, ataxia, memory impair **Notes:** Can cause retrograde amnesia; CYP3A4 substrate

Clonidine, Oral (Catapres) **Uses:** *HTN*; opioid, EtOH, & tobacco withdrawal **Action:** Centrally acting α-adrenergic stimulant **Dose:** *Adults.* 0.1 mg PO bid adjust daily by 0.1- to 0.2-mg increments (max 2.4 mg/d). **Peds.** 5–10 mcg/kg/d ÷ q8–12h (max 0.9 mg/d); ↓ in renal impair **Caution:** [C, +/–] Avoid w/ β-blocker; withdraw slowly **Contra:** Component sensitivity **Supplied:** Tabs 0.1, 0.2, 0.3 mg **SE:** Rebound HTN w/ abrupt cessation of doses >0.2 mg bid; drowsiness, orthostatic ↓ BP, xerostomia, constipation, bradycardia, dizziness **Notes:** More effective for HTN if combined w/ diuretics

Clonidine, Transdermal (Catapres TTS) Uses: *HTN* Action:
Centrally acting α-adrenergic stimulant **Dose:** Apply 1 patch q7d to hairless area (upper arm/torso); titrate to effect; ↓ in severe renal impair; do not D/C abruptly (rebound HTN) **Caution:** [C, +/−] Avoid w/ β-blocker, withdraw slowly **Contra:** Component sensitivity **Supplied:** TTS-1, TTS-2, TTS-3 (delivers 0.1, 0.2, 0.3 mg, respectively, of clonidine/d for 1 wk) **SE:** Drowsiness, orthostatic ↓ BP, xerostomia, constipation, bradycardia, dizziness **Notes:** Doses >2 TTS-3 usually not associated w/ ↑ efficacy; steady state in 2–3 d

Clopidogrel (Plavix) Uses: *Reduction of atherosclerotic events* Action:
↓ Plt aggregation **Dose:** 75 mg/d **Caution:** [B, ?] Active bleeding; risk of bleeding from trauma & other causes; TTP; liver Dz **Contra:** Active bleeding; intracranial bleeding **Supplied:** Tabs 75 mg **SE:** Prolongs bleeding time, GI intolerance, HA, dizziness, rash, thrombocytopenia, leukopenia **Notes:** Plt aggregation returns to baseline ≅5 d after D/C; plt transfusion reverses effects acutely; 300 mg PO × 1 dose can be used to load pts

Clorazepate (Tranxene) [C-IV] Uses: *Acute anxiety disorders, acute EtOH withdrawal Sxs, adjunctive therapy in partial Szs* Action: Benzodiazepine;
antianxiety agent **Dose:** *Adults.* 15–60 mg/d PO single or ÷ doses. *Elderly & debilitated pts:* Initial 7.5–15 mg/d in ÷ doses. *EtOH withdrawal:* Day 1: Initial 30 mg; then 30–60 mg in ÷ doses; Day 2: 45–90 mg in ÷ doses; Day 3: 22.5–45 mg in ÷ doses; Day 4: 15–30 mg in ÷ doses. *Peds.* 3.75–7.5 mg/dose bid to 60 mg/d max ÷ bid–tid **Caution:** [D, ?/−] Not OK for <9 y of age; elderly; Hx depression **Contra:** NA glaucoma **Supplied:** Tabs 3.75, 7.5, 15 mg; Tabs-SD (once-daily) 11.25, 22.5 mg **SE:** CNS depressant effects (drowsiness, dizziness, ataxia, memory impair), ↓ BP **Notes:** Monitor pts w/ renal/hepatic impair (drug may accumulate); avoid abrupt D/C; may cause dependence

Clotrimazole (Lotrimin, Mycelex) [OTC] Uses: *Candidiasis & tinea Infxns* Action: Antifungal; alters cell wall permeability. *Spectrum:* Oropha-
ryngeal candidiasis, dermatophytoses, superficial mycoses, cutaneous candidiasis, & vulvovaginal candidiasis **Dose:** *PO: Prophylaxis:* One troche dissolved in mouth tid *Rx:* One troche dissolved in mouth 5 ×/d for 14 d. *Vaginal 1% Cream:* 1 applicatorful hs for 7 d. *2% Cream:* 1 applicatorful hs for 3 d *Tabs:* 100 mg vaginally hs for 7 d or 200 mg (2 tabs) vaginally hs for 3 d or 500-mg tabs vaginally hs once. *Topical:* Apply bid for 10–14 d **Caution:** [B, (C if PO), ?] Not for systemic fungal Infxn; safety in children <3 y not established **Contra:** Allergy to any component **Supplied:** 1% cream; soln; lotion; troche 10 mg; vaginal tabs 100, 500 mg; vaginal cream 1%, 2% **SE:** *Topical:* Local irritation; *PO:* N/V, ↑ LFTs **Notes:** PO prophylaxis used for immunosuppressed pts

Clotrimazole & Betamethasone (Lotrisone) Uses: *Fungal skin Infxns* Action: Imidazole antifungal & antiinflammatory. *Spectrum:* Tinea pedis,

cruris, & corpora **Dose:** *Pts ≥17 y.* Apply & massage into area bid for 2–4 wk **Caution:** [C, ?] Varicella Infxn **Contra:** Children <12 y **Supplied:** Cream 15, 45 g; lotion 30 mL **SE:** Local irritation, rash **Notes:** Not for diaper dermatitis or under occlusive dressings

Clozapine (Clozaril)
WARNING: Myocarditis, agranulocytosis, Szs, & orthostatic ↓ BP associated w/ clozapine; ↑ mortality in elderly w/dementia-related psychosis **Uses:** *Refractory severe schizophrenia*; childhood psychosis **Action:** "Atypical" TCA **Dose:** 25 mg daily–bid initial; ↑ to 300–450 mg/d over 2 wk. Maintain at lowest dose possible; do not D/C abruptly **Caution:** [B, +/–] Monitor for psychosis & cholinergic rebound **Contra:** Uncontrolled epilepsy; comatose state; WBC ≤3500 cells/mm^3 before Rx or <3000 cells/mm^3 during Rx **Supplied:** Tabs 25, 100 mg **SE:** Tachycardia, drowsiness, weight gain, constipation, incontinence, rash, Szs, CNS stimulation, hyperglycemia **Notes:** Benign, self-limiting temperature elevations may occur during the 1st 3 wk of Rx, weekly CBC mandatory 1st 6 mo, then qowk

Cocaine [C-II]
Uses: *Topical anesthetic for mucous membranes* **Action:** Narcotic analgesic, local vasoconstrictor **Dose:** Apply lowest amount of topical soln that provides relief; 1 mg/kg max **Caution:** [C, ?] **Contra:** PRG **Supplied:** Topical soln & viscous preparations 4%, 10%; powder, soluble tabs (135 mg) for soln **SE:** CNS stimulation, nervousness, loss of taste/smell, chronic rhinitis **Notes:** Use only on mucous membranes of the PO, laryngeal, & nasal cavities; do not use on extensive areas of broken skin

Codeine [C-II]
Uses: *Mild–moderate pain; symptomatic relief of cough* **Action:** Narcotic analgesic; depresses cough reflex **Dose:** *Adults. Analgesic:* 15–60 mg PO or IM qid PRN. *Antitussive:* 10–20 mg PO q4h PRN; max 120 mg/d. *Peds. Analgesic:* 0.5–1 mg/kg/dose PO q4–6h PRN. *Antitussive:* 1–1.5 mg/kg/24 h PO ÷ q4h; max 30 mg/24 h; ↓ in renal/hepatic impair **Caution:** [C, (D if prolonged use or high doses at term), +] **Contra:** Component sensitivity **Supplied:** Tabs 15, 30, 60 mg; soln 15 mg/5 mL; inj 30, 60 mg/mL **SE:** Drowsiness, constipation **Notes:** Usually combined w/ APAP for pain or w/ agents (eg, terpin hydrate) as an antitussive; 120 mg IM = 10 mg IM morphine

Colchicine
Uses: *Acute gouty arthritis & prevention of recurrences; familial Mediterranean fever*; primary biliary cirrhosis **Action:** ↓ migration of leukocytes; ↓ leukocyte lactic acid production **Dose:** *Initial:* 0.5–1.2 mg PO, then 0.5–0.6 mg q1–2h until relief or GI SE develop (max 8 mg/d); do not repeat for 3 d. *IV:* 1–2 mg, then 0.5 mg q6h until relief (max 4 mg/d); do not repeat for 7 d. *Prophylaxis:* PO: 0.5–0.6 mg/d or 3–4 d/wk; ↓ renal impair; caution in elderly **Caution:** [D, +] In elderly **Contra:** Serious renal, GI, hepatic, or cardiac disorders; blood dyscrasias **Supplied:** Tabs 0.5, 0.6 mg; inj 1 mg/2 mL **SE:** N/V/D, abdominal pain, BM suppression, hepatotox; severe local irritation can occur following SQ/IM **Notes:** Colchicine 1–2 mg IV w/in 24–48 h of an acute attack diagnostic/therapeutic in monoarticular arthritis

Colesevelam (Welchol)
Uses: *Reduction of LDL & total cholesterol alone or in combo w/ an HMG-CoA reductase inhibitor* **Action:** Bile acid seques-

trant **Dose:** 3 tabs PO bid w/ meals **Caution:** [B, ?] Severe GI motility disorders; safety & efficacy not established in peds **Contra:** Bowel obstruction **Supplied:** Tabs 625 mg **SE:** Constipation, dyspepsia, myalgia, weakness **Notes:** May ↓ absorption of fat-soluble vitamins

Colestipol (Colestid) **Uses:** *Adjunct to ↓ serum cholesterol in primary hypercholesterolemia* **Action:** Binds intestinal bile acids to form insoluble complex **Dose:** Granules: 5–30 g/d ÷ 2–4 doses; tabs: 2–16 g/d daily–bid **Caution:** [C, ?] Avoid w/ high triglycerides, GI dysfunction **Contra:** Bowel obstruction **Supplied:** Tabs 1 g; granules 5, 300, 500 g **SE:** Constipation, abdominal pain, bloating, HA **Notes:** Do not use dry powder; mix w/ beverages, soups, cereals, etc; may ↓ absorption of other medications; may ↓ absorption of fat-soluble vitamins

Colfosceril Palmitate (Exosurf Neonatal) **Uses:** *Prophylaxis & Rx for RDS in infants* **Action:** Synthetic lung surfactant **Dose:** 5 mL/kg/dose through ET tube as soon after birth as possible & again at 12 & 24 h **Caution:** [?, ?] Pulmonary hemorrhaging **Supplied:** Inj 108 mg **SE:** Pulmonary hemorrher possible in infants weighing <700 g at birth; mucous plugging **Notes:** Monitor pulmonary compliance & oxygenation carefully; monitor ECG

Cortisone See Steroids, Tables 4 & 5 (pages 206 & 207)

Cromolyn Sodium (Intal, NasalCrom, Opticrom) **Uses:** *Adjunct to the Rx of asthma; prevent exercise-induced asthma; allergic rhinitis; ophth allergic manifestations*; food allergy **Action:** Antiasthmatic; mast cell stabilizer **Dose:** *Adults & Children >12 y.* *Inhal:* 20 mg (as powder in caps) inhaled qid or met-dose inhaler 2 puffs qid. *PO:* 200 mg qid 15–20 min ac, up to 400 mg qid. *Nasal instillation:* Spray once in each nostril 2–6×/d. *Ophth:* 1–2 gtt in each eye 4–6×/d. *Peds. Inhal:* 2 puffs qid of met-dose inhaler. *PO: Infants <2 y:* (not OK) 20 mg/kg/d in 4 ÷ doses. *2–12 y:* 100 mg qid ac **Caution:** [B, ?] **Contra:** Acute asthmatic attacks **Supplied:** PO conc 100 mg/5 mL; soln for neb 20 mg/2 mL; met-dose inhaler; nasal soln 40 mg/mL; ophth soln 4% **SE:** Unpleasant taste, hoarseness, coughing **Notes:** No benefit in acute Rx; 2–4 wk for maximal effect in perennial allergic disorders

Cyanocobalamin [Vitamin B₁₂] **Uses:** *Pernicious anemia & other vitamin B$_{12}$ deficiency states; ↑ requirements due to PRG; thyrotoxicosis; liver or kidney Dz* **Action:** Dietary vitamin B$_{12}$ supl **Dose:** *Adults.* 100 mcg IM or SQ qd for 5–10 d, then 100 mcg IM 2×/wk for 1 mo, then 100 mcg IM monthly. *Peds.* 100 mcg/d IM or SQ for 5–10 d, then 30–50 mcg IM q4wk **Caution:** [A (C if dose exceeds RDA), +] **Contra:** Allergy to cobalt; hereditary optic nerve atrophy; Leber Dz **Supplied:** Tabs 50, 100, 250, 500, 1000 mcg; inj 100, 1000 mcg/mL; gel 500 mcg/0.1 mL **SE:** Itching, D, HA, anxiety **Notes:** PO absorption erratic, altered by many drugs & not recommended; for use w/ hyperalimentation

Cyclobenzaprine (Flexeril) **Uses:** *Relief of muscle spasm* **Action:** Centrally acting skeletal muscle relaxant; reduces tonic somatic motor activity **Dose:** 10 mg PO bid–qid (2–3 wk max) **Caution:** [B, ?] Shares the toxic potential of the TCAs; urinary hesitancy or angle-closure glaucoma **Contra:** Do not use concomitantly or w/in 14 d of MAOIs; hyperthyroidism; heart failure; arrhythmias **Supplied:** Tabs 10 mg **SE:** Sedation & anticholinergic effects **Notes:** May inhibit mental alertness or physical coordination

Cyclopentolate (Cyclogyl) **Uses:** *Diagnostic procedures requiring cycloplegia & mydriasis* **Action:** Cycloplegic & mydriatic agent (can last up to 24 h) **Dose:** 1 gt then another in 5 min **Caution:** [C, ?] **Contra:** NA glaucoma **Supplied:** Soln, 0.5, 1, 2% **SE:** Blurred vision, ↑ sensitivity to light, tachycardia, restlessness

Cyclophosphamide (Cytoxan, Neosar) **Uses:** *Hodgkin Dz & NHLs; multiple myeloma; small-cell lung, breast, & ovarian CAs; mycosis fungoides; neuroblastoma; retinoblastoma; acute leukemias; & allogeneic & ABMT in high doses; severe rheumatologic disorders* **Action:** Converted to acrolein & phosphoramide mustard, the active alkylating moieties **Dose:** 500–1500 mg/m^2 as single dose at 2–4-wk intervals; 1.8 g/m^2 to 160 mg/kg (or ≅12 g/m^2 in a 75-kg individual) in the BMT setting (Per protocols); adjust in renal/hepatic impair **Caution:** [D, ?] w/ BM suppression **Contra:** Component sensitivity **Supplied:** Tabs 25, 50 mg; inj 100 mg **SE:** Myelosuppression (leukopenia & thrombocytopenia); hemorrhagic cystitis, SIADH, alopecia, anorexia; N/V; hepatotox & rarely interstitial pneumonitis; irreversible testicular atrophy possible; cardiotox rare; 2nd malignancies (bladder CA & acute leukemias); cumulative risk 3.5% at 8 y, 10.7% at 12 y **Notes:** Hemorrhagic cystitis prophylaxis: continuous bladder irrigation & mesna uroprotection; encourage hydration

Cyclosporine (Sandimmune, NeOral) **Uses:** *Organ rejection in kidney, liver, heart, & BMT w/ steroids; RA; psoriasis* **Action:** Immunosuppressant; reversible inhibition of immunocompetent lymphocytes **Dose:** *Adults & Peds.* PO: 15 mg/kg/d 12 h pretransplant; after 2 wk, taper by 5 mg/wk to 5–10 mg/kg/d. *IV:* If NPO, give ⅓ PO dose IV; ↓ in renal/hepatic impair **Caution:** [C, ?] Dose-related risk of nephrotox/hepatotox; live, attenuated vaccines may be less effective **Contra:** Abnormal renal Fxn; uncontrolled HTN **Supplied:** Caps 25, 50, 100 mg; PO soln 100 mg/mL; inj 50 mg/mL **SE:** May ↑ BUN & creatinine & mimic transplant rejection; HTN; HA; hirsutism **Notes:** Administer in glass container; many drug interactions; NeOral & Sandimmune not interchangeable; interaction w/ St. John's wort. Follow levels (Table 2, page 204)

Cyclosporine ophthalmic (Restasis) **Uses:** *↑ Tear production suppressed due to ocular inflammation* **Action:** Immune modulator, antiinflammatory **Dose:** 1 gt bid each eye 12 h apart. OK w/ artificial tears, allow 15 min between **Caution:** [C, –] **Contra:** Ocular Infxn, component allergy **Supplied:** Single-use vial 0.05% **SE:** Ocular burning/hyperemia **Notes:** Mix vial well

Cyproheptadine (Periactin) **Uses:** *Allergic Rxns; itching* **Action:** Phenothiazine antihistamine; serotonin antagonist **Dose:** *Adults.* 4–20 mg PO ÷ q8h; max 0.5 mg/kg/d. *Peds.* 2–6 y: 2 mg bid–tid (max 12 mg/24 h). 7–14 y: 4 mg bid–tid; ↓ in hepatic impair **Caution:** [B, ?] Symptomatic BPH **Contra:** Neonates or <2 y; NA glaucoma; BOO; acute asthma; GI obstruction **Supplied:** Tabs 4 mg; syrup 2 mg/5 mL **SE:** Anticholinergic, drowsiness, **Notes:** May stimulate appetite

Cytarabine [ARA-C] (Cytosar-U)
Uses: *Acute leukemias, CML, NHL; IT for leukemic meningitis or prophylaxis* **Action:** Antimetabolite; interferes w/ DNA synthesis **Dose:** 100–150 mg/m²/d for 5–10 d (low dose); 3 g/m² q12h for 8–12 doses (high dose); 1 mg/kg 1–2/wk (SQ maint regimens); 5–70 mg/m² up to 3/wk IT (Per protocols); ↓ in renal/hepatic impair **Caution:** [D, ?] w/ marked BM suppression, ↓ dosage by ↓ the number of days of administration **Contra:** Component sensitivity **Supplied:** Inj 100, 500 mg, 1, 2 g **SE:** Myelosuppression, N/V/D, stomatitis, flu-like syndrome, rash on palms/soles, hepatic dysfunction, cerebellar dysfunction, noncardiogenic pulmonary edema, neuropathy **Notes:** Little use in solid tumors; tox of high-dose regimens (conjunctivitis) ameliorated by corticosteroid ophth soln

Cytarabine Liposome (DepoCyt)
Uses: *Lymphomatous meningitis* **Action:** Antimetabolite; interferes w/ DNA synthesis **Dose:** 50 mg IT q14d for 5 doses, then 50 mg IT q28d for 4 doses; use dexamethasone prophylaxis **Caution:** [D, ?] May cause neurotox; blockage to CSF flow may ↑ the risk of neurotox; use in peds not established **Contra:** Active meningeal Infxn **Supplied:** IT inj 50 mg/5 mL **SE:** Neck pain/rigidity, HA, confusion, somnolence, fever, back pain, N/V, edema, neutropenia, thrombocytopenia, anemia **Notes:** Cytarabine liposomes are similar in microscopic appearance to WBCs; caution in interpreting CSF studies

Cytomegalovirus Immune Globulin [CMV-IG IV] (CytoGam)
Uses: *Attenuation of primary CMV Dz associated w/ transplantation* **Action:** Exogenous IgG antibodies to CMV **Dose:** 150 mg/kg/dose w/in 72 h of transplant, for 16 wk posttransplant; see insert for dosing schedule **Caution:** [C, ?] Anaphylactic Rxns; renal dysfunction **Contra:** Allergy to immunoglobulins; immunoglobulin A deficiency **Supplied:** Inj 50 mg/mL **SE:** Flushing, N/V, muscle cramps, wheezing, HA, fever **Notes:** IV use only; administer by separate line; do not shake

Dacarbazine (DTIC)
Uses: *Melanoma, Hodgkin Dz, sarcoma* **Action:** Alkylating agent; antimetabolite as a purine precursor; ↓ protein synthesis, RNA, & especially DNA **Dose:** 2–4.5 mg/kg/d for 10 consecutive d or 250 mg/m²/d for 5 d (Per protocols); ↓ in renal impair **Caution:** [C, ?] In BM suppression; renal/hepatic impair **Contra:** Component sensitivity **Supplied:** Inj 100, 200, 500 mg **SE:** Myelosuppression, severe N/V, hepatotox, flu-like syndrome, ↓ BP, photosensitivity, alopecia, facial flushing, facial paresthesias, urticaria, phlebitis at inj site **Notes:** Avoid extravasation

Daclizumab (Zenapax)
Uses: *Prevent acute organ rejection* **Action:** IL-2 receptor antagonist **Dose:** 1 mg/kg/dose IV; 1st dose pretransplant, then 4 doses 14 d apart posttransplant **Caution:** [C, ?] **Contra:** Component sensitivity **Supplied:** Inj 5 mg/mL **SE:** Hyperglycemia, edema, HTN, ↓ BP, constipation, HA, dizziness, anxiety, nephrotox, pulmonary edema, pain **Notes:** Administer w/in 4 h of preparation

Dactinomycin (Cosmegen) Uses: *Choriocarcinoma, Wilms' tumor, Kaposi sarcoma, Ewing sarcoma, rhabdomyosarcoma, testicular CA* Action: DNA intercalating agent Dose: 0.5 mg/d for 5 d; 2 mg/wk for 3 consecutive wk; 15 mcg/kg or 0.45 mg/m²/d (max 0.5 mg) for 5 d q3–8wk in ped sarcoma (Per protocols); ↓ in renal impair Caution: [C, ?] Contra: w/ concurrent or recent chickenpox or herpes zoster; infants <6 mo Supplied: Inj 0.5 mg SE: Myelo-/immunosuppression, severe N/V, alopecia, acne, hyperpigmentation, radiation recall phenomenon, tissue damage w/ extravasation, hepatotox

Dalteparin (Fragmin) Uses: *Unstable angina, non-Q-wave MI, prevention of ischemic complications due to clot formation in pts on concurrent ASA, prevention & Rx of DVT following surgery* Action: LMW heparin Dose: *Angina/MI:* 120 IU/kg (max 10,000 IU) SQ q12h w/ ASA. *DVT prophylaxis:* 2500–5000 IU SC 1–2 h preop, then qd for 5–10 d. *Systemic anticoagulation:* 200 IU/kg/d SQ or 100 IU/kg bid SQ; caution in renal/hepatic impair Caution: [B, ?] Active hemorrhage, cerebrovascular Dz, cerebral aneurysm, severe uncontrolled HTN Contra: HIT; allergy to pork products; Supplied: Inj 2500 IU (16 mg/0.2 mL), 5000 IU (32 mg/0.4 mL), 10,000 IU (64 mg/mL) SE: Bleeding, pain at inj site, thrombocytopenia Notes: Predictable antithrombotic effects eliminate need for lab monitoring; not for IM/IV use

Danaparoid (Orgaron) Uses: *Prophylaxis of DVT to prevent PE, in hip replacement surgery* Action: Antithrombotic; ↓ factor Xa & IIa Dose: 750 anti-Xa units bid SQ 1–4 h preop & starting no sooner than 2 h postop; ↓ in severe renal impair Caution: [B, ?/–] Contra: Active major bleeding, hemophilia, ITP, type II thrombocytopenia w/ a (+) antiplatelet Ab test Supplied: Amps & prefilled syringes 0.6 mL (750 anti-Xa units) SE: Bleeding, fever, inj site pain, ↑ risk of epidural/spinal hematoma w/epidural/spinal anesthesia Notes: aPTT monitoring not necessary

Dantrolene (Dantrium) Uses: *Rx clinical spasticity due to upper motor neuron disorders, (eg, spinal cord injuries, strokes, CP, MS); malignant hyperthermia* Action: Skeletal muscle relaxant Dose: *Adults. Spasticity:* Initial, 25 mg PO daily; ↑ 25 mg to effect to 100 mg max PO qid PRN. *Peds.* Initial, 0.5 mg/kg/dose bid; ↑ by 0.5 mg/kg to effect, to 3 mg/kg/dose max qid PRN. *Adults & Peds. Malignant hyperthermia:* Rx: Continuous rapid IV push, start 1 mg/kg until Sxs subside or 10 mg/kg is reached. *Postcrisis follow-up:* 4–8 mg/kg/d in 3–4 ÷ doses for 1–3 d to prevent recurrence Caution:[C, ?] Impaired cardiac/pulmonary Fxn Contra: Active hepatic Dz; where spasticity needed to maintain posture or balance Supplied: Caps 25, 50, 100 mg; powder for inj 20 mg/vial SE: Hepatotox w/↑ LFTs, drowsiness, dizziness, rash, muscle weakness, pleural effusion w/ pericarditis, D, blurred vision, hepatitis Notes: Monitor transaminases; avoid sunlight/EtOH/CNS depressants

Dapsone (Avlosulfon) Uses: *Rx & prevent PCP; toxoplasmosis prophylaxis; leprosy* Action: Unknown; bactericidal Dose: *Adults.* PCP prophylaxis

50–100 mg/d PO; Rx PCP 100 mg/d PO w/ TMP 15–20 mg/kg/d for 21 d. **Peds.** Prophylaxis of PCP 1–2 mg/kg/24 h PO daily; max 100 mg/d **Caution:** [C, +] G6PD deficiency; severe anemia **Contra:** Component sensitivity **Supplied:** Tabs 25, 100 mg **SE:** Hemolysis, methemoglobinemia, agranulocytosis, rash, cholestatic jaundice **Notes:** Absorption ↑ by an acidic environment; w/ leprosy, combine w/ rifampin & other agents

Daptomycin (Cubicin)   **Uses:** *Complicated skin/skin structure Infxns due to gram(+) organisms* **Action:** Cyclic lipopeptide, causes rapid membrane depolarization & bacterial death *Spectrum: Staphylococcus aureus* (including MRSA), *Streptococcus pyogenes, S. agalactiae, S. dysgalactiae* subsp *Equisimilis & Enterococcus faecalis* (vancomycin-susceptible strains only) **Dose:** 4 mg/kg IV daily × 7–14 d (over 30 min); w/ CrCl < 30 mL/min/dialysis: 4 mg/kg q48h **Caution:** [B, ?] Monitor CPK weekly **Supplied:** Inj 250, 500 mg/10 mL **SE:** Constipation, N/V/D, HA, rash, site Rxn, muscle pain/weakness, edema, cellulitis, hypo/hyperglycemia, ↑ alkaline phosphatase, cough, back pain, abdominal pain, ↓ K⁺, anxiety, chest pain, sore throat, Candida Infxns **Notes:** Consider suspending use of HMG-CoA reductase inhibitors (↑ myopathy risk)

Darbepoetin Alfa (Aranesp)   **Uses:** *Anemia associated w/ CRF* **Action:** ↑ Erythropoiesis, recombinant erythropoietin variant **Dose:** 0.45 mcg/kg single IV or SQ qwk; titrate, do not exceed target Hgb of 12 g/dL; see insert to convert from Epogen **Caution:** [C, ?] May ↑ risk of CV &/or neurologic SE in renal failure; HTN; w/ Hx Szs **Contra:** Uncontrolled HTN, component allergy **Supplied:** 25, 40, 60, 100 mcg/mL, in polysorbate or albumin excipient **SE:** May ↑ risk of cardiac events, CP, hypo/hypertension, N/V/D, myalgia, arthralgia, dizziness, edema, fatigue, fever, ↑ risk Infxn **Notes:** Longer ½-life than Epogen; weekly CBC until stable

Darifenacin (Enablex)   **Uses:** OAB **Action:** Muscarinic receptor antagonist **Dose:** 7.5 mg/d PO; 15 mg/d max (7.5 mg/d w/ moderate hepatic impair or w/ CYP3A4 inhibitors); w/ drugs metabolized by CYP2D (flecainide, thioridazine, TCAs);(swallow whole) **Caution:** [C, ?/–] **Contra:** Urinary/gastric retention, uncontrolled NA glaucoma **Supplied:** Tabs ER 7.5 mg **SE:** Xerostomia/eyes, constipation, dyspepsia, abdominal pain, retention, abnormal vision, dizziness, asthenia

Daunorubicin (Daunomycin, Cerubidine)   **WARNING:** Cardiac Fxn should be monitored due to potential risk for cardiac tox & CHF **Uses:** Acute leukemias **Action:** DNA intercalating agent; ↓ topoisomerase II; generates oxygen free radicals **Dose:** 45–60 mg/m²/d for 3 consecutive d; 25 mg/m²/wk (Per protocols); ↓ in renal/hepatic impair **Caution:** [D, ?] **Contra:** Component sensitivity **Supplied:** Inj 20 mg **SE:** Myelosuppression, mucositis, N/V, alopecia, radiation recall phenomenon, hepatotox (hyperbilirubinemia), tissue necrosis w/ extravasation, cardiotox (1–2% CHF risk w/ 550 mg/m² cumulative dose) **Notes:** Prevent cardiotox w/ dexrazoxane; administer allopurinol prior to Rx to prevent hyperuricemia

Delavirdine (Rescriptor) **Uses:** *HIV Infxn* **Action:** Nonnucleoside RT inhibitor **Dose:** 400 mg PO tid **Caution:** [C, ?] CDC recommends HIV-infected mothers not breast-feed due to risk of HIV transmission; renal/hepatic impair **Contra:** Concomitant use w/ drugs highly dependent on CYP3A for clearance (ie, alprazolam, ergot alkaloids, midazolam, pimozide, triazolam) **Supplied:** Tabs 100 mg **SE:** HA, fatigue, rash, ↑ transaminases, N/V/D **Notes:** Avoid antacids; ↓ cytochrome P-450 enzymes; numerous drug interactions; monitor LFTs

Demeclocycline (Declomycin) **Uses:** SIADH **Action:** Antibiotic, antagonizes ADH action on renal tubules **Dose:** 300–600 mg PO q12h on empty stomach; ↓ in renal failure; avoid antacids **Caution:** [D, +] Avoid in hepatic/renal dysfunction & children **Contra:** Allergy to tetracyclines **Supplied:** Tabs 150, 300 mg **SE:** D, abdominal cramps, photosensitivity, DI **Notes:** Avoid sunlight

Desipramine (Norpramin) **WARNING:** Closely monitor for worsening depression or emergence of suicidality **Uses:** *Endogenous depression,* chronic pain, & peripheral neuropathy **Action:** TCA; ↑ synaptic concentration of serotonin or norepinephrine in CNS **Dose:** 25–200 mg/d single or ÷ doses; usually a single hs dose (max 300 mg/d) **Caution:** [C, ?/–] CV Dz, Sz disorder, hypothyroidism **Contra:** Use of MAOIs w/in 14 d; during recovery phase of MI **Supplied:** Tabs 10, 25, 50, 75, 100, 150 mg; caps 25, 50 mg **SE:** Anticholinergic (blurred vision, urinary retention, xerostomia); orthostatic ↓ BP; prolongs QT interval, arrhythmias **Notes:** Numerous drug interactions; may cause blue-green urine; avoid sunlight

Desloratadine (Clarinex) **Uses:** *Symptoms of seasonal & perennial allergic rhinitis; chronic idiopathic urticaria* **Action:** Active metabolite of Claritin, H₁-antihistamine, blocks inflammatory mediators **Dose:** Adults & Peds >12 y. 5 mg PO qd; in hepatic/renal impair 5 mg PO qod **Caution:** [C, ?/–] RediTabs contain phenylalanine; safety not established for <12 y **Supplied:** Tabs & Reditabs (rapid dissolving) 5 mg **SE:** Allergy, anaphylaxis somnolence, HA, dizziness, fatigue, pharyngitis, xerostomia, nausea, dyspepsia, myalgia

Desmopressin (DDAVP, Stimate) **Uses:** *DI (intranasal & parenteral); bleeding due to uremia, hemophilia A, & type I von Willebrand Dz (parenteral), nocturnal enuresis* **Action:** Synthetic analog of vasopressin, a naturally occurring human ADH; ↑ factor VIII **Dose:** DI: Intranasal: Adults. 0.1–0.4 mL (10–40 mcg/d in 1–4 ÷ doses. Peds 3 mo–12 y. 0.05–0.3 mL/d in 1 or 2 doses. Parenteral: Adults. 0.5–1 mL (2–4 mcg/d in 2 ÷ doses); if converting from nasal to parenteral, use ⅒ nasal dose. PO: Adults. 0.05 bid; ↑ to max of 1.2 mg. Hemophilia A & von Willebrand Dz (type I): Adults & Peds >10 kg. 0.3 mcg/kg in 50 mL NS, inf over 15–30 min. Peds <10 kg. As above w/ dilution to 10 mL w/ NS. Nocturnal enuresis: Peds >6 y. 20 mcg intranasally hs **Caution:** [B, M] Avoid overhydration **Contra:** Hemophilia B; severe classic von Willebrand Dz; pts w/ factor VIII antibodies **Supplied:** Tabs 0.1, 0.2 mg; inj 4 mcg/mL; nasal soln 0.1, 1.5 mg/mL **SE:** Facial flushing, HA, dizziness, vulval pain, nasal congestion, pain at inj site,

↓ Na⁺, H₂O intox **Notes:** In very young & old pts, ↓ fluid intake to avoid H₂O intox & ↓ Na⁺

Dexamethasone, Nasal (Dexacort Phosphate Turbinaire)

Uses: *Chronic nasal inflammation or allergic rhinitis* **Action:** Antiinflammatory corticosteroid **Dose:** *Adult & Peds >12 y.* 2 sprays/nostril bid–tid, max 12 sprays/d. *Peds 6–12 y.* 1–2 sprays/nostril bid, max 8 sprays/d **Caution:** [C, ?] **Contra:** Untreated Infxn **Supplied:** Aerosol, 84 mcg/activation **SE:** Local irritation

Dexamethasone, Ophthalmic (AK-Dex Ophthalmic, Decadron Ophthalmic)

Uses: *Inflammatory or allergic conjunctivitis* **Action:** Antiinflammatory corticosteroid **Dose:** Instill 1–2 gtt tid–qid **Caution:** [C, ?/–] **Contra:** Active untreated bacterial, viral, & fungal eye Infxns **Supplied:** Susp & soln 0.1%; oint 0.05% **SE:** Long-term use associated w/ cataracts

Dexamethasone Systemic, Topical (Decadron) See Steroids,

Systemic, page 169, & Table 4, page 206, & Steroids, Topical, Table 5, page 207

Dexpanthenol (Ilopan-Choline PO, Ilopan)

Uses: *Minimize paralytic ileus, Rx postop distention* **Action:** Cholinergic agent **Dose:** *Adults.* Relief of gas: 2–3 tabs PO tid. *Prevent postop ileus:* 250–500 mg IM stat, repeat in 2 h, then q6h PRN. *Ileus:* 500 mg IM stat, repeat in 2 h, followed by doses q6h, PRN **Caution:** [C, ?] **Contra:** Hemophilia, mechanical obstruction **Supplied:** Inj; tabs 50 mg; cream **SE:** GI cramps

Dexrazoxane (Zinecard)

Uses: *Prevent anthracycline-induced (eg, doxorubicin) cardiomyopathy* **Action:** Chelates heavy metals; binds intracellular iron & prevents anthracycline-induced free radicals **Dose:** 10:1 ratio dexrazoxane:doxorubicin 30 min prior to each dose **Caution:** [C, ?] **Contra:** Component sensitivity **Supplied:** Inj 10 mg/mL **SE:** Myelosuppression (especially leukopenia), fever, Infxn, stomatitis, alopecia, N/V/D; mild ↑ transaminase, pain at inj site

Dextran 40 (Rheomacrodex)

Uses: *Shock, prophylaxis of DVT & thromboembolism, adjunct in peripheral vascular surgery* **Action:** Expands plasma volume; ↓ blood viscosity **Dose:** *Shock:* 10 mL/kg inf rapidly; 20 mL/kg max in the 1st 24 h; beyond 24 h 10 mL/kg max; D/C after 5 d. *Prophylaxis of DVT & thromboembolism:* 10 mL/kg IV day of surgery, then 500 mL/d IV for 2–3 d, then 500 mL IV q2–3d based on risk for up to 2 wk **Caution:** [C, ?] Inf Rxns; pts receiving corticosteroids **Contra:** Major hemostatic defects; cardiac decompensation; renal Dz w/ severe oliguria/anuria **Supplied:** 10% dextran 40 in 0.9% NaCl or 5% dextrose **SE:** Allergy/anaphylactoid Rxn (observe during 1st min of inf), arthralgia, cutaneous Rxns, ↓ BP, fever **Notes:** Monitor Cr & electrolytes; pts should be well hydrated

Dextromethorphan (Mediquell, Benylin DM, PediaCare 1, others) [OTC]

Uses: *Controlling nonproductive cough* **Action:** Depresses the cough center in the medulla **Dose:** *Adults.* 10–30 mg PO q4h PRN (max 120 mg/24 h). *Peds.* 7 mo–1 y: 2–4 mg q6–8h. 2–6 y: 2.5–7.5 mg q4–8h (max 30 mg/24 h). 7–12 y: 5–10 mg q4–8h (max 60 mg/24/h) **Caution:** [C, ?/–] Not for persistent or chronic cough **Supplied:** Caps 30 mg; lozenges 2.5, 5, 7.5, 15 mg; syrup 15 mg/15 mL, 10 mg/5 mL; liq 10 mg/15 mL, 3.5, 7.5, 15 mg/5 mL; sustained-action liq 30 mg/5 mL **SE:** GI disturbances **Notes:** May be found in combo OTC products w/ guaifenesin

Dezocine (Dalgan) Uses: *Moderate–severe pain* **Action:** Narcotic agonist–antagonist **Dose:** 5–20 mg IM or 2.5–10 mg IV q2–4h PRN; ↓ in renal impair **Caution:** [C, ?] **Contra:** Pts <18 y **Supplied:** Inj 5, 10, 15 mg/mL **SE:** Sedation, dizziness, vertigo, N/V, inj site Rxn **Notes:** Withdrawal possible in narcotic dependency

Diazepam (Valium) [C-IV] Uses: *Anxiety, EtOH withdrawal, muscle spasm, status epilepticus, panic disorders, amnesia, preop sedation* **Action:** Benzodiazepine **Dose:** *Adults. Status epilepticus:* 5–10 mg q10–20min to 30 mg max in 8-h period. *Anxiety, muscle spasm:* 2–10 mg PO bid–qid or IM/IV q3–4h PRN. *Preop:* 5–10 mg PO or IM 20–30 min or IV just prior to procedure. *EtOH withdrawal:* Initial 2–5 mg IV, then 5–10 mg q5–10min, 100 mg in 1 h max. May require up to 1000 mg in 24-h period for severe withdrawal. Titrate to agitation; avoid excessive sedation; may lead to aspiration or resp arrest. *Peds. Status epilepticus:* <5 y: 0.05–0.3 mg/kg/dose IV q15–30min up to a max of 5 mg. >5 y: Give up to max of 10 mg. *Sedation, muscle relaxation:* 0.04–0.3 mg/kg/dose q2–4h IM or IV to max of 0.6 mg/kg in 8 h, or 0.12–0.8 mg/kg/24 h PO ÷ tid–qid; ↓ in hepatic impair; avoid abrupt withdrawal **Caution:** [D, ?/–] **Contra:** Coma, CNS depression, resp depression, NA glaucoma, severe uncontrolled pain, PRG **Supplied:** Tabs 2, 5, 10 mg; soln 1, 5 mg/mL; inj 5 mg/mL; rectal gel 5 mg/mL **SE:** Sedation, amnesia, bradycardia, ↓ BP, rash, ↓ resp rate **Notes:** Do not exceed 5 mg/min IV in adults or 1–2 mg/min in peds because near arrest possible; IM absorption erratic

Diazoxide (Hyperstat, Proglycem) Uses: *Hypoglycemia due to hyperinsulinism (Proglycem); hypertensive crisis (Hyperstat)* **Action:** ↓ Pancreatic insulin release; antihypertensive **Dose:** *Hypertensive crisis:* 1–3 mg/kg IV (150 mg max in single inj); repeat in 5–15 min until BP controlled; repeat every 4–24 h; monitor BP closely. *Hypoglycemia: Adults & Peds.* 3–8 mg/kg/24 h PO ÷ q8–12h. *Neonates.* 8–15 mg/kg/24 h ÷ in 3 equal doses; maint 8–10 mg/kg/24 h PO in 2–3 equal doses **Caution:** [C, ?] ↓ effect w/ phenytoin; ↑ effect w/ diuretics, warfarin **Contra:** Allergy to thiazides or other sulfonamide-containing products; HTN associated w/ aortic coarctation, AV shunt, or pheochromocytoma **Supplied:** Inj 15 mg/mL; caps 50 mg; PO susp 50 mg/mL **SE:** Hyperglycemia, ↓ BP, dizziness, Na+ & H2O retention, N/V, weakness **Notes:** Can give false-negative insulin response to glucagons; treat extravasation w/ warm compress

Dibucaine (Nupercainal) Uses: *Hemorrhoids & minor skin conditions* **Action:** Topical anesthetic **Dose:** Insert PR w/ applicator bid & after each bowel movement; apply sparingly to skin **Caution:** [C, ?] **Contra:** Component sensitivity **Supplied:** 1% Oint w/ rectal applicator; 0.5% cream **SE:** Local irritation, rash

Diclofenac (Cataflam, Voltaren) WARNING: May ↑ risk of cardio vascular events & GI bleeding Uses: *Arthritis & pain* Action: NSAID Dose 50–75 mg PO bid; w/ food or milk Caution: [B (D 3rd tri or near delivery), ? CHF, HTN, renal/hepatic dysfunction, & Hx PUD Contra: Allergy to NSAIDs o aspirin; porphyria Supplied: Tabs 50 mg; tabs DR 25, 50, 75, 100 mg; XR tab 100 mg; ophthal soln 0.1% SE: Abdominal cramps, heartburn, GI ulceration, rash interstitial nephritis Notes: Do not crush; watch for GI bleed

Dicloxacillin (Dynapen, Dycill) Uses: *Rx of pneumonia, skin & sof tissue Infxns, & osteomyelitis caused by penicillinase-producing staphylococci* Action: Bactericidal; ↓ cell wall synthesis. Spectrum: S. aureus & Strep Dose Adults. 250–500 mg qid Peds <40 kg. 12.5–25 mg/kg/d ÷ qid; take on empty stom ach Caution: [B. ?] Contra: Component or PCN sensitivity Supplied: Caps 125 250, 500 mg; soln 62.5 mg/5 mL SE: N/D, abdominal pain Notes: Monitor PTT i pt on warfarin

Dicyclomine (Bentyl) Uses: *Functional IBSs* Action: Smooth muscle relaxant Dose: Adults. 20 mg PO qid; ↑ to 160 mg/d max or 20 mg IM q6h Peds Infants >6 mo: 5 mg/dose tid–qid. Children: 10 mg/dose tid–qid Caution: [B, – Contra: Infants < 6 mo, NA glaucoma, MyG, severe UC, BOO Supplied: Cap 10, 20 mg; tabs 20 mg; syrup 10 mg/5 mL; inj 10 mg/mL SE: Anticholinergic SE' may limit dose Notes: Take 30–60 min before meal; avoid EtOH

Didanosine [ddI] (Videx) WARNING: Allergy manifested as fever rash, fatigue, GI/resp Sxs reported; stop drug immediately & do not rechallenge lactic acidosis & hepatomegaly/steatosis reported Uses: *HIV Infxn in zidovudine intolerant pts* Action: Nucleoside antiretroviral agent Dose: Adults. >60 kg: 400 mg/d PO or 200 mg PO bid. <60 kg: 250 mg/d PO or 125 mg PO bid; adult should take 2 tabs/administration. Peds. Dose by following table; ↓ in renal impair

Peds Didanosine Dosing

BSA (m²)	Tablets (mg)	Powder (mg)
1.1–1.4	100 bid	125 bid
0.8–1	75 bid	94 bid
0.5–0.7	50 bid	62 bid
<0.4	25 bid	31 bid

Caution: [B, –] CDC recommends HIV-infected mothers not breast-feed due to risk of HIV transmission Contra: Component sensitivity Supplied: Chew tabs 25 50, 100, 150, 200 mg; powder packets 100, 167, 250, 375 mg; powder for soln 2 4 g SE: Pancreatitis, peripheral neuropathy, D, HA Notes: Do not take w/ meals thoroughly chew tablets, do not mix w/ fruit juice or other acidic beverages; reconstitute powder w/ H_2O

Diflunisal (Dolobid) **WARNING:** May ↑ risk of cardiovascular events & GI bleeding **Uses:** *Mild–moderate pain; osteoarthritis* **Action:** NSAID **Dose:** *Pain:* 500 mg PO bid. *Osteoarthritis:* 500–1500 mg PO in 2–3 ÷ doses; ↓ in renal impair, take w/ food/milk **Caution:** [C (D 3rd tri or near delivery), ?] CHF, HTN, renal/hepatic dysfunction, & Hx PUD. **Contra:** Allergy to NSAIDs or aspirin, active GI bleed **Supplied:** Tabs 250, 500 mg **SE:** May ↑ bleeding time; HA, abdominal cramps, heartburn, GI ulceration, rash, interstitial nephritis, fluid retention

Digoxin (Lanoxin, Lanoxicaps) **Uses:** *CHF, AF & flutter, & PAT* **Action:** Positive inotrope; ↑ AV node refractory period **Dose:** *Adults. PO digitalization:* 0.5–0.75 mg PO, then 0.25 mg PO q6–8h to total 1–1.5 mg. *IV or IM digitalization:* 0.25–0.5 mg IM or IV, then 0.25 mg q4–6h to total ≅1 mg. *Daily maint:* 0.125–0.5 mg/d PO, IM, or IV (average daily dose 0.125–0.25 mg). *Peds. Preterm infants:* Digitalization: 30 mcg/kg PO or 25 mcg/kg IV; give ½ of dose initial, then ¼ of dose at 8–12-h intervals for 2 doses. *Maint:* 5–7.5 mcg/kg/24 h PO or 4–6 mcg/ kg/24 h IV ÷ q12h. *Term infants:* Digitalization: 25–35 mcg/kg PO or 20–30 mcg/kg IV; give ½ the dose initial, then ⅓ of dose at 8–12 h. *Maint:* 6–10 mcg/kg/24 h PO or 5–8 mcg/kg/24 h ÷ q12h. *1 mo–2 y:* Digitalization: 35–60 mcg/kg PO or 30–50 mcg/kg IV; give ½ the initial dose, then ⅓ dose at 8–12-h intervals for 2 doses. *Maint:* 10–15 mcg/kg/24 h PO or 7.5–15 mcg/kg/24 h IV ÷ q12h. *2–10 y:* Digitalization: 30–40 mcg/kg PO or 25 mcg/kg IV; give ½ initial dose, then ⅓ of the dose at 8–12-h intervals for 2 doses. *Maint:* 8–10 mcg/kg/24 h PO or 6–8 mcg/kg/24 h IV ÷ q12h. *>10 y:* Same as for adults; ↓ in renal impair, follow serum levels **Caution:** [C, +] **Contra** AV block; idiopathic hypertrophic subaortic stenosis; constrictive pericarditis **Supplied:** Caps 0.05, 0.1, 0.2 mg; tabs 0.125, 0.25, 0.5 mg; elixir 0.05 mg/mL; inj 0.1, 0.25 mg/mL **SE:** Can cause heart block; ↓ K⁺ potentiates tox; N/V, HA, fatigue, visual disturbances (yellow-green halos around lights), cardiac arrhythmias **Notes:** Multiple drug interactions; IM inj painful, has erratic absorption & should not be used; Levels, Table 2, page 200.

Digoxin Immune Fab (Digibind) **Uses:** *Life-threatening digoxin intox* **Action:** Antigen-binding fragments bind & inactivate digoxin **Dose:** *Adults & Peds.* Based on serum level & pt's weight; see charts provided w/ drug **Caution:** [C, ?] **Contra:** Allergy to sheep products **Supplied:** Inj 38 mg/vial **SE:** Worsening of cardiac output or CHF, ↓ K⁺, facial swelling, & redness **Notes:** Each vial binds ≅ 0.6 mg of digoxin; renal failure may need redosing in several days

Diltiazem (Cardizem, Cardizem CD, Cardizem SR, Cartia XT, Dilacor XR, Diltia XT, Tiamate, Tiazac) **Uses:** *Angina, prevention of reinfarction, HTN, AF or flutter, & PAT* **Action:** CCB **Dose:** *PO:* Initial, 30 mg PO qid; ↑ to 180–360 mg/d in 3–4 ÷ doses PRN. *SR:* 60–120 mg PO bid; ↑ to 360 mg/d max. *CD or XR:* 120–360 mg/d (max 480 mg/d). *IV:* 0.25 mg/kg IV bolus over 2 min; may repeat in 15 min at 0.35 mg/kg; begin inf of 5–15 mg/h

Caution: [C, +] ↑ effect w/ amiodarone, cimetidine, fentanyl, lithium, cyclosporine, digoxin, β-blockers, cisapride, theophylline **Contra:** SSS, AV block, ↓ BP, AMI, pulmonary congestion **Supplied:** *Cardizem CD:* Caps 120, 180, 240, 300, 360 mg; *Cardizem SR:* caps 60, 90, 120 mg; *Cardizem:* Tabs 30, 60, 90, 120 mg; *Cartia XT:* Caps 120, 180, 240, 300 mg; *Dilacor XR:* Caps 180, 240 mg; *Diltia XT:* Caps 120, 180, 240 mg; *Tiazac:* Caps 120, 180, 240, 300, 360, 420 mg; *Tiamate (XR):* Tabs 120, 180, 240 mg; inj 5 mg/mL **SE:** Gingival hyperplasia, bradycardia, AV block, ECG abnormalities, peripheral edema, dizziness, HA **Notes:** Cardizem CD, Dilacor XR, & Tiazac not interchangeable

Dimenhydrinate (Dramamine, others) Uses: *Prevention & Rx of N/V, dizziness, or vertigo of motion sickness* **Action:** Antiemetic **Dose:** *Adults.* 50–100 mg PO q4–6h, max 400 mg/d; 50 mg IM/IV PRN. *Peds.* 5 mg/kg/24 h PO or IV ÷ qid (max 300 mg/d) **Caution:** [B, ?] **Contra:** Component sensitivity **Supplied:** Tabs 50 mg; chew tabs 50 mg; liq 12.5 mg/4 mL, 12.5 mg/5 mL, 15.62 mg/5 mL; inj 50 mg/mL **SE:** Anticholinergic side effects

Dimethyl Sulfoxide [DMSO] (Rimso 50) Uses: *Interstitial cystitis* **Action:** Unknown **Dose:** Intravesical, 50 mL, retain for 15 min; repeat q2wk until relief **Caution:** [C, ?] **Contra:** Component sensitivity **Supplied:** 50% soln in 50 mL **SE:** Cystitis, eosinophilia, GI, & taste disturbance

Dinoprostone (Cervidil Vaginal Insert, Prepidil Vaginal Gel) Uses: *Induce labor; terminate PRG (12–28 wk); evacuate uterus in missed abortion or fetal death* **Action:** prostaglandin, changes consistency, dilatation, & effacement of the cervix; induces uterine contraction **Dose:** *Gel:* 0.5 mg; if no cervical/uterine response, repeat 0.5 mg q6h (max 24-h dose 1.5 mg). *Vaginal insert:* 1 insert (10 mg = 0.3 mg dinoprostone/h over 12 h); remove w/ onset of labor or 12 h after insertion. *Vaginal supp:* 20 mg repeated every 3–5 h; adjust PRN supp: 1 high in vagina, repeat at 3–5-h intervals until abortion (240 mg max) **Caution:** [X, ?] **Contra:** Ruptured membranes, allergy to prostaglandins, placenta previa or unexplained vaginal bleeding during PRG, when oxytocic drugs contraindicated or if prolonged uterine contractions are inappropriate (Hx C-section or major uterine surgery, presence of cephalopelvic disproportion, etc) **Supplied:** *Endocervical gel:* 0.5 mg in 3-g syringes (each package contains a 10-mm & 20-mm shielded catheter) *Vaginal gel:* 0.5 mg/3 g *Vaginal supp:* 20 mg *Vaginal insert, CR:* 0.3 mg/h **SE:** N/V/D, dizziness, flushing, HA, fever

Diphenhydramine (Benadryl) [OTC] Uses: *Rx & prevent allergic Rxns, motion sickness, potentiate narcotics, sedation, cough suppression, & Rx of extrapyramidal Rxns* **Action:** Antihistamine, antiemetic **Dose:** *Adults.* 25–50 mg PO, IV, or IM bid–tid. *Peds.* 5 mg/kg/24 h PO or IM ÷ qid (max 300 mg/d); ↑ dosing interval in moderate–severe renal failure **Caution:** [B, –] **Contra:** Do not use in acute asthma attack **Supplied:** Tabs & caps 25, 50 mg; chew tabs 12.5 mg; elixir 12.5 mg/5 mL; syrup 12.5 mg/5 mL; liq 6.25 mg/5 mL, 12.5 mg/5 mL; inj 50 mg/mL **SE:** Anticholinergic side effects (xerostomia, urinary retention, sedation)

Diphenoxylate + Atropine (Lomotil) [C-V] Uses: *D* Action: Constipating meperidine congener, reduces GI motility Dose: *Adults.* Initial, 5 mg PO tid–qid until under control, then 2.5–5 mg PO bid. *Peds >2 y:* 0.3–0.4 mg/kg/24 h (of diphenoxylate) bid–qid Caution: [C, +] Contra: Obstructive jaundice, diarrhea due to bacterial Infxn; children <2 y Supplied: Tabs 2.5 mg of diphenoxylate/0.025 mg of atropine; liq 2.5 mg diphenoxylate/0.025 mg atropine/5 mL SE: Drowsiness, dizziness, xerostomia, blurred vision, urinary retention, constipation

Diphtheria, Tetanus Toxoids, & Acellular pertussis adsorbed, Hepatitis B (Recombinant), & Inactivated Poliovirus Vaccine [IPV] combined (Pediarix) Uses: *Vaccine against diphtheria, tetanus, pertussis, HBV, polio (types 1, 2, 3) as a 3-dose primary series in infants & children <7, born to HBsAg– mothers* Actions: Active immunization Dose: *Infants:* Three 0.5-mL doses IM, at 6–8-wk intervals, start at 2 mo; child given 1 dose of hep B vaccine, same; child previously vaccinated w/ one or more doses IPV, use to complete series Caution: [C, N/A] Contra: If HbsAG+ mother, adults, children >7 y, immunosuppressed, allergy to yeast, neomycin, or polymyxin B, Hx allergy to any component, encephalopathy, or progressive neurologic disorders; caution in bleeding disorders. Supplied: Single-dose vials 0.5 mL SE: Drowsiness, restlessness, fever, fussiness, ↓ appetite, nodule redness, pain/swelling at inj site Notes: Give IM only

Dipivefrin (Propine) Uses: *Open-angle glaucoma* Action: α-Adrenergic agonist Dose: 1 gt into eye q12h Caution: [B, ?] Contra: Closed-angle glaucoma Supplied: 0.1% soln SE: HA, local irritation, blurred vision, photophobia, HTN

Dipyridamole (Persantine) Uses: *Prevent postop thromboembolic disorders, often in combo w/ ASA or warfarin (eg, CABG, vascular graft); w/ warfarin after artificial heart valve; chronic angina; w/ ASA to prevent coronary artery thrombosis; dipyridamole IV used in place of exercise stress test for CAD* Action: Anti-plt activity; coronary vasodilator Dose: *Adults.* 75–100 mg PO tid–qid; stress test 0.14 mg/kg/min (max 60 mg over 4 min). *Peds >12 y.* 3–6 mg/kg/d divided tid Caution: [B. ?/–] Caution w/ other drugs that affect coagulation Contra: Component sensitivity Supplied: Tabs 25, 50, 75 mg; inj 5 mg/mL SE: HA, ↓ BP, nausea, abdominal distress, flushing rash, dyspnea Notes: IV use can worsen angina

Dipyridamole & Aspirin (Aggrenox) Uses: *↓ Reinfarction after MI; prevent occlusion after CABG; ↓ risk of stroke* Action: ↓ Plt aggregation (both agents) Dose: 1 cap PO bid Caution: [C, ?] Contra: Ulcers, bleeding diathesis Supplied: Dipyridamole (XR) 200 mg/aspirin 25 mg SE: ASA component: allergic Rxns, skin Rxns, ulcers/GI bleed, bronchospasm; dipyridamole component: dizziness, HA, rash Notes: Swallow capsule whole

Dirithromycin (Dynabac) Uses: *Bronchitis, community-acquired pneumonia, & skin & skin structure Infxns* Action: Macrolide antibiotic. Spectrum:

M. catarrhalis, Streptococcus pneumoniae, Legionella, H. influenzae, S. pyogenes, S. aureus **Dose:** 500 mg/d PO; w/ food **Caution:** [C, M] **Contra:** w/ pimozide **Supplied:** Tabs 250 mg **SE:** Abdominal discomfort, HA, rash, ↑ K⁺ **Notes:** Swallow whole

Disopyramide (Norpace, NAPamide)

Uses: *Suppression & prevention of VT* **Action:** Class 1A antiarrhythmic **Dose:** *Adults.* 400–800 mg/d ÷ q6h for regular & q12h for SR. *Peds.* <1 y: 10–30 mg/kg/24 h PO (÷ qid). 1–4 y: 10–20 mg/kg/24 h PO (÷ qid). 4–12 y: 10–15 mg/kg/24 h PO (÷ qid). 12–18 y: 6–15 mg/kg/24 h PO (÷ qid); ↓ in renal/hepatic impair **Caution:** [C, +] **Contra:** AV block, cardiogenic shock **Supplied:** Caps 100, 150 mg; SR caps 100, 150 mg **SE:** Anticholinergic SEs; negative inotrope, may induce CHF **Notes:** See Drug Levels, Table 2, page 200.

Dobutamine (Dobutrex)

Uses: *Short-term use in cardiac decompensation secondary to depressed contractility* **Action:** Positive inotrope **Dose:** *Adults & Peds.* Cont IV inf of 2.5–15 mcg/kg/min; rarely, 40 mcg/kg/min may be required; titrate to response **Caution:** [C, ?] **Contra:** Sensitivity to sulfites, idiopathic hypertrophic subaortic stenosis **Supplied:** Inj 250 mg/20 mL **SE:** Chest pain, HTN, dyspnea **Notes:** Monitor PWP & cardiac output if possible; check ECG for ↑ heart rate, ectopic activity; follow BP

Docetaxel (Taxotere)

Uses: *Breast (anthracycline-resistant), ovarian, lung CAs, & CAP* **Action:** Antimitotic agent; promotes microtubular aggregation; semisynthetic taxoid **Dose:** 100 mg/m² over 1 h IV q3wk (Per protocols); start dexamethasone 8 mg bid prior & continue for 3–4 d; ↓ dose w/ ↑ bilirubin levels **Caution:** [D, –] **Contra:** Component sensitivity **Supplied:** Inj 20, 40, 80 mg/mL **SE:** Myelosuppression, neuropathy, N/V, alopecia, fluid retention syndrome; cumulative doses of 300–400 mg/m² w/o steroid prep & posttreatment & 600–800 mg/m² w/ steroid prep; allergy possible, but rare w/ steroid prep

Docusate Calcium (Surfak)/Docusate Potassium (Dialose)/Docusate Sodium (DOSS, Colace)

Uses: *Constipation; adjunct to painful anorectal conditions (hemorrhoids)* **Action:** Stool softener **Dose:** *Adults.* 50–500 mg PO ÷ daily–qid. *Peds. Infants–3 y:* 10–40 mg/24 h ÷ daily–qid. *3–6 y:* 20–60 mg/24 h ÷ daily–qid. *6–12 y:* 40–150 mg/24 h ÷ daily–qid **Caution:**[C, ?] **Contra:** Concomitant use of mineral oil; intestinal obstruction, acute abdominal pain, N/V **Supplied:** *Ca:* Caps 50, 240 mg. *K:* Caps 100, 240 mg. *Na:* Caps 50, 100 mg; syrup 50, 60 mg/15 mL; liq 150 mg/15 mL; soln 50 mg/mL **SE:** No significant side effects, rare abdominal cramping, D; no laxative action **Notes:** Take w/ full glass of H₂O; do not use >1 wk

Dofetilide (Tikosyn)

WARNING: To minimize the risk of induced arrhythmia, pts initiated or reinitiated on Tikosyn should be placed for a minimum of 3 d in a facility that can provide calculations of CrCl, continuous ECG monitoring, & cardiac resuscitation **Uses:** *Maintain normal sinus rhythm in AF/A flutter after conversion* **Action:** Type III antiarrhythmic **Dose:** 125–500 mcg PO bid based on

CrCl & QTc (see insert) **Caution:** [C, –] **Contra:** Baseline QTc is > 440 ms (500 ms w/ ventricular conduction abnormalities) or CrCl < 20 mL/min; concomitant use of verapamil, cimetidine, trimethoprim, or ketoconazole **Supplied:** Caps 125, 250, 500 mcg **SE:** Ventricular arrhythmias, HA, CP, dizziness **Notes:** Avoid w/ other drugs that prolong the QT interval; hold class I or III antiarrhythmics for at least 3 ½-lives prior to dofetilide; amiodarone level should be < 0.3 mg/L prior to dosing

Dolasetron (Anzemet) **Uses:** *Prevent chemo-associated N/V* **Action:** 5-HT$_3$ receptor antagonist **Dose:** *Adults & Peds. IV:* 1.8 mg/kg IV as single dose 30 min prior to chemo *Adults. PO:* 100 mg PO as a single dose 1 h prior to chemo *Peds. PO:* 1.8 mg/kg PO to max 100 mg as single dose **Caution:** [B, ?] **Contra:** Component sensitivity **Supplied:** Tabs 50, 100 mg; inj 20 mg/mL **SE:** Prolongs QT interval, HTN, HA, abdominal pain, urinary retention, transient ↑ LFTs

Dopamine (Intropin) **Uses:** *Short-term use in cardiac decompensation secondary to ↓ contractility; ↑ organ perfusion (at low dose)* **Action:** Positive inotropic agent w/ dose response: 2–10 mcg/kg/min β-effects (↑ CO & renal perfusion); 10–20 mcg/kg/min β-effects (peripheral vasoconstriction, pressor). >20 mcg/kg/min peripheral & renal vasoconstriction **Dose:** *Adults & Peds.* 5 mcg/kg/min by cont inf, ↑ increments of 5 mcg/kg/min to 50 mcg/kg/min max based on effect **Caution:** [C, ?] **Contra:** Pheochromocytoma, VF, sulfite sensitivity **Supplied:** Inj 40, 80, 160 mg/mL **SE:** Tachycardia, vasoconstriction, ↓ BP, HA, N/V, dyspnea **Notes:** Dosage >10 mcg/kg/min may ↓ renal perfusion; monitor urinary output; monitor ECG for ↑ in heart rate, BP, & ectopic activity; monitor PCWP & cardiac output if possible

Dornase Alfa (Pulmozyme) **Uses:** *↓ Frequency of resp Infxns in CF* **Action:** Enzyme that selectively cleaves DNA **Dose:** Inhal 2.5 mg/d **Caution:** [B, ?] **Contra:** Allergy to Chinese hamster products **Supplied:** Soln for inhal 1 mg/mL **SE:** Pharyngitis, voice alteration, CP, rash **Notes:** Use w/ recommended nebulizer

Dorzolamide (Trusopt) **Uses:** *Glaucoma* **Action:** Carbonic anhydrase inhibitor **Dose:** 1 gt in eye(s) tid **Caution:** [C, ?] **Contra:** Component sensitivity **Supplied:** 2% soln **SE:** Local irritation, bitter taste, superficial punctate keratitis, ocular allergic Rxn

Dorzolamide & Timolol (Cosopt) **Uses:** *Glaucoma* **Action:** Carbonic anhydrase inhibitor w/ β-adrenergic blocker **Dose:** 1 gt in eye(s) bid **Caution:** [C, ?] **Contra:** Component sensitivity **Supplied:** Soln dorzolamide 2% & timolol 0.5% **SE:** Local irritation, bitter taste, superficial punctate keratitis, ocular allergic Rxn

Doxazosin (Cardura) **Uses:** *HTN & symptomatic BPH* **Action:** α$_1$-Adrenergic blocker; relaxes bladder neck smooth muscle **Dose:** *HTN:* Initial 1 mg/d PO; may be ↑ to 16 mg/d PO. *BPH:* Initial 1 mg/d PO, may be ↑ to 8 mg/d PO **Caution:** [B, ?] **Contra:** Component sensitivity **Supplied:** Tabs 1, 2, 4, 8 mg **SE:** Dizziness, HA, drowsiness, sexual dysfunction, doses >4 mg ↑ likelihood of postural ↓ BP **Notes:** First dose hs; syncope may occur w/in 90 mins of initial dose

Doxepin (Sinequan, Adapin)   **WARNING:** Closely monitor for worsening depression or emergence of suicidality **Uses:** *Depression, anxiety, chronic pain* **Action:** TCA; ↑ synaptic CNS conc of serotonin or norepinephrine **Dose:** 25–150 mg/d PO, usually hs but can be in ÷ doses; ↓ in hepatic impair **Caution:** [C, ?/–] **Contra:** NA glaucoma **Supplied:** Caps 10, 25, 50, 75, 100, 150 mg; PO conc 10 mg/mL **SE:** Anticholinergic SEs, ↓ BP, tachycardia, drowsiness, photosensitivity

Doxepin, Topical (Zonalon)   **Uses:** *Short-term Rx pruritus (atopic dermatitis or lichen simplex chronicus)* **Action:** Antipruritic; H_1- & H_2-receptor antagonism **Dose:** Apply thin coating qid for max 8 d **Caution:** [C, ?/–] **Contra:** Component sensitivity **Supplied:** 5% cream **SE:** ↓ BP, tachycardia, drowsiness, photosensitivity **Notes:** Limit application area to avoid systemic tox

Doxorubicin (Adriamycin, Rubex)   **Uses:** *Acute leukemias; Hodgkin Dz & NHLs; breast CA; soft tissue & osteosarcomas; Ewing sarcoma; Wilms tumor; neuroblastoma; bladder, ovarian, gastric, thyroid, & lung CAs* **Action:** Intercalates DNA; ↓ DNA topoisomerases I & II **Dose:** 60–75 mg/m² q3wk; ↓ cardiotox w/ weekly (20 mg/m²/wk) or cont inf (60–90 mg/m² over 96 h); (Per protocols) **Caution:** [D, ?] **Contra:** Severe CHF, cardiomyopathy, preexisting myelosuppression, previous Rx w/ complete cumulative doses of doxorubicin, idarubicin, daunorubicin **Supplied:** Inj 10, 20, 50, 75, 200 mg **SE:** Myelosuppression, venous streaking & phlebitis, N/V/D, mucositis, radiation recall phenomenon, cardiomyopathy rare but dose-related; limit of 550 mg/m² cumulative dose (400 mg/m² if prior mediastinal irradiation) **Notes:** Dexrazoxane may limit cardiac tox; extravasation leads to tissue damage; discolors urine red/orange

Doxycycline (Vibramycin)   **Uses:** *Broad-spectrum antibiotic activity* **Action:** Tetracycline; interferes w/ protein synthesis. *Spectrum: Rickettsia* sp, *Chlamydia*, & *M. pneumoniae* **Dose:** *Adults.* 100 mg PO q12h on 1st day, then 100 mg PO daily–bid or 100 mg IV q12h. *Peds >8y.* 5 mg/kg/24 h PO, to a max of 200 mg/d ÷ daily–bid **Supplied:** Tabs 50, 100 mg; caps 20, 50, 100 mg; syrup 50 mg/5 mL; susp 25 mg/5 mL; inj 100, 200 mg/vial **Caution:** [D, +] **Contra:** Children <8 y, severe hepatic dysfunction **SE:** D, GI disturbance, photosensitivity **Notes:** ↓ effect w/ antacids; tetracycline of choice in renal impair

Dronabinol (Marinol) [C-II]   **Uses:** *N/V associated w/ CA chemo; appetite stimulation* **Action:** *Antiemetic;* ↓ vomiting center in the medulla **Dose:** *Adults & Peds.* Antiemetic: 5–15 mg/m²/dose q4–6h PRN. *Adults.* Appetite stimulant: 2.5 mg PO before lunch & dinner **Caution:** [C, ?] **Contra:** Hx schizophrenia **Supplied:** Caps 2.5, 5, 10 mg **SE:** Drowsiness, dizziness, anxiety, mood change, hallucinations, depersonalization, orthostatic ↓ BP, tachycardia **Notes:** Principal psychoactive substance present in marijuana

Droperidol (Inapsine)   **Uses:** *N/V; anesthetic premedication* **Action:** Tranquilizer, sedation, & antiemetic **Dose:** *Adults. Nausea:* 2.5–5 mg IV or IM q3–4h PRN. *Premed:* 2.5–10 mg IV, 30–60 min preop. *Peds. Premed:* 0.1–0.15

mg/kg/dose **Caution:** [C, ?] **Contra:** Component sensitivity **Supplied:** Inj 2.5 mg/mL **SE:** Drowsiness, moderate ↓ BP, occasional tachycardia & extrapyramidal Rxns, QT interval prolongation, arrhythmias **Notes:** Give IVP slowly over 2–5 min

Drotrecogin Alfa (Xigris) Uses: *↓ Mortality in adults w/ severe sepsis (associated w/ acute organ dysfunction) at high risk of death (eg, as determined by APACHE II)* **Action:** Recombinant human activated protein C; mechanism unknown **Dose:** 24 mcg/kg/h, total of 96 h **Caution:** [C, ?] **Contra:** Active bleeding, recent stroke or CNS surgery, head trauma, epidural catheter, CNS lesion w/ herniation risk **Supplied:** 5-, 20-mg vials **SE:** Bleeding **Notes:** W/ single organ dysfunction & recent surgery may not be at high risk of death irrespective of APACHE II score & therefore not among the indicated population. *Percutaneous procedures:* Stop inf 2 h before the procedure & resume 1 h after; major surgery: stop inf 2 h before surgery & resume 12 h after surgery in absence of bleeding

Duloxetine (Cymbalta) **WARNING:** Antidepressants may ↑ risk of suicidality; consider risks/benefits of use. Closely monitor clinical worsening, suicidality, or behavior changes **Uses:** *Depression, DM peripheral neuropathic pain* **Action:** Selective serotonin & norepinephrine reuptake inhibitor (SSNRI) **Dose:** *Depression:* 40–60 mg/d PO ÷ bid. *DM neuropathy:* 60 mg/d PO; **Caution:** [C, ?/–]; use in 3rd tri; avoid if CrCl < 30 mL/min; NA glaucoma; w/fluvoxamine, inhibitors of CYP2D6, TCAs, phenothiazines, type 1C antiarrhythmics **Contra:** MAOI use w/in 14 d, w/ thioridazine, NA glaucoma, hepatic insuff **Supplied:** Caps delayed-release 20, 30, 60 mg **SE:** N, dizziness, somnolence, fatigue, sweating, xerostomia, constipation, decreased appetite, sexual dysfunction, urinary hesitancy, ↑ LFTs, HTN **Notes:** Swallow whole; monitor BP, avoid abrupt D/C

Dutasteride (Avodart) Uses: *Symptomatic BPH* **Action:** 5α-Reductase inhibitor **Dose:** 0.5 mg PO daily **Caution:** [X, –] Hepatic impair; pregnant women should not handle pills **Contra:** Women & children **Supplied:** Caps 0.5 mg **SE:** ↓ PSA levels, impotence, ↓ libido, gynecomastia **Notes:** Do not donate blood until 6 mo after D/C drug

Echothiophate Iodine (Phospholine Ophthalmic) Uses: *Glaucoma* **Action:** Cholinesterase inhibitor **Dose:** 1 gt eye(s) bid w/ one dose hs **Caution:** [C, ?] **Contra:** Active uveal inflammation or any inflammatory Dz of iris/ciliary body; glaucoma associated w/ iridocyclitis **Supplied:** Powder to reconstitute 1.5 mg/0.03%; 3 mg/0.06%; 6.25 mg/0.125%; 12.5 mg/0.25% **SE:** Local irritation, myopia, blurred vision, ↓ BP, bradycardia

Econazole (Spectazole) Uses: *Tinea, cutaneous Candida, & tinea versicolor Infxns* **Action:** Topical antifungal **Dose:** Apply to areas bid (daily for tinea versicolor) for 2–4 wk **Caution:** [C, ?] **Contra:** Component sensitivity **Supplied:** Topical cream 1% **SE:** Local irritation, pruritus, erythema **Notes:** Symptom/clinical improvement seen early in Rx, must carry out course of therapy to avoid recurrence

Edrophonium (Tensilon) Uses: *Diagnosis of MyG; acute MyG crisis; curare antagonist* **Action:** Anticholinesterase **Dose:** *Adults. Test for MyG:* 2 mg

IV in 1 min; if tolerated, give 8 mg IV; (+) test is brief ↑ in strength. **Peds.** *Test for MyG:* Total dose 0.2 mg/kg; 0.04 mg/kg test dose; if no Rxn, give remainder in 1-mg increments to 10 mg max; ↓ in renal impair **Caution:** [C, ?] **Contra:** GI or GU obstruction; allergy to sulfite **Supplied:** Inj 10 mg/mL **SE:** N/V/D, excessive salivation, stomach cramps, ↑ aminotransferases **Notes:** Can cause severe cholinergic effects; keep atropine available

Efalizumab (Raptiva)   **WARNING:** Associated w/ serious Infxns, malignancy, thrombocytopenia **Uses:** Chronic moderate–severe plaque psoriasis **Action:** MoAb **Dose:** *Adults.* 0.7 mg/kg SQ conditioning dose, followed by 1 mg/kg/wk; single doses should not exceed 200 mg **Caution:** [C, +/–] **Contra:** Admin of most vaccines **Supplied:** 125-mg vial **SE:** First-dose Rxn, HA, worsening psoriasis, ↑ LFT, immunosuppressive-related Rxns (see warning) **Notes:** Minimize 1st-dose Rxn by administering conditioning dose; monitor plts monthly, then every 3 mo & dose ↑; pts may be trained in self-admin

Efavirenz (Sustiva)   **Uses:** *HIV Infxns* **Action:** Antiretroviral; nonnucleoside RTI **Dose:** *Adults.* 600 mg/d PO q hs. **Peds.** See insert; avoid high-fat meals **Caution:** [C, ?] CDC recommends HIV-infected mothers not breast-feed due to risk of HIV transmission **Contra:** Component sensitivity **Supplied:** Caps 50, 100, 200 mg **SE:** Somnolence, vivid dreams, dizziness, rash, N/V/D **Notes:** Monitor LFT, cholesterol

Eletriptan (Relpax)   **Uses:** Acute Rx of migraine **Action:** Selective serotonin receptor (5-HT$_1$B/$_1$D) agonist **Dose:** 20–40 mg PO, may repeat in 2 h; 80 mg/24h max **Caution:** [C, +] **Contra:** Hx ischemic heart Dz, coronary artery spasm, stroke or TIA, peripheral vascular Dz, IBD, uncontrolled HTN, hemiplegic or basilar migraine, severe hepatic impair, w/in 24 h of another 5-HT$_1$ agonist or ergot, w/in 72 h of CYP3A4 inhibitors **Supplied:** Tabs 20, 40 mg **SE:** Dizziness, somnolence, N, asthenia, xerostomia, paresthesias; pain, pressure, or tightness in chest, jaw or neck; serious cardiac events

Emedastine (Emadine)   **Uses:** *Allergic conjunctivitis* **Action:** Antihistamine; selective H$_1$-antagonist **Dose:** 1 gt in eye(s) up to qid **Caution:** [B, ?] **Contra:** Allergy to ingredients (preservatives benzalkonium, tromethamine) **Supplied:** 0.05% soln **SE:** HA, blurred vision, burning/stinging, corneal infiltrates/staining, dry eyes, foreign body sensation, hyperemia, keratitis, tearing, pruritus, rhinitis, sinusitis, asthenia, bad taste, dermatitis, discomfort **Notes:** Do not use contact lenses if eyes are red

Emtricitabine (Emtriva)   **WARNING:** Class warning for lipodystrophy, lactic acidosis, & severe hepatomegaly **Uses:** HIV-1 Infxn **Action:** Nucleoside RT inhibitor (NRTI) **Dose:** 200 mg PO daily; ↓ dose for renal impair **Caution:** [B, –] **Contra:** Component sensitivity **Supplied:** 200 mg caps **SE:** HA, D, nausea, rash, rare hyperpigmentation of feet & hands, Posttreatment exacerbation of hepatitis **Notes:** First NRTI with once-daily dosing

Enalapril (Vasotec)   **Uses:** *HTN, CHF, LVD,* DN **Action:** ACE inhibitor **Dose:** *Adults.* 2.5–40 mg/d PO; 1.25 mg IV q6h. **Peds.** 0.05–0.08 mg/kg/dose PO q12–24h; ↓ in renal impair **Caution** [C (1st tri; D 2nd & 3rd tri), +] Use with NSAIDs, K+ supls **Contra:** Bilateral renal artery stenosis, angioedema **Supplied:** Tabs 2.5, 5, 10, 20 mg; IV 1.25 mg/mL (1, 2 mL) **SE:** Symptomatic ↓ BP with initial dose (especially with concomitant diuretics), ↑ K+, nonproductive cough, angioedema **Notes:** Monitor BP; D/C diuretic for 2–3 d prior to initiation

Enfuvirtide (Fuzeon) **WARNING:** Rarely causes allergy; never rechallenge **Uses:** *W/ antiretroviral agents for HIV-1 Infxn in treatment-experienced pts with evidence of viral replication despite ongoing antiretroviral therapy* **Action:** Fusion inhibitor **Dose:** 90 mg (1 mL) SQ bid in upper arm, anterior thigh, or abdomen **Caution:** [B, –] **Contra:** Previous allergy to drug **Supplied:** 90 mg/mL on reconstitution; dispensed as pt convenience kit with monthly supplies **SE:** Inj site reactions (in nearly all pts); pneumonia, D, nausea, fatigue, insomnia, peripheral neuropathy **Notes:** Rotate inj site; available only via restricted drug distribution system; immediately administer on reconstitution or refrigerate for up to 24 h prior

Enoxaparin (Lovenox) **WARNING:** Recent or anticipated epidural/spinal anesthesia ↑ risk of spinal/epidural hematoma w/ subsequent paralysis **Uses:** *Prevention & Rx of DVT; Rx PE; unstable angina & non-Q-wave MI* **Action:** LMW heparin **Dose:** *Adults. Prevention:* 30 mg SQ bid or 40 mg SQ q24h. *DVT/PE Rx:* 1 mg/kg SQ q12h or 1.5 mg/kg SQ q24h. *Angina:* 1 mg/kg SQ q12h. *Peds. Prevention:* 0.5 mg/kg SQ q12h. *DVT/PE Rx:* 1 mg/kg SQ q12h; ↓ dose w/ CrCl < 30 ml/min **Caution** [B, ?] Not thromboprophylaxis in prosthetic heart valves **Contra:** Active bleeding, HIT Ab(+) **Supplied:** Inj 10 mg/0.1 mL (30-, 40-, 60-, 80-, 100-, 120-, & 150-mg syringes) **SE:** Bleeding, hemorrhage, bruising, thrombocytopenia, pain/hematoma at site, ↑ AST/ALT **Notes:** Does not significantly affect bleeding time, plt Fxn, PT, or aPTT; monitor plt, bleeding; may monitor anti-factor Xa

Entacapone (Comtan) **Uses:** *Parkinson Dz* **Action:** Selective & reversible carboxymethyl transferase inhibitor **Dose:** 200 mg with each levodopa/carbidopa dose; max 1600 mg/d; ↓ levodopa/carbidopa dose by 25% if levodopa dose >800 mg **Caution:** [C, ?] Hepatic impair **Contra:** Concurrent use with nonselective MAOI **Supplied:** Tabs 200 mg **SE:** Dyskinesia, hyperkinesia, nausea, dizziness, hallucinations, orthostatic ↓ BP, brown-orange urine, D **Notes:** Monitor LFT; do not D/C abruptly

Ephedrine **Uses:** *Acute bronchospasm, bronchial asthma, nasal congestion,* ↓ BP, narcolepsy, enuresis, & MyG **Action:** Sympathomimetic; stimulates α- & β-receptors; bronchodilator **Dose:** *Adults.* 25–50 mg IM or IV q10min to a max of 150 mg/d or 25–50 mg PO q3–4h PRN. *Peds.* 0.2–0.3 mg/kg/dose IM/IV q4–6h PRN **Caution:** [C, ?/–] **Contra:** Cardiac arrhythmias; angle-closure glaucoma **Supplied:** Inj 50 mg/mL; caps 25 mg; nasal spray 0.25% **SE:** CNS stimulation (nervousness, anxiety, trembling), tachycardia, arrhythmia, HTN, xerostomia, painful urination **Notes:** Protect from light; monitor BP, HR, urinary output; can cause false(+) amphetamine EMIT; take last dose 4–6h before hs

Epinephrine (Adrenalin, Sus-Phrine, EpiPen, others) Uses: *Cardiac arrest, anaphylactic Rxn, bronchospasm, open-angle glaucoma* **Action:** β-adrenergic agonist, some α-effects **Dose:** *Adults.* ACLS: 0.5–1 mg (5–10 mL of 1:10,000) IV q 5 min to response. *Anaphylaxis:* 0.3–0.5 mg SQ of 1:1000 dilution, may repeat q5–15min to a max of 1 mg/dose & 5 mg/d. *Asthma:* 0.1–0.5 mL SQ of 1:1000 dilution, repeated at 20-min to 4-h intervals or 1 inhal (met-dose) repeat in 1–2 min or susp 0.1–0.3 mL SQ for extended effect. *Peds.* ACLS: 1st dose 0.1 mL/kg IV of 1:10,000 dilution, then 0.1 mL/kg IV of 1:1000 dilution q3–5min to response. *Anaphylaxis:* 0.001mg/kg SQ q15min ×2 doses, then q4h PRN. *Asthma:* 0.01 mL/kg SQ of 1:1000 dilution q8–12h. **Caution:** [C, ?] ↓ bronchodilation with β-blockers **Contra:** Cardiac arrhythmias, angle-closure glaucoma **Supplied:** Inj 1:1000, 1:2000, 1:10,000, 1:100,000; susp for inj 1:200; aerosol 220 mcg/spray; soln for inhal 1% **SE:** CV (tachycardia, HTN, vasoconstriction), CNS stimulation (nervousness, anxiety, trembling), ↓ renal blood flow **Notes:** Can give via ET tube if no central line (use 2–2.5 × IV dose)

Epinastine (Elestat) Uses: *Itching w/ allergic conjunctivitis* **Action:** Antihistamine **Dose:** 1 gt bid **Caution:** [C, ?/–] **Supplied:** Soln 0.05% **SE:** Burning, folliculosis, hyperemia, pruritus, URI, HA, rhinitis, sinusitis, cough, pharyngitis **Notes:** Remove contacts before, reinsert in 10 min

Epirubicin (Ellence) Uses: *Adjuvant therapy with evidence of axillary nodal involvement following resection of primary breast CA* **Actions:** Anthracycline cytotoxic agent **Dose:** Per protocols; ↓ dose with hepatic impair. **Caution:** [D, –] **Contra:** Baseline neutrophil count < 1500 cells/mm³, severe myocardial insuff, recent MI, severe arrhythmias, severe hepatic dysfunction, previous Rx with anthracyclines up to max cumulative dose **Supplied:** Inj 50 mg/25 mL, 200 mg/100 mL **SE:** Mucositis, N/V/D, alopecia, myelosuppression, cardiotox, secondary AML, tissue necrosis w/ extravasation

Eplerenone (Inspra) Uses: *HTN* **Action:** Selective aldosterone antagonist **Dose:** *Adults:* 50 mg PO daily–bid, doses >100 mg no benefit w/ ↑ K⁺; ↓ to 25 mg PO qd if giving w/ CYP3A4 inhibitors **Caution:** [B, +/–] Use of CYP3A4 inhibitors (ketoconazole, itraconazole, erythromycin, fluconazole, verapamil, saquinavir); monitor K⁺ with ACE inhibitor, ARBs, NSAIDs, K⁺-sparing diuretics; grapefruit juice, St. John's wort **Contra:** K⁺ >5.5 mEq/L; NIDDM w/ microalbuminuria; SCr >2 mg/dL (males), >1.8 mg/dL (females); CrCl <50 mL/min; concurrent K⁺ supls/K⁺-sparing diuretics **Supplied:** Tabs 25, 50, 100 mg **SE:** Hypertriglyceridemia, ↑ K⁺, HA, dizziness, gynecomastia, hypercholesterolemia, D, orthostatic ↓ BP **Notes:** May take 4 wk to see full effect

Epoetin Alfa [Erythropoietin, EPO] (Epogen, Procrit) Uses: *CRF associated anemia* zidovudine Rx in HIV-infected pts, CA chemo; ↓ transfusions associated with surgery **Action:** Induces erythropoiesis **Dose:** *Adults & Peds.* 50–150 units/kg IV/SQ 3×/wk; adjust dose q4–6wk PRN. *Surgery:* 300 units/kg/d × 10 d prior to surgery to 4 d after; ↓ dose if Hct approaches 36% or Hgb,

↑ >4 points in 2-wk period **Caution:** [C, +] **Contra:** Uncontrolled HTN **Supplied:** Inj 2000, 3000, 4000, 10,000, 20,000, 40,000 units/mL **SE:** HTN, HA, fatigue, fever, tachycardia, N/V **Notes:** Store in refrigerator; monitor baseline & posttreatment Hct/Hgb, BP, ferritin

Epoprostenol (Flolan) Uses: *Pulmonary HTN* Action: Dilates pulmonary/systemic arterial vascular beds; ↓ plt aggregation **Dose:** Initial 2 ng/kg/min; ↑ by 2 ng/kg/min q15min until dose-limiting SE (CP, dizziness, N/V, HA, ↓ BP, flushing); IV cont inf 4 ng/kg/min < maximum-tolerated rate; adjust based on response; see package insert guidelines **Caution:** [B, ?] ↑ tox w/diuretics, vasodilators, acetate in dialysis fluids, anticoagulants **Contra:** Chronic use in CHF 2nd-deg severe LVSD **Supplied:** Inj 0.5, 1.5 mg **SE:** Flushing, tachycardia, HA, fever, chills, nervousness, HA, N/V/D, jaw pain, flu-like Sxs **Notes:** Abrupt D/C can cause rebound pulmonary HTN; monitor bleeding if using other antiplatelet/anticoagulants; watch ↓ BP effects with other vasodilators/diuretics

Eprosartan (Teveten) Uses: *HTN,* DN, CHF Action: ARB **Dose:** 400–800 mg/d single dose or bid **Caution:** [C (1st tri); D (2nd & 3rd tri), –] Lithium, ↑ K+ with K+-sparing diuretics/supls/high-dose trimethoprim **Contra:** Bilateral renal artery stenosis, 1st-deg aldosteronism **Supplied:** Tabs 400, 600 mg **SE:** Fatigue, depression, hypertriglyceridemia, URI, UTI, abdominal pain, rhinitis/pharyngitis/cough

Eptifibatide (Integrilin) Uses: *ACS, PCI* Action: Glycoprotein IIb/IIIa inhibitor **Dose:** 180 mcg/kg IV bolus, then 2 mcg/kg/min cont inf; ↓ in renal impair (SCr >2 mg/dL, <4 mg/dL: 135 mcg/kg bolus & 0.5 mcg/kg/min inf) **Caution:** [B, ?] Monitor bleeding with other anticoagulants **Contra:** Other GPIIb/IIIa inhibitors, Hx abnormal bleeding, hemorrhagic stroke (within 30 d), severe HTN, major surgery (within 6 wk), plt count <100,000 cells/mm³, renal dialysis **Supplied:** Inj 0.75, 2 mg/mL **SE:** Bleeding, ↓ BP, inj site Rxn, thrombocytopenia **Notes:** Monitor bleeding, coags, plts, SCr, activated coagulation time (ACT) with prothrombin consumption index (maintain ACT between 200–300 s)

Erlotinib (Tarceva) Uses: *NSCLC after failure of 1 chemo agent* Action: HER1/EGFR tyrosine kinase inhibitor **Dose:** 150 mg/d PO 1 h ac or 2 h pc; ↓ (in 50-mg decrements) w/severe Rxn or w/ CYP3A4 (page 220) inhibitors; Per protocols **Caution:** [D, ?/–]; use w/ CYP3A4 (page 220) inhibitors **Supplied:** Tabs 25, 100, 150 mg **SE:** Rash, N/V/D, anorexia, abdominal pain, fatigue, cough, dyspnea, stomatitis, conjunctivitis, pruritus, dry skin, Infxn, ↑ LFT , interstitial lung disease **Notes:** May ↑ INR w/warfarin, monitor INR

Ertapenem (Invanz) Uses: *Complicated intraabdominal, acute pelvic, & skin Infxns, pyelonephritis, community-acquired pneumonia* Action: A carbapenem; β-lactam antibiotic, ↓ cell wall synthesis. *Spectrum:* Good gram(+/–) & anaerobic coverage, but not *Pseudomonas,* PCN-resistant pneumococci, MRSA, *Enterococcus,* β-lactamase(+) *H. influenza, Mycoplasma, Chlamydia* **Dose:** *Adults.* 1 g IM/IV qd; 500 mg/d in CrCl <30 mL/min **Caution:** [C, ?/–] Probenecid ↓ renal clearance **Contra:** <18 y, PCN allergy **Supplied:** Inj 1 g/vial **SE:** HA, N/V/D, inj site Rxns, thrombocytosis, ↑ LFTs **Notes:** Can give IM × 7 d, IV × 14 d; 137 mg Na⁺(6 mEq)/g ertapenem

Erythromycin (E-Mycin, E.E.S., Ery-Tab) Uses: *Bacterial Infxns; bowel decontamination*; GI motility; *acne vulgaris* **Action:** Bacteriostatic; interferes with protein synthesis. *Spectrum:* Group A streptococci (*S. pyogenes*), *S. pneumoniae*, *N. meningitides*, *N. gonorrhea* (in PCN-allergic pts), *Legionella*, *M. pneumoniae* **Dose:** *Adults.* Base 250–500 mg PO q6–12h or ethylsuccinate 400–800 mg q6–12h; 500 mg–1 g IV q6h. *Prokinetic:* 250 mg PO tid 30 mins ac. *Peds.* 30–50 mg/kg/d PO ÷ q6–8h or 20–40 mg/kg/d IV ÷ q6h, max 2 g/d **Caution:** [B, +] ↑ tox of carbamazepine, cyclosporine, digoxin, methylprednisolone, theophylline, felodipine, warfarin, simvastatin/lovastatin **Contra:** Hepatic impair, pre-existing liver Dz (estolate), use with pimozide **Supplied:** *Powder for inj as lactobionate:* 500 mg, 1 g. *Base:* Tabs 250, 333, 500 mg; caps 250 mg. *Estolate:* Susp 125, 250 mg/5 mL. *Stearate:* Tabs 250, 500 mg. *Ethylsuccinate:* Chew tabs 200 mg; tabs 400 mg; susp 200, 400 mg/5 mL **SE:** HA, abdominal pain, N/V/D; [QT prolongation, torsades de pointes, ventricular arrhythmias/tachycardias (rarely)]; cholestatic jaundice (estolate) **Notes:** 400 mg ethylsuccinate = 250 mg base/state/estolate; w/ food to minimize GI upset; lactobionate salt contains benzyl alcohol (caution in neonates)

Erythromycin & Benzoyl Peroxide (Benzamycin) Uses: Topical Rx of *acne vulgaris* **Action:** Macrolide antibiotic with keratolytic **Dose:** Apply bid (AM & PM) **Caution:** [C, ?] **Contra:** Component sensitivity **Supplied:** Gel erythromycin 30 mg/benzoyl peroxide 50 mg/g **SE:** Local irritation, dryness

Erythromycin & Sulfisoxazole (Eryzole, Pediazole) Uses: *Upper & lower resp tract; bacterial Infxns; otitis media in children due to H. influenzae* **Action:** Macrolide antibiotic w sulfonamide **Dose:** Based on erythromycin content. *Adults.* 400 mg erythromycin/1200 mg sulfisoxazole PO q6h. *Peds >2 mo.* 40–50 mg/kg/d erythromycin & 150 mg/kg/d sulfisoxazole PO ÷ q6h; max 2 g/d erythromycin or 6 g/d sulfisoxazole × 10 d; ↓ in renal impair **Caution:** [C (D if given near term), +] PO anticoagulants, MRX, hypoglycemics, phenytoin, cyclosporine **Contra:** Infants <2 mo **Supplied:** Susp erythromycin ethylsuccinate 200 mg/sulfisoxazole 600 mg/5 mL (100, 150, 200 mL) **SE:** GI disturbance

Erythromycin, Ophthalmic (Ilotycin Ophthalmic) Uses: *Conjunctival/corneal Infxns* **Action:** Macrolide antibiotic **Dose:** ½ in. 2–6 ×/d **Caution:** [B, +] **Contra:** Erythromycin hypersensitivity **Supplied:** 0.5% oint **SE:** Local irritation

Erythromycin, Topical (A/T/S, Eryderm, Erycette, T-Stat) Uses: *Acne vulgaris* **Action:** Macrolide antibiotic **Dose:** Wash & dry area, apply 2% product over area bid **Caution:** [B, +] **Contra:** Component sensitivity **Supplied:** Soln 1.5%, 2%; gel 2%; impregnated pads & swabs 2% **SE:** Local irritation

Escitalopram (Lexapro) **WARNING:** Closely monitor for worsening depression or emergence of suicidality, particularly in ped pts **Uses:** Depression, anxiety **Action:** SSRI **Dose:** *Adults.* 10–20 mg PO qd; 10 mg/d in elderly & hepatic impair **Caution:** [C, +/–] ↑ Risk of serotonin syndrome with other SSRI, tramadol, linezolid, sumatriptan **Contra:** With or w/in 14 d of MAOI **Supplied:** Tabs 5, 10, 20 mg; soln 1 mg/mL **SE:** N/V/D, sweating, insomnia, dizziness, xerostomia, sexual dysfunction **Notes:** Full effects may take 3 wk

Esmolol (Brevibloc) **Uses:** *SVT & noncompensatory sinus tachycardia, AF/flutter* **Action:** β₁-Adrenergic blocker; class II antiarrhythmic **Dose:** *Adults & Peds.* Initiate Rx with 500 mcg/kg load over 1 min, then 50 mcg/kg/min × 4 min; if inadequate response, repeat the loading dose & maint inf of 100 mcg/kg/min × 4 min; titrate by repeating load, then incremental ↑ in the maint dose of 50 mcg/kg/min for 4 min until desired heart rate reached or ↓ BP; average dose 100 mcg/kg/min **Caution:** [C (1st tri; D 2nd or 3rd tri), ?] **Contra:** Sinus bradycardia, heart block, uncompensated CHF, cardiogenic shock, ↓ BP **Supplied:** Inj 10, 250 mg/mL; premix inf 10 mg/mL **SE:** ↓ BP (↓ or discontinuing inf reverses ↓ BP in 30 min); bradycardia, diaphoresis, dizziness, pain on inj **Notes:** Hemodynamic effects back to baseline w/in 20–30 mins after D/C inf

Esomeprazole (Nexium) **Uses:** *Short-term (4–8 wk) for erosive esophagitis/GERD; H. pylori Infxn in combo with antibiotics* **Action:** Proton pump inhibitor, ↓ gastric acid **Dose:** *Adults. GERD/erosive gastritis:* 20–40 mg/d PO × 4–8 wk; *Maint:* 20 mg/d PO. *H. pylori Infxn:* 40 mg/d PO, plus clarithromycin 500 mg PO bid & amoxicillin 1000 mg/bid for 10 d; **Caution:** [B, ?/–] **Contra:** Component sensitivity **Supplied:** Caps 20, 40 mg **SE:** HA, D, abdominal pain **Notes:** Do not chew; may open capsule & sprinkle on applesauce

Estazolam (ProSom) [C-IV] **Uses:** *Short-term management of insomnia* **Action:** Benzodiazepine **Dose:** 1–2 mg PO qhs PRN; ↓ in hepatic impair/elderly/debilitated **Caution:** [X, –] ↑ effects w/ CNS depressants **Contra:** PRG **Supplied:** Tabs 1, 2 mg **SE:** Somnolence, weakness, palpitations **Notes:** May cause psychological/physical dependence; avoid abrupt D/C after prolonged use

Esterified Estrogens (Estratab, Menest) **WARNING:** Do not use in the prevention of CV Dz **Uses:** *Vasomotor Sxs or vulvar/vaginal atrophy associated with menopause*; female hypogonadism **Action:** Estrogen supl **Dose:** *Menopause:* 0.3–1.25 mg/d, cyclically 3 wk on, 1 wk off. *Hypogonadism:* 2.5–7.5 mg/d PO × 20 d, off × 10 d **Caution:** [X, –] **Contra:** Genital bleeding of unknown cause, breast CA, estrogen-dependent tumors, thromboembolic disorders, thrombophlebitis, recent MI, PRG, severe hepatic Dz **Supplied:** Tabs 0.3, 0.625, 1.25, 2.5 mg **SE:** Nausea, HA, bloating, breast enlargement/tenderness, edema, venous thromboembolism, hypertriglyceridemia, gallbladder Dz **Notes:** Use lowest dose for shortest time; refer to Women's Health Initiatives (WHI) data

Esterified Estrogens + Methyltestosterone (Estratest, Estratest HS) Uses: *Vasomotor Sxs*; postpartum breast engorgement **Action:** Estrogen & androgen supl **Dose:** 1 tab/d × 3 wk, 1 wk off **Caution:** [X, –] **Contra:** Genital bleeding of unknown cause, breast CA, estrogen-dependent tumors, thromboembolic disorders, thrombophlebitis, recent MI, PRG **Supplied:** Tabs (estrogen/methyltestosterone) 0.625 mg/1.25 mg (hs), 1.25 mg/2.5 mg **SE:** Nausea, HA, bloating, breast enlargement/tenderness, edema, ↑ triglycerides, venous thromboembolism, gallbladder Dz **Notes:** Use lowest dose for shortest time

Estradiol (Estrace) Uses: *Atrophic vaginitis, vasomotor Sxs associated w/ menopause, osteoporosis* **Action:** Estrogen supl **Dose:** *PO:* 1–2 mg/d, adjust PRN to control Sxs. *Vaginal cream:* 2–4 g/d × 2 wk, then 1 g 1–3×/wk **Caution:** [X, –] **Contra:** Genital bleeding of unknown cause, breast CA, estrogen-dependent tumors, thromboembolic disorders, thrombophlebitis; recent MI; hepatic impair **Supplied:** Tabs 0.5, 1, 2 mg; vaginal cream 0.1 mg/g **SE:** Nausea, HA, bloating, breast enlargement/tenderness, edema, ↑ triglycerides, venous thromboembolism, gallbladder Dz

Estradiol Cypionate & Medroxyprogesterone Acetate (Lunelle) WARNING: Cigarette smoking ↑ risk of serious CV side effects from contraceptives containing estrogen. This risk ↑ with age & with heavy smoking (> 15 cigarettes/d) & is quite marked in women > 35 y. Women who use Lunelle should be strongly advised not to smoke Uses: *Contraceptive* **Action:** Estrogen & progestin **Dose:** 0.5 mL IM (deltoid, ant thigh, buttock) monthly, do not exceed 33 d **Caution:** [X, M] HTN, gallbladder Dz, ↑ lipids, migraines, sudden HA, valvular heart Dz with complications **Contra:** PRG, heavy smokers >35 y, DVT, PE, cerebro/CV Dz, estrogen-dependent neoplasm, undiagnosed abnormal uterine bleeding, hepatic tumors, cholestatic jaundice **Supplied:** Estradiol cypionate (5 mg), medroxyprogesterone acetate (25 mg) single-dose vial or prefilled syringe (0.5 mL) **SE:** Arterial thromboembolism, HTN, cerebral hemorrhage, MI, amenorrhea, acne, breast tenderness **Notes:** Start w/in 5 d of menstruation

Estradiol, Transdermal (Estraderm, Climara, Vivelle) Uses: *Severe menopausal vasomotor Sxs; female hypogonadism* **Action:** Estrogen supl **Dose:** 0.1 mg/d patch 1–2×/wk depending on product; adjust PRN to control Sxs **Caution:** [X, –] (See estradiol) **Contra:** PRG, undiagnosed genital bleeding, carcinoma of breast, estrogen-dependent tumors, Hx thrombophlebitis, thrombosis, **Supplied:** TD patches (deliver mg/24 h) 0.025, 0.0375, 0.05, 0.075, 0.1 **SE:** Nausea, bloating, breast enlargement/tenderness, edema, HA, hypertriglyceridemia, gallbladder Dz **Notes:** Do not apply to breasts, place on trunk of body & rotate sites

Estramustine Phosphate (Estracyt, Emcyt) Uses: *Advanced CAP* **Action:** Antimicrotubule agent; weak estrogenic & antiandrogenic activity **Dose:** 14 mg/kg/d in 3–4 ÷ doses; take on empty stomach, do not take with milk/milk products **Caution:** [NA, not used in females] **Contra:** Active thrombophlebitis or thromboembolic disorders **Supplied:** Caps 140 mg **SE:** N/V, exacerbation of preexisting CHF, thrombophlebitis, MI, PE, gynecomastia in 20–100%

Estrogen, Conjugated (Premarin) **WARNING:** Should not be used for the prevention of CV Dz. The WHI reported ↑ risk of MI, stroke, breast CA, PE, & DVT when combined with methoxyprogesterone over 5 y of Rx; ↑ risk of endometrial CA **Uses:** *Moderate–severe menopausal vasomotor Sxs; atrophic vaginitis; palliative for advanced prostatic carcinoma; prevention & Rx of estrogen deficiency osteoporosis* **Action:** Hormonal replacement **Dose:** 0.3–1.25 mg/d PO cyclically; prostatic carcinoma requires 1.25–2.5 mg PO tid; **Caution:** [X, –] **Contra:** Severe hepatic impair, genital bleeding of unknown cause, breast CA, estrogen-dependent tumors, thromboembolic disorders, thrombosis, thrombophlebitis, recent MI **Supplied:** Tabs 0.3, 0.625, 0.9, 1.25, 2.5 mg; inj 25 mg/mL **SE:** ↑ Risk of endometrial carcinoma, gallbladder Dz, thromboembolism, HA, & possibly breast CA; generic products not equivalent

Estrogen, Conjugated-Synthetic (Cenestin) **Uses:** *Rx of moderate–severe vasomotor Sxs associated with menopause* **Action:** Hormonal replacement **Dose:** 0.625–1.25 mg PO daily **Caution:** [X, –] **Contra:** See estrogen, conjugated **Supplied:** Tabs 0.625, 0.9, 1.25 mg **SE:** Associated with an ↑ risk of endometrial CA, gallbladder Dz, thromboembolism, & possibly breast CA

Estrogen, Conjugated + Medroxyprogesterone (Prempro, Premphase) **WARNING:** Should not be used for the prevention of CV Dz; the WHI study reported ↑ risk of MI, stroke, breast CA, PE, & DVT over 5 y of Rx **Uses:** *Moderate–severe menopausal vasomotor Sxs; atrophic vaginitis; prevent postmenopausal osteoporosis* **Action:** Hormonal replacement **Dose:** Prempro 1 tab PO daily; Premphase 1 tab PO daily **Caution:** [X, –] **Contra:** Severe hepatic impair, genital bleeding of unknown cause, breast CA, estrogen-dependent tumors, thromboembolic disorders, thrombosis, thrombophlebitis **Supplied:** (expressed as estrogen/medroxyprogesterone) *Prempro:* Tabs 0.625/2.5, 0.625/5 mg *Premphase:* Tabs 0.625/0 (days 1–14) & 0.625/5 mg (days 15–28) **SE:** Gallbladder Dz, thromboembolism, HA, breast tenderness

Estrogen, Conjugated + Methylprogesterone (Premarin + Methylprogesterone) **Uses:** *Menopausal vasomotor Sxs; osteoporosis* **Action:** Estrogen & androgen combo **Dose:** 1 tab/d **Caution:** [X, –] **Contra:** Severe hepatic impair, genital bleeding of unknown cause, breast CA, estrogen-dependent tumors, thromboembolic disorders, thrombosis, thrombophlebitis **Supplied:** Tabs 0.625 mg estrogen, conjugated, & 2.5 or 5 mg of methylprogesterone **SE:** Nausea, bloating, breast enlargement/tenderness, edema, HA, hypertriglyceridemia, gallbladder Dz

Estrogen, Conjugated + Methyltestosterone (Premarin + Methyltestosterone) **Uses:** *Moderate–severe menopausal vasomotor Sxs*; postpartum breast engorgement **Action:** Estrogen & androgen combo **Dose:** 1 tab/d × 3 wk, then 1 wk off **Caution:** [X, –] **Contra:** Severe hepatic impair, genital bleeding of unknown cause, breast CA, estrogen-dependent tumors, thromboembolic disorders, thrombosis, thrombophlebitis **Supplied:** Tabs (estrogen/methyltestosterone) 0.625 mg/5 mg, 1.25 mg/10 mg **SE:** Nausea, bloating, breast enlargement/tenderness, edema, HA, hypertriglyceridemia, gallbladder Dz

Eszopiclone (Lunesta) [C-IV] Uses: *Insomnia* **Action:** Nonbenzodiazepine hypnotic **Dose:** 2–3 mg/d hs *Elderly:* 1–2 mg/d hs; hepatic impair/use w/ CYP3A4 inhibitor: 1 mg/d hs **Caution:** [C, ?/–] **Supplied:** Tabs 1-, 2-, 3-mg **SE:** HA, xerostomia, dizziness, somnolence, hallucinations, rash, Infxn, unpleasant taste **Notes:** High-fat meals slows absorption

Etanercept (Enbrel) Uses: *Reduces Sxs of RA in pts who fail other DMARD,* Crohn Dz **Action:** Binds TNF **Dose:** *Adults.* 25 mg SQ 2×/wk (separated by at least 72–96 h). *Peds 4–17 y.* 0.4 mg/kg SQ 2×/wk (max 25 mg) **Caution:** [B, ?] conditions that predispose to Infxn (ie, DM) **Contra:** Active Infxn; **Supplied:** Inj 25 mg/vial **SE:** HA, rhinitis, inj site Rxn, URI, rhinitis **Notes:** Rotate inj sites

Ethambutol (Myambutol) Uses: *Pulmonary TB* & other mycobacterial Infxns, MAC **Action:** ↓ RNA synthesis **Dose:** *Adults & Peds >12 y.* 15–25 mg/kg/d PO as a single dose; ↓ in renal impair, take w/ food, avoid antacids **Caution:** [B, +] **Contra:** Optic neuritis **Supplied:** Tabs 100, 400 mg **SE:** HA, hyperuricemia, acute gout, abdominal pain, ↑ LFTs, optic neuritis, GI upset

Ethinyl Estradiol (Estinyl, Feminone) Uses: *Menopausal vasomotor Sxs; female hypogonadism* **Action:** Estrogen supl **Dose:** 0.02–1.5 mg/d ÷ daily–tid **Caution:** [X, –] **Contra:** Severe hepatic impair; genital bleeding of unknown cause, breast CA, estrogen-dependent tumors, thromboembolic disorders, thrombosis, thrombophlebitis **Supplied:** Tabs 0.02, 0.05, 0.5 mg **SE:** Nausea, bloating, breast enlargement/tenderness, edema, HA, hypertriglyceridemia, gallbladder Dz

Ethinyl Estradiol & Levonorgestrel (Preven) Uses: *Emergency contraceptive* ("morning-after pill"); prevent PRG after contraceptive failure or unprotected intercourse **Actions:** Estrogen & progestin; interferes with implantation **Dose:** 4 tabs, take 2 tabs q12h × 2 (w/in 72 h of intercourse) **Caution:** [X, M] **Contra:** Known/suspected PRG, abnormal uterine bleeding **Supplied:** Kit: ethinyl estradiol (0.05), levonorgestrel (0.25) blister pack with 4 pills & urine PRG test **SE:** Peripheral edema, N/V/D, bloating, abdominal pain, fatigue, HA, & menstrual changes **Notes:** Will not induce abortion; may ↑ risk of ectopic PRG

Ethinyl Estradiol & Norelgestromin (Ortho Evra) Uses: *Contraceptive patch* **Action:** Estrogen & progestin **Dose:** Apply patch to abdomen, buttocks, upper torso (not breasts), or upper outer arm at the beginning of the menstrual cycle; new patch is applied weekly for 3 wk; week 4 is patch-free **Caution:** [X, M] **Contra:** Thrombophlebitis, undiagnosed vaginal bleeding, PRG, carcinoma of breast, estrogen-dependent tumor **Supplied:** 20 cm² patch (6 mg norelgestromin (active metabolite norgestirate) & 0.75 mg of ethinyl estradiol) **SE:** Breast discomfort, HA, site Rxns, nausea, menstrual cramps; thrombosis risks similar to OCP **Notes:** Less effective in women >90 kg

Ethosuximide (Zarontin) Uses: *Absence (petit mal) Szs* Action: Anticonvulsant; ↑ Sz threshold Dose: *Adults.* Initial, 250 mg PO ÷ bid; ↑ by 250 mg/d q4–7d PRN (max 1500 mg/d). *Peds 3–6 y.* Initial: 15 mg/kg/d PO ÷ bid. *Maint:* 15–40 mg/kg/d ÷ bid, max 1500 mg/d Caution: [C, +] in renal/hepatic impair Contra: Component sensitivity Supplied: Caps 250 mg; syrup 250 mg/5 mL SE: Blood dyscrasias, GI upset, drowsiness, dizziness, irritability

Etidronate Disodium (Didronel) Uses: *↑ Ca^{2+} of malignancy, Paget Dz, & heterotopic ossification* Action: ↓ Nl & abnormal bone resorption Dose: *Paget Dz:* 5–10 mg/kg/d PO ÷ doses (for 3–6 mo). ↑ Ca^{2+}: 7.5 mg/kg/d IV inf over 2 h × 3 d, then 20 mg/kg/d PO on last day of inf × 1–3 mo Caution: [B PO (C parenteral), ?] Contra: SCr >5 mg/dL Supplied: Tabs 200, 400 mg; inj 50 mg/mL SE: GI intolerance (↓ by ÷ daily doses); hypophosphatemia, hypomagnesemia, bone pain, abnormal taste, fever, convulsions, nephrotox Notes: Take PO on empty stomach 2 h before any meal

Etodolac (Lodine) WARNING: May ↑ risk of cardiovascular events & GI bleeding Uses: *Osteoarthritis & pain,* RA Action: NSAID Dose: 200–400 mg PO bid–qid (max 1200 mg/d) Caution: [C (D 3rd tri), ?] ↑ bleeding risk with aspirin, warfarin; ↑ nephrotox w/ cyclosporine; Hx CHF, HTN, renal/hepatic impair, PUD Contra: Active GI ulcer Supplied: Tabs 400, 500 mg; ER tabs 400, 500, 600 mg; caps 200, 300 mg SE: N/V/D, gastritis, abdominal cramps, dizziness, HA, depression, edema, renal impair Notes: Do not crush tabs

Etonogestrel/Ethinyl Estradiol (NuvaRing) Uses: *Contraceptive* Action: Estrogen & progestin combo Dose: Rule out PRG first; insert ring vaginally for 3 wk, remove for 1 wk; insert new ring 7 d after last removed (even if still bleeding) at same time of day ring removed. First day of menses is day 1, insert prior to day 5 even if still bleeding. Use other contraception for first 7 d of starting therapy. See insert if converting from other contraceptive; after delivery or 2nd tri abortion insert 4 wk postpartum (if not breast-feeding) Caution: [X, ?/–] HTN, gallbladder Dz, ↑ lipids, migraines, sudden HA Contra: PRG, heavy smokers >35 y, DVT, PE, cerebro-/CV Dz, estrogen-dependent neoplasm, undiagnosed abnormal genital bleeding, hepatic tumors, cholestatic jaundice Supplied: Intravaginal ring: ethinyl estradiol 0.015 mg/d & etonogestrel 0.12 mg/d Notes: If ring accidentally removed, rinse with cool/lukewarm H_2O (not hot) & reinsert ASAP; if not reinserted w/in 3 h, effectiveness ↓; do not use with diaphragm

Etoposide [VP-16] (VePesid, Toposar) Uses: *Testicular CA, non-small-cell lung CA, Hodgkin Dz & NHLs, ped ALL, & allogeneic/autologous BMT in high doses* Action: Topoisomerase II inhibitor Dose: 50 mg/m²/d IV for 3–5 d; 50 mg/m²/d PO for 21 d (PO bioavailability = 50% of the IV form); 2–6 g/m² or 25–70 mg/kg used in BMT (Per protocols); ↓ in renal/hepatic impair Caution: [D, –] Contra: IT administration Supplied: Caps 50 mg; inj 20 mg/mL SE: Myelosuppression, N/V, alopecia, ↓ BP if infused rapidly, anorexia, anemia, leukopenia, potential for secondary leukemias Notes: Emesis in 10–30%

Exemestane (Aromasin) Uses: *Advanced breast CA in post-menopausal women whose Dz has progressed following tamoxifen therapy* **Action:** An irreversible, steroidal aromatase inhibitor; ↓ circulating estrogens **Dose:** 25 mg PO daily after a meal **Caution:** [D, ?/–] **Contra:** Component sensitivity **Supplied:** Tabs 25 mg **SE:** Hot flashes, nausea, fatigue

Exenatide (Byetta) Uses: Type 2 DM combined w/ metformin &/or sulfonylurea **Action:** An incretin mimetic: ↑ insulin release, ↓ glucagon secretion, ↓ gastric emptying, promotes satiety **Dose:** 5 mcg SQ bid w/in 60 min before AM & PM meals; ↑ to 10 mcg SQ bid after 1 mo PRN; do not give pc **Caution:** [C, ?/–] may ↓ absorption of other oral drugs (take antibiotics/contraceptives 1 h before) **Contra:** Component sensitivity **Supplied:** Soln 5, 10 mcg/dose (prefilled pen) **SE:** Hypoglycemia, N/V/D, dizziness, HA, dyspepsia, ↓ appetite, jittery **Notes:** Consider ↓ sulfonylurea to ↓ risk of hypoglycemia; discard pen 30 d after 1st use

Ezetimibe (Zetia) Uses: *Primary hypercholesterolemia alone or in combo with an HMG-CoA reductase inhibitor* **Action:** ↓ intestinal absorption of cholesterol & phytosterols **Dose:** *Adults & Peds >10 y.* 10 mg/d PO **Caution:** [C, +/–] Bile acid sequestrants ↓ bioavailability **Contra:** Hepatic impair **Supplied:** Tabs 10 mg **SE:** HA, D, abdominal pain, ↑ transaminases in combo with an HMG-CoA reductase inhibitor

Ezetimibe/Simvastatin (Vytorin) Uses: *Hypercholesterolemia* **Action:** ↓ Absorption of cholesterol & phytosterols w/HMG-CoA-reductase inhibitor **Dose:** 10/10–10/80 mg/d PO; w/cyclosporine or danazol:10/10 mg/d max; w/ amiodarone or verapamil: 10/20 mg/d max; ↓ in severe renal insuff **Caution:** [X, –]; w/ CYP3A4 inhibitors, gemfibrozil, niacin > 1 g/d, danazol, amiodarone, verapamil **Contra:** PRG/lactation; liver disease or ↑ LFTs **Supplied:** Tabs (ezetimibe/simvastatin) 10/10, 10/20, 10/40, 10/80 mg **SE:** HA, GI upset, myalgia, myopathy manifested as muscle pain, weakness or tenderness w/ creatine kinase 10 × ULN, rhabdomyolysis, hepatitis, Infxn **Notes:** Monitor LFTs

Famciclovir (Famvir) Uses: *Acute herpes zoster (shingles) & genital herpes* **Action:** ↓ viral DNA synthesis **Dose:** *Zoster:* 500 mg PO q8h ×7 d. *Simplex:* 125–250 mg PO bid; ↓ in renal impair **Caution:** [B, –] **Contra:** Component sensitivity **Supplied:** Tabs 125, 250, 500 mg **SE:** Fatigue, dizziness, HA, pruritus, N/D **Notes:** Best given w/in 72 h of initial lesion

Famotidine (Pepcid) Uses: *Short-term Rx of active duodenal ulcer & benign gastric ulcer; maint for duodenal ulcer, hypersecretory conditions, GERD, & heartburn* **Action:** H₂-antagonist; ↓ gastric acid secretion **Dose:** *Adults. Ulcer:* 20 mg IV q12h or 20–40 mg PO qhs × 4–8 wk. *Hypersecretion:* 20–160 mg PO q6h. *GERD:* 20 mg PO bid ×6 wk; maint: 20 mg PO hs. *Heartburn:* 10 mg PO PRN q12h. *Peds.* 0.5–1 mg/kg/d; ↓ in severe renal insuff **Caution:** [B, M] **Contra:** Component sensitivity **Supplied:** Tabs 10, 20, 40 mg; chew tabs 10 mg; susp 40 mg/5 mL; inj 10 mg/2 mL **SE:** Dizziness, HA, constipation, D, thrombocytopenia **Notes:** Chewable tabs contain phenylalanine

Felodipine (Plendil) Uses: *HTN & CHF* Action: CCB Dose: 2.5–10 mg PO daily; ↓ in hepatic impair Caution: [C, ?] ↑ effect with azole antifungals, erythromycin, grapefruit juice Contra: Component sensitivity Supplied: ER tabs 2.5, 5, 10 mg SE: Peripheral edema, flushing, tachycardia, HA, gingival hyperplasia Notes: Follow BP in elderly & in impaired hepatic Fxn; swallow whole

Fenofibrate (Tricor) Uses: *Hypertriglyceridemia* Action: ↓ Triglyceride synthesis Dose: 48–145 mg daily; ↓ in renal impair, w/ meals Caution: [C, ?] Contra: Hepatic/severe renal insuff, 1st-deg biliary cirrhosis, unexplained persistent ↑ LFTs, gallbladder Dz Supplied: Tabs 48, 145 mg SE: GI disturbances, cholecystitis, arthralgia, myalgia, dizziness Notes: Monitor LFTs

Fenoldopam (Corlopam) Uses: *Hypertensive emergency* Action: Rapid vasodilator Dose: Initial 0.03–0.1 mcg/kg/min IV inf, titrate q15min in 0.05–0.1 mcg/kg/min increments Caution: [B, ?] ↓ BP w/ β-blockers Contra: Allergy to sulfites Supplied: Inj 10 mg/mL SE: ↓ BP, edema, facial flushing, N/V/D, atrial flutter/fibrillation, ↑ intraocular pressure Notes: Avoid concurrent β-blockers

Fenoprofen (Nalfon) WARNING: May ↑ risk of cardiovascular events and GI bleeding Uses: *Arthritis & pain* Action: NSAID Dose: 200–600 mg q4–8h, to 3200 mg/d max; take with food Caution: [B (D 3rd tri), +/–] CHF, HTN, renal/hepatic impair, Hx PUD Contra: NSAID sensitivity Supplied: Caps 200, 300 mg; tabs 600 mg SE: GI disturbance, dizziness, HA, rash, edema, renal impair, hepatitis Notes: Swallow whole

Fentanyl (Sublimaze) [C-II] Uses: *Short-acting analgesic* in anesthesia & PCA Action: Narcotic analgesic Dose: *Adults.* 25–100 mcg/kg/dose IV/IM titrated to effect. *Peds.* 1–2 mcg/kg IV/IM q1–4h titrated to effect; ↓ in renal impair Caution: [B, +] Contra: ↑ ICP, resp depression, severe renal/hepatic impair Supplied: Inj 0.05 mg/mL SE: ↓ BP, bradycardia, constipation, nausea, resp depression, miosis Notes: 0.1 mg of fentanyl = 10 mg of morphine IM

Fentanyl, Transdermal (Duragesic) [C-II] Uses: *Chronic pain* Action: Narcotic Dose: Apply patch to upper torso q72hr; dose calculated from narcotic requirements in previous 24 h; ↓ in renal impair Caution: [B, +] Contra: ↑ ICP, resp depression, severe renal/hepatic impair Supplied: TD patches 25, 50, 75, 100 mcg/h SE: Sedation, ↓ BP, bradycardia, constipation, nausea, resp depression, miosis Notes: 0.1 mg of fentanyl = 10 mg of morphine IM

Fentanyl, Transmucosal System (Actiq) [C-II] Uses: *Induction of anesthesia; breakthrough CA pain* Action: Narcotic analgesic Dose: *Adults. Anesthesia:* 5–15 mcg/kg. *Pain:* 200 mcg over 15 min, titrate to effect; ↓ in renal impair Caution: [B, +] Contra: ↑ ICP, resp depression, severe renal/hepatic impair Supplied: Lozenges on stick 200, 400, 600, 800, 1200, 1600 mcg SE: Sedation, ↓ BP, bradycardia, constipation, nausea, resp depression, miosis Notes: 0.1 mg of fentanyl = 10 mg of morphine IM

Ferrous Gluconate (Fergon) Uses: *Iron deficiency anemia* & Fe supl Action: Dietary supl Dose: *Adults.* 100–200 mg of elemental Fe/d ÷ doses. *Peds.*

4–6 mg/kg/d ÷ doses; take on empty stomach (OK w/ meals if GI upset occurs); avoid antacids **Caution:** [A, ?] **Contra:** Hemochromatosis, hemolytic anemia **Supplied:** Tabs 300 (34 mg Fe), 325 mg (36 mg Fe) **SE:** GI upset, constipation, dark stools, discoloration of urine, may stain teeth **Notes:** 12% elemental Fe; false + stool guaiac

Ferrous Gluconate Complex (Ferrlecit)   **Uses:** *Iron deficiency anemia or supl to erythropoietin therapy* **Action:** Fe Supl **Dose:** Test dose: 2 mL (25 mg Fe) infused over 1 h. If no reaction, 125 mg (10 mL) IV over 1 h. Usual cumulative dose 1 g Fe over 8 sessions (until favorable Hct) **Caution:** [B, ?] **Contra:** Anemia not due to Fe deficiency; CHF; Fe overload **Supplied:** Inj 12.5 mg/mL Fe **SE:** ↓ BP, serious allergic Rxns, GI disturbance, inj site Rxn **Notes:** Dose expressed as mg Fe; may infuse during dialysis

Ferrous Sulfate   **Uses:** *Fe deficiency anemia & Fe supl* **Action:** Dietary supl **Dose:** *Adults.* 100–200 mg elemental Fe/d in ÷ doses. *Peds.* 1–6 mg/kg/d ÷ daily–tid; on empty stomach (OK w/ meals if GI upset occurs); avoid antacids **Caution:** [A, ?] ↑ absorption w/ vitamin C; ↓ absorption w/ tetracycline, fluoroquinolones, antacids, H_2-blockers, proton pump inhibitors **Contra:** Hemochromatosis, hemolytic anemia **Supplied:** Tabs 187 (60 mg Fe), 200 (65 mg Fe), 324 (65 mg Fe), 325 mg (65 mg Fe); SR caplets & tabs 160 mg (50 mg Fe), 200 mg (65 mg Fe); gtt 75 mg/0.6 mL (15 mg Fe/0.6 mL); elixir 220 mg/5 mL (44 mg Fe/5 mL); syrup 90 mg/5 mL (18 mg Fe/5 mL) **SE:** GI upset, constipation, dark stools, discolored urine

Fexofenadine (Allegra, Allegra-D)   **Uses:** *Allergic rhinitis* **Action:** Antihistamine **Dose:** *Adults & Peds >12 y.* 60 mg PO bid or 180 mg/d; ↓ in renal impair **Caution:** [C, ?] **Contra:** Component sensitivity **Supplied:** Caps 60 mg; tabs 30, 60, 180 mg; Allegra-D (60 mg fexofenadine/120 mg pseudoephedrine) **SE:** Drowsiness (uncommon)

Filgrastim [G-CSF] (Neupogen)   **Uses:** *↓ Incidence of Infxn in febrile neutropenic pts; Rx chronic neutropenia* **Action:** Recombinant G-CSF **Dose:** *Adults & Peds.* 5 mcg/kg/d SQ or IV single daily dose; D/C therapy when ANC >10,000 **Caution:** [C, ?] Interactions w/ drugs that potentiate release of neutrophils (eg, lithium) **Contra:** Allergy to *E. coli*-derived proteins or G-CSF **Supplied:** Inj 300 mcg/mL **SE:** Fever, alopecia, N/V/D, splenomegaly, bone pain, HA, rash **Notes:** Monitor CBC & plt; monitor for cardiac events; no benefit w/ ANC >10,000/mm^3

Finasteride (Proscar, Propecia)   **Uses:** *BPH & androgenetic alopecia* **Action:** ↓ 5α-Reductase **Dose:** *BPH:* 5 mg/d PO. *Alopecia:* 1 mg/d PO; food may ↓ absorption **Caution:** [X, –] Hepatic impair **Contra:** Pregnant women should avoid handling pills **Supplied:** Tabs 1 mg (Propecia), 5 mg (Proscar) **SE:** ↓ PSA levels (↓ by ≈ 50%) ; ↓ libido, impotence (rare) **Notes:** Reestablish PSA baseline at 6 mo; 3–6 mo for effect on urinary Sxs; continue therapy to maintain new hair

Flavoxate (Urispas)   **Uses:** *Relief of Sx of dysuria, urgency, nocturia, suprapubic pain, urinary frequency, incontinence* **Action:** Antispasmotic **Dose:**

100–200 mg PO tid–qid **Caution:** [B, ?] **Contra:** Pyloric or duodenal obstruction, GI hemorrhage, GI obstruction, ileus, achalasia, BPH **Supplied:** Tabs 100 mg **SE:** Drowsiness, blurred vision, xerostomia

Flecainide (Tambocor) **Uses:** Prevent AF/flutter & PSVT, *prevent/suppress life-threatening ventricular arrhythmias* **Action:** Class 1C antiarrhythmic **Dose:** *Adults.* 100 mg PO q12h; ↑ by 50 mg q12h q4d to max 400 mg/d. *Peds.* 3–6 mg/kg/d in 3 ÷ doses; ↓ in renal impair, **Caution:** [C, +] monitor in hepatic impair ↑ conc with amiodarone, digoxin, quinidine, ritonavir/amprenavir, BB, verapamil **Contra:** 2nd-/3rd-degree AV block, RBBB w/ bifascicular or trifascicular block, cardiogenic shock, CAD, ritonavir/amprenavir, alkalinizing agents **Supplied:** Tabs 50, 100, 150 mg **SE:** Dizziness, visual disturbances, dyspnea, palpitations, edema, tachycardia, CHF, HA, fatigue, rash, nausea **Notes:** May cause new/worsened arrhythmias; initiate Rx in hospital; dose q8h if pt is intolerant/condition is uncontrolled at 12-h intervals

Floxuridine (FUDR) **Uses:** *GI adenoma, liver, renal cell carcinoma*; colon & pancreatic CAs **Action:** Inhibits thymidylate synthase; ↓ DNA synthesis (S-phase specific) **Dose:** 0.1–0.6 mg/kg/d for 1–6 wk (Per protocols) **Caution:** [D, –] Drug interaction w/ live & rotavirus vaccine **Contra:** BM suppression, poor nutritional status, potentially serious Infxn **Supplied:** Inj 500 mg **SE:** Myelosuppression, anorexia, abdominal cramps, N/V/D, mucositis, alopecia, skin rash, & hyperpigmentation; rare neurotox (blurred vision, depression, nystagmus, vertigo, & lethargy); intraarterial catheter-related problems (ischemia, thrombosis, bleeding, & Infxn) **Notes:** Need effective birth control; palliative Rx for inoperable/incurable pts

Fluconazole (Diflucan) **Uses:** *Candidiasis (esophageal, oropharyngeal, urinary tract, vaginal, prophylaxis); cryptococcal meningitis* **Action:** Antifungal; ↓ fungal cytochrome P-450 sterol demethylation. *Spectrum:* All *Candida* sp except *C. krusei* **Dose:** *Adults.* 100–400 mg PO or IV. *Vaginitis:* 150 mg PO qd. *Crypto:* 400 mg day 1, then 200 mg × 10–12wk after CSF (–). *Peds.* 3–6 mg/kg/d PO or IV; ↓ in renal impair **Caution:** [C, –] **Contra:** w/ terfenadine **Supplied:** Tabs 50, 100, 150, 200 mg; susp 10, 40 mg/mL; inj 2 mg/mL **SE:** HA, rash, GI upset, ↓ K+, ↑ LFTs **Notes:** PO use produces the same levels as IV; PO preferred

Fludarabine Phosphate (Flamp, Fludara) **Uses:** *Autoimmune hemolytic anemia, CLL, cold agglutinin hemolysis,* low-grade lymphoma, mycosis fungoides **Action:** ↓ Ribonucleotide reductase; blocks DNA polymerase-induced DNA repair **Dose:** 18–30 mg/m²/d for 5 d, as a 30-min inf (Per protocols) **Caution:** [D, –] Give cytarabine before fludarabine (↓ its metabolism) **Contra:** Severe Infxns **Supplied:** Inj 50 mg **SE:** Myelosuppression, N/V/D, ↑ LFT, edema, CHF, fever, chills, fatigue, dyspnea, nonproductive cough, pneumonitis, severe CNS tox rare in leukemia **Notes:** Not OK in CrCl <30 mL/min

Fludrocortisone Acetate (Florinef) **Uses:** *Adrenocortical insuff, Addison Dz, salt-wasting syndrome* **Action:** Mineralocorticoid replacement **Dose:**

Adults. 0.1–0.2 mg/d PO. *Peds.* 0.05–0.1 mg/d PO **Caution:** [C, ?] **Contra:** Systemic fungal Infxns; known allergy **Supplied:** Tabs 0.1 mg **SE:** HTN, edema, CHF, HA, dizziness, convulsions, acne, rash, bruising, hyperglycemia, HPA suppression, cataracts **Notes:** For adrenal insuff, use w/ glucocorticoid; dosage changes based on plasma renin activity

Flumazenil (Romazicon) Uses: *Reverse sedative effects of benzodiazepines & general anesthesia* **Action:** Benzodiazepine receptor antagonist **Dose:** *Adults.* 0.2 mg IV over 15 s; repeat PRN, to 1 mg max (3 mg max in benzodiazepine OD). *Peds.* 0.01 mg/kg (0.2 mg/dose max) IV over 15 s; repeat 0.005 mg/kg at 1-min intervals to max 1 mg total; ↓ in hepatic impair **Caution:** [C, ?] **Contra:** In TCA OD; if pts given benzodiazepines to control life-threatening conditions (ICP/status epilepticus) **Supplied:** Inj 0.1 mg/mL **SE:** N/V, palpitations, HA, anxiety, nervousness, hot flashes, tremor, blurred vision, dyspnea, hyperventilation, withdrawal syndrome **Notes:** Does not reverse narcotic Sx or amnesia

Flunisolide (AeroBid, Nasal* Uses: *Asthma in pts requiring chronic steroid therapy; relieve seasonal/perennial allergic rhinitis* **Action: Topical steroid **Dose:** *Adults. Met-dose inhal:* 2 inhal bid (max 8/d). *Nasal:* 2 sprays/nostril bid (max 8/d). *Peds >6 y. Met-dose inhal:* 2 inhal bid (max 4/d). *Nasal:* 1–2 sprays/nostril bid (max 4/d) **Caution:** [C, ?] **Contra:** Status asthmaticus **Supplied:** Aerosol 250 mg/actuation; nasal spray 0.025% **SE:** Tachycardia, bitter taste, local effects, oral candidiasis **Notes:** Not for acute asthma

Fluorouracil [5-FU] (Adrucil) Uses: *Colorectal, gastric, pancreatic, breast, basal cell,* head, neck, bladder, CAs **Action:** Inhibitor of thymidylate synthetase (interferes with DNA synthesis, S-phase specific) **Dose:** 370–1000 mg/m²/d for 1–5 d IV push to 24-h cont inf; protracted venous inf of 200–300 mg/m²/d (Per protocol) **Caution:** [D, ?] ↑ tox w/ allopurinol; do not give MRX before 5-FU **Contra:** Poor nutritional status, depressed BM Fxn, thrombocytopenia, major surgery w/in past mo, DPD enzyme deficiency, PRG, serious Infxn, bilirubin >5 mg/dL **Supplied:** Inj 50 mg/mL **SE:** Stomatitis, esophagopharyngitis, N/V/D, anorexia, myelosuppression (leukocytopenia, thrombocytopenia, & anemia), rash/dry skin/photosensitivity, tingling in hands/feet w/pain (palmar–plantar erythrodysesthesia), phlebitis/discoloration at inj sites **Notes:** ↑ Thiamine intake; sun sensitivity; daily doses > 800 mg not OK; contraception recommended

Fluorouracil, Topical [5-FU] (Efudex) Uses: *Basal cell carcinoma; actinic/solar keratosis* **Action:** Inhibitor of thymidylate synthetase (↓ DNA synthesis, S-phase specific) **Dose:** Apply 5% cream bid × 3–6 wk **Caution:** [D, ?] Irritant chemo **Contra:** Component sensitivity **Supplied:** Cream 1, 5%; soln 1, 2, 5% **SE:** Rash, dry skin, photosensitivity **Notes:** Healing may not be evident for 1–2 mo; wash hands thoroughly; avoid occlusive dressings; do not overuse

Fluoxetine (Prozac, Sarafem) **WARNING:** Closely monitor for worsening depression or emergence of suicidality, particularly in ped pts Uses: *Depression, OCD, panic disorder, bulimia, PMDD* (Sarafem) **Action:** SSRI **Dose:**

20 mg/d PO (max 80 mg/d ÷); weekly regimen 90 mg/wk after 1–2 wk of standard dose. *Bulimia:* 60 mg q AM. *Panic disorder:* 20 mg/d. *OCD:* 20–80 mg/d. *PMDD:* 20 mg/d or 20 mg intermittently, start 14 d prior to menses, repeat with each cycle; ↓ in hepatic failure **Caution:** [B, ?/–] Serotonin syndrome w/ MAOI, SSRI, serotonin agonists, linezolid; risk of QT prolongation w/ phenothiazines **Contra:** MAOI/thioridazine (wait 5 wk after D/C before starting MAOI) **Supplied:** *Prozac:* Caps 10, 20, 40 mg; scored tabs 10 mg; SR cap 90 mg; soln 20 mg/5 mL. *Sarafem:* Caps 10, 20 mg **SE:** Nausea, nervousness, weight loss, HA, insomnia

Fluoxymesterone (Halotestin) Uses: Androgen-responsive metastatic *breast CA, hypogonadism* Action: ↓ Secretion of LH & FSH (feedback inhibition) Dose: *Breast CA:* 10–40 mg/d ÷ × 1–3 mo. *Hypogonadism:* 5–20 mg/d Caution: [X, ?/–] ↑ effect w/ anticoagulants, cyclosporine, insulin, lithium, narcotics Contra: Serious cardiac, liver, or kidney Dz; PRG Supplied: Tabs 2, 5, 10 mg SE: Virilization, amenorrhea & menstrual irregularities, hirsutism, alopecia, acne, nausea, & cholestasis. *Hematologic tox:* Suppression of clotting factors II, V, VII, & X & polycythemia; ↑ libido, HA, & anxiety Notes: Radiographic exam of hand/wrist q6mo in prepubertal children; ↓ total T_4 levels

Fluphenazine (Prolixin, Permitil) Uses: *Schizophrenia* Action: Phenothiazine antipsychotic; blocks postsynaptic mesolimbic dopaminergic brain receptors Dose: 0.5–10 mg/d in ÷ doses PO q6–8h, average maint 5 mg/d; or 1.25 mg IM, then 2.5–10 mg/d in ÷ doses q6–8h PRN; ↓ in elderly Caution: [C, ?/–] Contra: Severe CNS depression, coma, subcortical brain damage, blood dyscrasias, hepatic Dz, w/ caffeine, tannic acid, or pectin-containing products Supplied: Tabs 1, 2.5, 5, 10 mg; conc 5 mg/mL; elixir 2.5 mg/5 mL; inj 2.5 mg/mL; depot inj 25 mg/mL SE: Drowsiness, extrapyramidal effects Notes: Monitor LFTs; less sedative/hypotensive than chlorpromazine

Flurazepam (Dalmane) [C-IV] Uses: *Insomnia* Action: Benzodiazepine Dose: *Adults & Peds >15 y.* 15–30 mg PO qhs PRN; ↓ in elderly Caution: [X, ?/–] Elderly, low albumin, hepatic impair Contra: NA glaucoma; PRG Supplied: Caps 15, 30 mg SE: "Hangover" due to accumulation of metabolites, apnea Notes: May cause dependency

Flurbiprofen (Ansaid) WARNING: May ↑ risk of cardiovascular events and GI bleeding Uses: *Arthritis* Action: NSAID Dose: 50–300 mg/d ÷ bid–qid, max 300 mg/d w/ food Caution: [B (D in 3rd tri), +] Contra: PRG (3rd tri); aspirin allergy Supplied: Tabs 50, 100 mg SE: Dizziness, GI upset, peptic ulcer Dz

Flutamide (Eulexin) WARNING: Liver failure & death reported. Measure LFT before, monthly, & periodically after; D/C immediately if ALT 2× upper limits of nl or jaundice develops Uses: Advanced *CAP* (in combo with LHRH agonists, eg, leuprolide or goserelin), with radiation & GnRH for localized CAP Action: Nonsteroidal antiandrogen Dose: 250 mg PO tid (750 mg total) Caution: [D, ?] Contra: Severe hepatic impair Supplied: Caps 125 mg SE: Hot flashes, loss of libido, impotence, N/V/D, gynecomastia

Fluticasone, Nasal (Flonase) Uses: *Seasonal allergic rhinitis* Action: Topical steroid Dose: *Adults & Adolescents.* Nasal: 2 sprays/nostril/d. *Peds 4–11 y.* Nasal: 1–2 sprays/nostril/d Caution: [C, M] Contra: Primary Rx of status asthmaticus Supplied: Nasal spray 50 mcg/actuation SE: HA, dysphonia, oral candidiasis

Fluticasone, Oral (Flovent, Flovent Rotadisk) Uses: Chronic *asthma* Action: Topical steroid Dose: *Adults & Adolescents.* 2–4 puffs bid. *Peds 4–11 y.* 50 mcg bid Caution: [C, M] Contra: Primary Rx of status asthmaticus Supplied: Met-dose inhal 44, 110, 220 mcg/activation; Rotadisk dry powder: 50, 100, 250 mcg/activation SE: HA, dysphonia, oral candidiasis Notes: Risk of thrush; counsel on use of device

Fluticasone Propionate & Salmeterol Xinafoate (Advair Diskus) Uses: *Maint therapy for asthma* Action: Corticosteroid w/ long-acting bronchodilator Dose: *Adults & Peds >12 y.* 1 inhal bid q 12 h Caution: [C, M] Contra: Not for acute attack or in conversion from PO steroids or status asthmaticus Supplied: Met-dose inhal powder (fluticasone/salmeterol in mcg) 100/50, 250/50, 500/50 SE: Upper resp Infxn, pharyngitis, HA Notes: Combo of Flovent & Serevent; do not use with spacer, do not wash mouthpiece, do not exhale into device

Fluvastatin (Lescol) Uses: *Atherosclerosis, primary hypercholesterolemia, hypertriglyceridemia* Action: HMG-CoA reductase inhibitor Dose: 20–80 mg PO qhs; ↓ w/ hepatic impair Caution: [X, –] Contra: Active liver Dz, ↑ LFTs, PRG, breast-feeding Supplied: Caps 20, 40 mg; XL 80 mg SE: HA, dyspepsia, N/D, abdominal pain

Fluvoxamine (Luvox) WARNING: Closely monitor for worsening depression or emergence of suicidality, particularly in ped pts Uses: *OCD* Action: SSRI Dose: Initial 50 mg single qhs dose, ↑ to 300 mg/d in ÷ doses; ↓ in elderly/hepatic impair, titrate slowly Caution: [C, ?/–] Numerous interactions (MAOIs, phenothiazines, SSRIs, serotonin agonists) Contra: MAOI w/in 14 days Supplied: Tabs 25, 50, 100 mg SE: HA, nausea, D, somnolence, insomnia Notes: ÷ doses >100 mg

Folic Acid Uses: *Megaloblastic anemia; folate deficiency* Action: Dietary supl Dose: *Adults.* Supl: 0.4 mg/d PO. PRG: 0.8 mg/d PO. *Folate deficiency:* 1 mg PO qd–tid. *Peds.* Supl: 0.04–0.4 mg/24 h PO, IM, IV, or SQ. *Folate deficiency:* 0.5–1 mg/24 h PO, IM, IV, or SQ Caution: [A, +] Contra: Pernicious, aplastic, normocytic anemias Supplied: Tabs 0.4, 0.8, 1 mg; inj 5 mg/mL SE: Well tolerated Notes: OK for all women of childbearing age; ↓ fetal neural tube defects by 50%; no effect on normocytic anemias

Fondaparinux (Arixtra) WARNING: When epidural/spinal anesthesia or spinal puncture is used, pts anticoagulated or scheduled to be anticoagulated with LMW heparins, heparinoids, or fondaparinux for prevention of thromboembolic complications are at risk for epidural or spinal hematoma, which can result in long-term or permanent paralysis Uses: *DVT prophylaxis* in hip fracture or replacement or knee replacement **Action:** Synthetic, specific inhibitor of activated factor X; a LMW heparin **Dose:** 2.5 mg SQ qd, up to 5–9 d; start at least 6 h postop **Caution:** [B, ?] ↑ bleeding risk w/ anticoagulants, antiplatelets, drotrecogin alfa, NSAIDs **Contra:** Wt <50 kg, CrCl <30 mL/min, active bleeding, bacterial endocarditis, thrombocytopenia associated w/ antiplatelet Ab **Supplied:** Prefilled syringes 2.5 mg/0.5mL **SE:** Thrombocytopenia, anemia, fever, nausea **Notes:** D/C if plts <100,000 mm³; only give SQ; may monitor anti-factor Xa levels

Formoterol (Foradil Aerolizer) **Uses:** Maint Rx of *asthma & prevention of bronchospasm* with reversible obstructive airway Dz; exercise-induced bronchospasm **Action:** Long-acting β₂-adrenergic agonist, bronchodilator **Dose:** *Adults & Peds >5 y. Asthma:* Inhale one 12-mcg cap q12h w/ aerolizer, 24 mcg/d max. *Adults & Peds > 12 y. Exercise-induced bronchospasm:* 1 inhal 12-mcg cap 15 min before exercise **Caution:** [C, ?] **Contra:** Need for acute bronchodilation; use w/in 2 wk of MAOI **Supplied:** 12-mcg blister pack for use in aerolizer **SE:** Paradoxical bronchospasm; URI, pharyngitis, back pain **Notes:** Do not swallow caps—for use only with inhaler; do not start with significantly worsening or acutely deteriorating asthma

Fosamprenavir (Lexiva) **WARNING:** Do not use with severe liver dysfunction, reduce dose with mild–moderate liver impair (fosamprenavir 700 mg bid w/o ritonavir) **Uses:** HIV Infxn **Action:** Protease inhibitor **Dose:** 1400 mg bid w/o ritonavir; if w/ritonavir, fosamprenavir 1400 mg + ritonavir 200 mg qd or fosamprenavir 700 mg + ritonavir 100 mg bid. If w/ efavirenz & ritonavir: fosamprenavir 1400 mg + ritonavir 300 mg qd **Caution:** [C, ?/–] **Contra:** w/ergot alkaloids, midazolam, triazolam, or pimozide; avoid if sulfa allergy **Supplied:** Tabs 700 mg **SE:** N/V/D, HA, fatigue, rash **Notes:** Numerous drug interactions because of hepatic metabolism

Foscarnet (Foscavir) **Uses:** *CMV retinitis*; acyclovir-resistant *herpes Infxns* **Action:** ↓ Viral DNA polymerase & RT **Dose:** *CMV retinitis: Induction:* 60 mg/kg IV q8h or 100 mg/kg q12h × 14–21 d. *Maint:* 90–120 mg/kg/d IV (Monday–Friday). *Acyclovir-resistant HSV induction:* 40 mg/kg IV q8–12h × 14–21 d. ↓ with renal impair **Caution:** [C, –] ↑ Sz potential w/ flouroquinolones; avoid nephrotoxic Rx (cyclosporine, aminoglycosides, ampho B, protease inhibitors) **Contra:** Significant renal impair (CrCl <0.4 mL/min/kg) **Supplied:** Inj 24 mg/mL **SE:** Nephrotox, electrolyte abnormalities **Notes:** Sodium loading (500 mL 0.9% NaCl) before & after helps minimize nephrotox; monitor ionized calcium; administer through central line

Fosfomycin (Monurol) **Uses:** *Uncomplicated UTI* **Action:** ↓ bacterial cell wall synthesis. *Spectrum:* Gram(+) (staph, pneumococci); gram(–) (*E. coli, Enterococcus, Salmonella, Shigella, H. influenzae, Neisseria,* indole-negative *Proteus, Providencia*). *B. fragilis* & anaerobic gram(–) cocci are resistant **Dose:** 3 g PO dissolved in 90–120 mL of H₂O single dose; ↓ in renal impair **Caution:** [B, ?] ↓ absorption w/ antacids/Ca salts **Contra:** Component sensitivity **Supplied:** Granule packets 3 g **SE:** HA, GI upset **Notes:** May take 2–3 d for Sxs to improve

Fosinopril (Monopril) Uses: **HTN, CHF,* DN* Action: ACE inhibitor Dose: 10 mg/d PO initial; max 40 mg/d PO; ↓ in elderly; ↓ in renal impair Caution: [D, +] ↑ K+ w/ K+ supls, ARBs, K+-sparing diuretics; ↑ renal AE w/ NSAIDs, diuretics, hypovolemia Contra: Hereditary/idiopathic angioedema or angioedema with ACE inhibitor, bilateral renal artery stenosis Supplied: Tabs 10, 20, 40 mg SE: Nonproductive cough, dizziness, angioedema, ↑ K+

Fosphenytoin (Cerebyx) Uses: **Status epilepticus** Action: ↓ Sz spread in motor cortex Dose: Dose as phenytoin equivalents (PE). *Load:* 15–20 mg PE/kg. *Maint:* 4–6 mg PE/kg/d; ↓ dosage, monitor levels in hepatic impair Caution: [D, +] May ↑ phenobarbital Contra: Sinus bradycardia, SA block, 2nd/3rd-degree AV block, Adams–Stokes syndrome, rash during Rx Supplied: Inj 75 mg/mL SE: ↓ BP, dizziness, ataxia, pruritus, nystagmus Notes: 15 min to convert fosphenytoin to phenytoin; admin <150 mg PE/min to prevent ↓ BP; administer with BP monitoring

Frovatriptan (Frova) See Table 11, page 218

Fulvestrant (Faslodex) Uses: *Hormone receptor(+) metastatic *breast CA** in postmenopausal women with Dz progression following antiestrogen therapy Action: Estrogen receptor antagonist Dose: 250 mg IM monthly, either a single 5-mL inj or two concurrent 2.5-mL IM inj into buttocks Caution: [X, ?/–] ↑ effects w/ CYP3A4 inhibitors w/ hepatic impair Contra: PRG Supplied: Prefilled syringes 50 mg/mL (single 5 mL, dual 2.5 mL) SE: N/V/D, constipation, abdominal pain, HA, back pain, hot flushes, pharyngitis, inj site Rxns Notes: Only use IM

Furosemide (Lasix) Uses: **CHF, HTN, edema,* ascites* Action: Loop diuretic; ↓ Na & Cl reabsorption in ascending loop of Henle & distal tubule Dose: *Adults.* 20–80 mg PO or IV bid. *Peds.* 1 mg/kg/dose IV q6–12h; 2 mg/kg/dose PO q12–24h (max 6 mg/kg/dose) Caution: [C, +] ↓ K+, ↑ risk of digoxin tox; ↑ risk of ototox w/ aminoglycosides, cisplatinum (esp in renal dysfunction) Contra: Allergy to sulfonylureas; anuria; hepatic coma/severe electrolyte depletion Supplied: Tabs 20, 40, 80 mg; soln 10 mg/mL, 40 mg/5 mL; inj 10 mg/mL SE: ↓ BP, hyperglycemia, ↓ K+ Notes: Monitor electrolytes, renal Fxn; high doses IV may cause ototox

Gabapentin (Neurontin) Uses: *Adjunct therapy in the Rx of *partial Szs; postherpetic neuralgia (PHN)*; chronic pain syndromes* Action: Anticonvulsant Dose: *Anticonvulsant:* 300–1200 mg PO tid (max 3600 mg/d). *PHN:* 300 mg day 1, 300 mg bid day 2, 300 mg tid day 3, titrate (1800–3600 mg/d); ↓ in renal impair Caution: [C, ?] Contra: Component sensitivity Supplied: Caps 100, 300, 400 mg; soln 250 mg/5mL; tab 600, 800 mg SE: Somnolence, dizziness, ataxia, fatigue Notes: Not necessary to monitor levels

Galantamine (Reminyl) Uses: **Alzheimer Dz** Action: Acetylcholinesterase inhibitor Dose: 4 mg PO bid, ↑ to 8 mg bid after 4 wk; may ↑ to 12 mg bid in 4 wk Caution: [B, ?] ↑ effect w/ succinylcholine, amiodarone, diltiazem, verapamil, NSAIDs, digoxin; ↓ effect w/ anticholinergics Contra: Severe renal/hepatic impair Supplied: Tabs 4, 8, 12 mg; soln 4 mg/mL SE: GI disturbances, weight loss, sleep disturbances, dizziness, HA **Notes:** Caution w/ urinary outflow obstruction, Parkinson Dz, severe asthma/COPD, severe heart Dz or ↓ BP

Gallium Nitrate (Ganite) **Uses:** *↑ Ca²⁺ of malignancy*; bladder CA **Action:** ↓ bone resorption of Ca²⁺ **Dose:** ↑ *Ca²⁺:* 200 mg/m²/day × 5 d. *CA:* 350 mg/m² cont inf × 5 d to 700 mg/m² rapid IV inf q2wk in antineoplastic settings (Per protocols) **Caution:** [C, ?] Do not give with live vaccines or rotavirus vaccine **Contra:** SCr >2.5 mg/dL **Supplied:** Inj 25 mg/mL **SE:** Renal insuff, ↓ Ca²⁺, hypophosphatemia, ↓ bicarbonate, <1% acute optic neuritis **Notes:** Bladder CA: use in combo with vinblastine & ifosfamide

Ganciclovir (Cytovene, Vitrasert) **Uses:** *Rx & prevent CMV retinitis, prevent CMV Dz* in transplant recipients **Action:** ↓ viral DNA synthesis **Dose:** *Adults & Peds. IV:* 5 mg/kg IV q12h for 14–21 d, then maint 5 mg/kg/d IV × 7 d/wk or 6 mg/kg/d IV × 5 d/wk. *Ocular implant:* One implant q5–8mo. *Adults. PO:* Following induction, 1000 mg PO tid. *Prevention:* 1000 mg PO tid; with food; ↓ in renal impair **Caution:** [C, –] ↑ effect w/ immunosuppressives, imipenem/ cilastatin, zidovudine, didanosine, other nephrotoxic Rx **Contra:** ANC <500, plt <25,000), intravitreal implant **Supplied:** Caps 250, 500 mg; inj 500 mg; ocular implant 4.5 mg **SE:** Granulocytopenia & thrombocytopenia, fever, rash, GI upset **Notes:** Not a cure for CMV; handle inj w/ cytotox cautions; implant confers no systemic benefit

Gatifloxacin (Tequin, Zymar Ophthalmic) **Uses:** *Bronchitis, sinusitis, community-acquired pneumonia, UTI, uncomplicated skin/soft tissue Infxn* **Action:** Quinolone antibiotic, ↓ DNA-gyrase. *Spectrum:* Gram(+) (except MRSA, *Listeria*), gram(–) (not *Pseudomonas*), atypicals, some anaerobes (*Clostridium*, not *C. difficile*) **Dose:** 400 mg/d PO or IV; *Ophth:* Day 1 & 2 one gt q2h in eye while awake (8 ×/day max) day 3–7, one gt 4×d while awake; (↓ in renal impair) **Caution:** [C, M] **Contra:** Prolonged QT interval, uncorrected ↓ K⁺, w/ other Rx that prolong QT interval (Class Ia & III antiarrhythmics, erythromycin, antipsychotics, TCA) children <18 y or in PRG/lactating women **Supplied:** Tabs 200, 400 mg; inj 10 mg/mL; premixed infuse D₅W 200 mg, 400 mg; ophth soln 0.3% **SE:** Prolonged QT interval, HA, N/D, tendon rupture, photosensitivity **Notes:** Reliable activity against *S. pneumoniae;* take 4 h after antacids containing Mg, Al, Fe, or Zn; drink plenty of fluids; avoid direct sunlight

Gefitinib (Iressa) **Uses:** *Rx locally advanced or metastatic non-small-cell lung CA after failure of both platinum-based & docetaxel chemotherapies* **Action:** ↓ intracellular phosphorylation of tyrosine kinases **Dose:** 250 mg/d PO **Caution:** [D, –] **Supplied:** Tabs 250 mg **SE:** D, rash, acne, dry skin, N/V, interstitial lung Dz, ↑d liver transaminases **Notes:** Follow LFTs

Gemcitabine (Gemzar) **Uses:** *Pancreatic CA, brain mets, NSCLC,* gastric CA **Action:** Antimetabolite; ↓ ribonucleotide reductase; produces false nucleotide base-inhibiting DNA synthesis **Dose:** 1000 mg/m² over 30 min–1 h IV inf/wk × 3–4 wk or 6–8 wk; dose modifications based on hematologic Fxn (Per protocol) **Caution:** [D, ?/–] **Contra:** PRG **Supplied:** Inj 200 mg, 1 g **SE:** Myelosuppression, N/V/D, drug fever, skin rash **Notes:** Reconstituted soln concn 38 mg/mL (not 40 mg/mL as earlier labeling); monitor hepatic/renal Fxn prior & during Rx

Gemfibrozil (Lopid)
Uses: *Hypertriglyceridemia, coronary heart Dz* **Action:** Fibric acid **Dose:** 1200 mg/d PO ÷ bid 30 min ac AM & PM **Caution:** [C, ?] Enhances the effect of warfarin, sulfonylureas; ↑ risk of rhabdomyopathy w/ HMG-CoA reductase inhibitors; ↓ effects w/ cyclosporine **Contra:** Renal/hepatic impair (SCr >2.0 mg/dL), gallbladder Dz, primary biliary cirrhosis **Supplied:** Tabs 600 mg **SE:** Cholelithiasis, GI upset **Notes:** Avoid concurrent use with the HMG-CoA reductase inhibitors; monitor LFTs & serum lipids

Gemifloxacin (Factive)
Uses: Community-acquired pneumonia, acute exacerbation of chronic bronchitis **Action:** ↓ DNA gyrase & topoisomerase IV; **Spectrum:** *S. pneumoniae* (including MDR strains), *H. influenzae, H. parainfluenzae, M. catarrhalis, M. pneumoniae, Chlamydia pneumoniae, K. pneumoniae* **Dose:** 320 mg PO qd; CrCl < 40 mL/min: 160 mg PO qd **Caution:** [C, ?/–]; children < 18 y; Hx of ↑ QTc interval, electrolyte disorders, w/ Class IA/III antiarrhythmics, erythromycin, TCAs, antipsychotics **Contra:** Fluoroquinolone allergy **Supplied:** Tab 320 mg **SE:** Rash, N/V/D, abdominal pain, dizziness, xerostomia, arthralgia, allergy/anaphylactic reactions, peripheral neuropathy, tendon rupture **Notes:** Take 3 h before or 2 h after: Al/Mg-containing antacids, Fe, Z or other metal cations

Gemtuzumab Ozogamicin (Mylotarg)
WARNING: Can cause severe allergic Rxns & other infusion-related reactions including severe pulmonary events; hepatotox, including severe hepatic venoocclusive Dz (VOD) reported **Uses:** *Relapsed CD33+ AML in pts > 60 who are poor candidates for chemo* **Action:** MoAb linked to calicheamicin; selective for myeloid cells **Dose:** Per protocol **Caution:** [D,?/–] **Contra:** Component sensitivity **Supplied:** 5 mg/20 mL vial **SE:** Myelosuppression, allergy (including anaphylaxis), inf Rxns (chills, fever, N/V, HA), pulmonary events, hepatotox **Notes:** Only use as single agent, not in combo w/ other agents; premedicate (diphenhydramine & acetaminophen)

Gentamicin (Garamycin, G-Mycitin, others)
Uses: *Serious Infxns* caused by *Pseudomonas, Proteus, E. coli, Klebsiella, Enterobacter, & Serratia* & initial Rx of gram(–) sepsis **Action:** Bactericidal; ↓ protein synthesis. **Spectrum:** Synergy w/ PCNs; gram(–) (not *Neisseria, Legionella, Acinetobacter*) **Dose:** *Adults.* 3–7 mg/kg/24h IV ÷ q8–24h. *Synergy:* 1 mg/kg q8h. *Peds. Infants <7 d <1200 g:* 2.5 mg/kg/dose q18–24h. *Infants >1200 g:* 2.5 mg/kg/dose q12–18h. *Infants >7 d:* 2.5 mg/kg/dose IV q8–12h. *Children:* 2.5 mg/kg/d IV q8h; ↓ with renal insuff **Caution:** [C, +/–] Avoid other nephrotoxic Rxs **Contra:** Aminoglycoside sensitivity **Supplied:** Premixed infus 40, 60, 70, 80, 90, 100, 120 mg; ADD-Vantage inj vials 10 mg/mL; inj 40 mg/mL; IT preservative-free 2 mg/mL **SE:** Nephrotox/ototox/neurotox **Notes:** Follow CrCl, SCr & serum concn

for dose adjustments (Table 2, page 200); once daily dosing popular; follow; use IBW to dose (use adjusted if obese >30% IBW)

Gentamicin & Prednisolone, Ophthalmic (Pred-G Ophthalmic)

Uses: *Steroid-responsive ocular & conjunctival Infxns* sensitive to gentamicin **Action:** Bactericidal; ↓ protein synthesis plus antiinflammatory **Spectrum:** *Staphylococcus, E. coli, H. influenzae, Klebsiella, Neisseria, Pseudomonas, Proteus,* & *Serratia* sp **Dose:** *Oint:* ½ in. in conjunctival sac daily–tid. *Susp:* 1 gt bid–qid, up to 1 gt/h for severe Infxns **Contra:** Aminoglycoside sensitivity **Caution:** [C, ?] **Supplied:** *Oint, ophth:* Prednisolone acetate 0.6% & gentamicin sulfate 0.3% (3.5 g). *Susp, ophth:* Prednisolone acetate 1% & gentamicin sulfate 0.3% (2, 5, 10 mL) **SE:** Local irritation

Gentamicin, Ophthalmic (Garamycin, Genoptic, Gentacidin, Gentak, others)

Uses: *Conjunctival Infxns* **Action:** Bactericidal; ↓ protein synthesis **Dose:** *Oint:* Apply ½ in. bid–tid. *Soln:* 1–2 gtt q2–4h, up to 2 gtt/h for severe Infxn **Caution:** [C, ?] **Contra:** Aminoglycoside sensitivity **Supplied:** Soln & oint 0.3% **SE:** Local irritation **Notes:** Do not use other eye drops w/in 5–10 mins; do not touch dropper to eye

Gentamicin, Topical (Garamycin, G-Mycitin)

Uses: *Skin Infxns* caused by susceptible organisms **Action:** Bactericidal; ↓ protein synthesis **Dose:** *Adults & Peds >1 y.* Apply tid–qid **Caution:** [C, ?] **Contra:** Aminoglycoside sensitivity **Supplied:** Cream & oint 0.1% **SE:** Irritation

Glimepiride (Amaryl)

Uses: *Type 2 DM* **Action:** Sulfonylurea; ↑ pancreatic insulin release; ↑ peripheral insulin sensitivity; ↓ hepatic glucose output & production **Dose:** 1–4 mg/d, max 8 mg **Caution:** [C, –] **Contra:** DKA **Supplied:** Tabs 1, 2, 4 mg **SE:** HA, nausea, hypoglycemia **Notes:** Give w/ 1st meal of day

Glipizide (Glucotrol, Glucotrol XL)

Uses: *Type 2 DM* **Action:** Sulfonylurea; ↑ pancreatic insulin release; ↑ peripheral insulin sensitivity; ↓ hepatic glucose output & production; ↓ intestinal absorption of glucose **Dose:** 5 mg initial, ↑ by 2.5–5 mg/d as needed; XL max 20 mg; 30 min ac; hold if pt NPO **Caution:** [C, ?/–] Severe liver Dz **Contra:** DKA, Type 1 DM, sensitivity to sulfonamides **Supplied:** Tabs 5, 10 mg; XL tabs 2.5, 5, 10 mg **SE:** HA, anorexia, N/V/D, constipation, fullness, rash, urticaria, photosensitivity **Notes:** Counsel pt about diabetes management; wait several days before adjusting dose; monitor glucose

Glucagon

Uses: Severe *hypoglycemic* Rxns in DM with sufficient liver glycogen stores or β-blocker OD **Action:** Accelerates liver gluconeogenesis **Dose:** *Adults.* 0.5–1 mg SQ, IM, or IV; repeat in 20 min PRN. β-Blocker OD: 3–10 mg IV; repeat in 10 min PRN; may give cont infus 1–5 mg/h. *Peds. Neonates:* 0.3 mg/kg/dose SQ, IM, or IV q4h PRN. *Children:* 0.025–0.1 mg/kg/dose SQ, IM, or IV; repeat in 20 min PRN **Caution:** [B, M] **Contra:** Known pheochromocytoma **Supplied:** Inj 1 mg **SE:** N/V, ↓ BP **Notes:** Administration of glucose IV necessary; ineffective in starvation, adrenal insuff, or chronic hypoglycemia

Glyburide (DiaBeta, Micronase, Glynase)

Uses: *Type 2 DM* **Action:** Sulfonylurea; ↑ pancreatic insulin release; ↑ peripheral insulin sensitivity;

↓ hepatic glucose output & production; ↓ intestinal absorption of glucose **Dose:** 1.25–10 mg qd–bid, max 20 mg/d. *Micronized:* 0.75–6 mg qd–bid, max 12 mg/d **Caution:** [C, ?] Renal impair **Contra:** DKA, Type I DM **Supplied:** Tabs 1.25, 2.5, 5 mg; micronized tabs 1.5, 3, 6 mg **SE:** HA, hypoglycemia **Notes:** Not OK for CrCl <50 mL/min; hold dose if pt NPO

Glyburide/Metformin (Glucovance) Uses: *Type 2 DM* **Action:** *Sulfonylurea:* ↑ Pancreatic insulin release. *Metformin:* ↑ Peripheral insulin sensitivity; ↓ hepatic glucose output & production; ↓ intestinal absorption of glucose **Dose:** 1st line (naive pts), 1.25/250 mg PO daily–bid; 2nd line, 2.5/500 mg or 5/500 mg bid (max 20/2000 mg); take w/ meals, ↑ dose gradually hold prior to & 48 h after ionic contrast media **Caution:** [C, –] **Contra:** SCr >1.4 in females or >1.5 in males; hypoxemic conditions (CHF, sepsis, recent MI); alcoholism; metabolic acidosis; liver Dz; **Supplied:** Tabs 1.25/250 mg, 2.5/500 mg, 5/500 mg **SE:** HA, hypoglycemia, lactic acidosis, anorexia, N/V, rash **Notes:** Avoid EtOH; hold dose if NPO; monitor folate levels for megaloblastic anemia

Glycerin Suppository Uses: *Constipation* **Action:** Hyperosmolar laxative **Dose:** *Adults.* 1 adult supp PR PRN. *Peds.* 1 infant supp PR daily–bid PRN **Caution:** [C, ?] **Supplied:** Supp (adult; infant); liq 4 mL/applicatorful **SE:** Can cause D

Gonadorelin (Lutrepulse) Uses: *Primary hypothalamic amenorrhea* **Action:** Stimulates pituitary release of LH & FSH **Dose:** 5 mcg IV q 90 min × 21 d using Lutrepulse pump kit **Caution:** [B, M] ↑ levels w/ androgens, estrogens, progestins, glucocorticoids, spironolactone, levodopa; ↓ levels w/ OCP, digoxin, dopamine antagonists **Contra:** Any condition exacerbated by PRG, ovarian cysts, causes of anovulation other than hypothalamic, conditions worsened by reproductive hormones, hormonally dependent tumor **Supplied:** Inj 100 mcg **SE:** Risk of multiple pregnancies; inj site pain **Notes:** Monitor LH, FSH

Goserelin (Zoladex) Uses: Advanced *CAP* & w/ radiation for localized high-risk CAP, *endometriosis, breast CA* **Action:** LHRH agonist, ↓ LH, resulting in ↓ testosterone **Dose:** 3.6 mg SQ (implant) q 28d or 10.8 mg SQ q3mo; usually into lower abdominal wall **Caution:** [X, –] **Contra:** PRG, breast-feeding, 10.8-mg implant not for women **Supplied:** SQ implant 3.6 (1 mo), 10.8 (3 mo) **SE:** Hot flashes, ↓ libido, gynecomastia, & transient exacerbation of CA-related bone pain ("flare reaction") 7–10 d after 1st dose) **Notes:** Inject SQ into fat in abdominal wall; do not aspirate; females must use contraception

Granisetron (Kytril) Uses: *Prevention of N/V* **Action:** Serotonin receptor antagonist **Dose:** *Adults & Peds.* 10 mcg/kg/dose IV 30 min prior to chemo *Adults.* 2 mg PO 1 h prior to chemo, then 12 h later. *Postop N/V:* 1 mg IV before end of OR case **Caution:** [B, +/–] St. John's wort ↓ levels **Contra:** Liver Dz, children <2 y **Supplied:** Tabs 1 mg; inj 1 mg/mL; soln 2 mg/10 mL **SE:** HA, constipation

Guaifenesin (Robitussin, others) Uses: *Relief of dry, nonproductive cough* **Action:** Expectorant **Dose:** *Adults.* 200–400 mg (10–20 mL) PO q4h (max

2.4 g/d). **Peds.** <2 y: 12 mg/kg/d in 6 ÷ doses. 2–5 y: 50–100 mg (2.5–5 mL) PO q4h (max 600 mg/d). 6–11 y: 100–200 mg (5–10 mL) PO q4h (max 1.2 g/d) **Caution:** [C, ?] **Supplied:** Tabs 100, 200; SR tabs 600, 1200 mg; caps 200 mg; SR caps 300 mg; liq 100 mg/5 mL **SE:** GI upset **Notes:** Give w/ large amount of H_2O; some dosage forms contain EtOH

Guaifenesin & Codeine (Robitussin AC, Brontex, others) [C-V] Uses: *Relief of dry, nonproductive cough* Action: Antitussive w/ expectorant Dose: Adults. 5–10 mL or 1 tab PO q6–8h (max 60 mL/24 h). Peds. 2–6 y: 1–1.5 mg/kg codeine/d ÷ dose q4–6h (max 30 mg/24 h). 6–12 y: 5 mL q4h (max 30 mL/24 h) Caution: [C, +] Supplied: Brontex tab 10 mg codeine/300 mg guaifenesin; liq 2.5 mg codeine/75 mg guaifenesin/5 mL; others 10 mg codeine/100 mg guaifenesin/5 mL SE: Somnolence

Guaifenesin & Dextromethorphan (many OTC brands) Uses: *Cough* due to upper resp tract irritation Action: Antitussive w/ expectorant Dose: Adults & Peds >12 y. 10 mL PO q6–8h (max 40 mL/24 h). Peds. 2–6 y: Dextromethorphan 1–2 mg/kg/24 h ÷ 3–4 × d (max 10 mL/d). 6–12 y: 5 mL q6–8h (max 20 mL/d) Caution: [C, +] Contra: Administration w/ MAOI Supplied: Many OTC formulations SE: Somnolence Notes: Give with plenty of fluids

Haemophilus B Conjugate Vaccine (ActHIB, HibTITER, PedvaxHIB, Prohibit, others) Uses: Routine *immunization* of children against H. influenzae type B Dzs Action: Active immunization against Haemophilus B Dose: Peds. 0.5 mL (25 mg) IM in deltoid or vastus lateralis Caution: [C, +] Contra: Febrile illness, immunosuppression, allergy to thimerosal Supplied: Inj 7.5, 10, 15, 25 mcg/0.5 mL SE: Observe for anaphylaxis; edema, ↑ risk of Haemophilus B Infxn the week after vaccination Notes: Booster not required; report all serious adverse Rxn to VAERS: 1-800-822-7967

Haloperidol (Haldol) Uses: *Psychotic disorders, agitation, Tourette disorders, & hyperactivity in children* Action: Antipsychotic, neuroleptic Dose: Adults. Moderate Sxs: 0.5–2 mg PO bid–tid. Severe Sxs/agitation: 3–5 mg PO bid–tid or 1–5 mg IM q4h PRN (max 100 mg/d). Peds. 3–6 y: 0.01–0.03 mg/kg/24 h PO qd. 6–12 y: Initial, 0.5–1.5 mg/24 h PO qd; ↑ by 0.5 mg/24 h to maintenance of 2–4 mg/d (0.05–0.1 mg/kg/24 h) or 1–3 mg/dose IM q4–8h to 0.1 mg/kg/24 h max; Tourette Dz may require up to 15 mg/24 h PO; ↓ in elderly Caution: [C, ?] ↑ effects w/ SSRIs, CNS depressants, TCA, indomethacin, metoclopramide; avoid levodopa (↓ antiparkinsonian effects) Contra: NA glaucoma, severe CNS depression, coma, Parkinson Dz, BM suppression, severe cardiac/hepatic Dz Supplied: Tabs 0.5, 1, 2, 5, 10, 20 mg; conc liq 2 mg/mL; inj 5 mg/mL; decanoate inj 50, 100 mg/mL SE: Extrapyramidal Sxs (EPS), ↓ BP, anxiety, dystonias Notes: Do not give decanoate IV; dilute PO conc liq w/ H_2O/juice; monitor for EPS

Haloprogin (Halotex) Uses: *Topical Rx of tinea pedis, tinea cruris, tinea corporis, tinea manus* Action: Topical antifungal Dose: Adults. Apply bid for ≤ 2 wk; intertriginous may require ≤ 4 wk Caution: [B, ?] Contra: Component

sensitivity **Supplied:** 1% cream; soln **SE:** Local irritation **Notes:** Avoid contact w eyes; improvement should occur w/in 4 wk

Heparin Uses: *Rx & prevention of DVT & PE,* unstable angina, AF w/ em boli formation, & acute arterial occlusion **Action:** Acts w/ antithrombin III to inac tivate thrombin & ↓ thromboplastin formation **Dose:** *Adults. Prophylaxis* 3000–5000 units SQ q8–12h. *Thrombosis Rx:* Load 50–80 units/kg IV, then 10–2 units/kg IV qh (adjust based on PTT). *Peds. Infants:* Load 50 units/kg IV bolus then 20 units/kg IV by cont inf. *Children:* Load 50 units/kg IV, then 15–2 units/kg cont inf or 100 units/kg/dose q4h IV intermittent bolus (adjust based o PTT) **Caution:** [B, +] ↑ risk of hemorrhage w/ anticoagulants, aspirin, an tiplatelets, cephalosporins w/ MTT side chain **Contra:** Uncontrolled bleeding, se vere thrombocytopenia, suspected ICH **Supplied:** Inj 10, 100, 1000, 2000, 2500 5000, 7500, 10,000, 20,000, 40,000 units/mL **SE:** Bruising, bleeding, thrombocy topenia **Notes:** Follow PTT, thrombin time, or activated clotting time to monitor little PT effect; therapeutic PTT 1.5–2 × control for most conditions; monitor fo HIT; follow plt counts

Hepatitis A Vaccine (Havrix, Vaqta) Uses: *Prevent hepatitis A* i high-risk individuals (eg, travelers, certain professions, or high-risk behaviors) **Ac tion:** Provides active immunity **Dose:** (Expressed as ELISA units [EL.U.]) *Havri Adults.* 1440 EL.U. single IM dose. *Peds >2 y.* 720 EL.U. single IM dose. *Vaqta Adults.* 50 units single IM dose. *Peds.* 25 units single IM dose **Caution:** [C, + **Contra:** Allergy to any component of formulation **Supplied:** Inj 720 EL.U./0. mL, 1440 EL.U./1 mL; 50 units/mL **SE:** Fever, fatigue, pain at inj site, HA **Notes** Booster OK 6–12 mo after primary; report serious adverse Rxns to VAERS: 1-800 822-7967

Hepatitis A (Inactivated) & Hepatitis B (Recombinant) Va cine (Twinrix) Uses: *Active immunization against hepatitis A/B* **Action** Active immunity **Dose:** 1 mL IM at 0, 1, & 6 mo **Caution:** [C, +] **Contra:** Compo nent sensitivity **Supplied:** Single-dose vials, syringes **SE:** Fever, fatigue, pain site, HA **Notes:** Booster OK 6–12 mo after vaccination; report all serious advers Rxns to VAERS: 1-800-822-7967

Hepatitis B Immune Globulin (HyperHep, H-BIG) Uses: *Ex posure to HBsAg(+) materials,* eg, blood, plasma, or serum (accidental needle stick, mucous membrane contact, or PO ingestion) **Action:** Passive immunization **Dose:** *Adults & Peds.* 0.06 mL/kg IM to a max of 5 mL; w/in 24 h of exposure w/in 14 d of sexual contact; repeat 1 & 6 mo after exposure **Caution:** [C, ?] **Con tra:** Allergies to γ-globulin or antiimmunoglobulin Ab; allergies to thimerosal; IgA deficiency **Supplied:** Inj **SE:** Pain at site, dizziness **Notes:** Administered IM i gluteal or deltoid; if exposure continues, pt should also receive hepatitis B vaccine

Hepatitis B Vaccine (Engerix-B, Recombivax HB) Uses: *Pre vention of hepatitis B* **Action:** Active immunization; recombinant DNA technol ogy **Dose:** *Adults.* 3 IM doses of 1 mL each; 1st 2 doses 1 mo apart; the 3rd 6 m after the 1st. *Peds.* 0.5 mL IM given on adult schedule **Caution:** [C, +] ↓ effect w/ immunosuppressives **Contra:** Yeast allergy **Supplied:** *Engerix-B:* Inj 20 mcg/mL; peds inj 10 mcg/0.5 mL. *Recombivax HB:* Inj 10 & 40 mcg/mL; peds inj 5 mcg/0.5 mL **SE:** Fever, inj site soreness **Notes:** IM inj for adults & older peds in the deltoid; in other peds, administer in the anterolateral thigh

Hetastarch (Hespan) Uses: *Plasma volume expansion* as adjunct in shock & leukapheresis **Action:** Synthetic colloid; action similar to albumin **Dose:** *Volume expansion:* 500–1000 mL (1500 mL/d max) IV (20 mL/kg/h max rate). *Leukapheresis:* 250–700 mL; ↓ in renal failure **Caution:** [C, +] **Contra:** Severe bleeding disorders, CHF, or oliguric/anuric renal failure **Supplied:** Inj 6 g/100 mL **SE:** Bleeding (prolongs PT, PTT, bleed time, etc) **Notes:** Not blood or plasma substitute

Hydralazine (Apresoline, others) Uses: *Moderate–severe HTN; CHF* (w/ Isordil) **Action:** Peripheral vasodilator **Dose:** *Adults.* Initial 10 mg PO qid, ↑ to 25 mg qid 300 mg/d max. *Peds.* 0.75–3 mg/kg/24 h PO ÷ q6–12h; ↓ in renal impair; check CBC & ANA before starting **Caution:** [C, +] ↑ hepatic Fxn & CAD; ↑ tox w/ MAOI, indomethacin, β-blockers **Contra:** Dissecting aortic aneurysm, mitral valve rheumatic heart Dz **Supplied:** Tabs 10, 25, 50, 100 mg; inj 20 mg/mL **SE:** SLE-like syndrome w/ chronic high doses; SVT following IM route, peripheral neuropathy **Notes:** Compensatory sinus tachycardia eliminated w/ β-blocker

Hydrochlorothiazide (HydroDIURIL, Esidrix, others) Uses: *Edema, HTN* **Action:** Thiazide diuretic; ↓ Na reabsorption in the distal tubule **Dose:** *Adults.* 25–100 mg/d PO single or ÷ doses. *Peds. <6 mo:* 2–3 mg/kg/d in 2 ÷ doses. *>6 mo:* 2 mg/kg/d in 2 ÷ doses **Caution:** [D, +] **Contra:** Anuria, sulfonamide allergy, renal decompensation **Supplied:** Tabs 25, 50, 100 mg; caps 12.5 mg; PO soln 50 mg/5 mL **SE:** ↓ K^+, hyperglycemia, hyperuricemia, ↓ Na^+ **Notes:** May cause sun sensitivity

Hydrochlorothiazide & Amiloride (Moduretic) Uses: *HTN* **Action:** Combined thiazide & a K^+-sparing diuretic **Dose:** 1–2 tabs/d PO **Caution:** [D, ?] **Contra:** w/renal failure, sulfonamide allergy **Supplied:** Tabs (amiloride/HCTZ) 5 mg/50 mg **SE:** ↓ BP, photosensitivity, ↑ K^+/↓ K^+, hyperglycemia, ↓ Na^+, hyperlipidemia, hyperuricemia

Hydrochlorothiazide & Spironolactone (Aldactazide) Uses: *Edema, HTN* **Action:** Combined thiazide & K^+-sparing diuretic **Dose:** 25–200 mg each component/d, ÷ doses **Caution:** [D, +] **Contra:** Sulfonamide allergy **Supplied:** Tabs (HCTZ/spironolactone) 25 mg/25 mg, 50 mg/50 mg **SE:** Photosensitivity, ↓ BP, ↑ or ↓ K^+, ↓ Na^+, hyperglycemia, hyperlipidemia, hyperuricemia

Hydrochlorothiazide & Triamterene (Dyazide, Maxzide) Uses: *Edema & HTN* **Action:** Combined thiazide & K^+-sparing diuretic **Dose:** *Dyazide:* 1–2 caps PO qd–bid. *Maxzide:* 1 tab/d PO **Caution:** [D, +/–] **Contra:** Sulfonamide allergy **Supplied:** (Triamterene/HCTZ) 37.5 mg/25 mg, 50 mg/25 mg, 75 mg/50 mg

SE: Photosensitivity, ↓ BP, ↑ or ↓ K^+, ↓ Na^+, hyperglycemia, hyperlipidemia, hyperuricemia **Notes:** HCTZ component in Maxzide more bioavailable than in Dyazide

Hydrocodone & Acetaminophen (Lorcet, Vicodin, others) [C-III] **Uses:** *Moderate–severe pain*; **Action:** Narcotic analgesic w/ nonnarcotic analgesic; hydrocodone is antitussive **Dose:** 1–2 caps or tabs PO q4–6h PRN **Caution:** [C, M] **Contra:** CNS depression, severe resp depression **Supplied:** Many formulations; specify hydrocodone/APAP dose; caps 5/500; tabs 2.5/500, 5/400, 5/500, 7.5/400, 10/400, 7.5/500, 7.5/650, 7.5/750, 10/325, 10/400, 10/500, 10/650; elixir & soln (fruit punch) 2.5 mg hydrocodone/167 mg APAP/5 mL **SE:** GI upset, sedation, fatigue **Notes:** Do not exceed >4 g acetaminophen/d

Hydrocodone & Aspirin (Lortab ASA, others) [C-III] **Uses:** *Moderate–severe pain* **Action:** Narcotic analgesic with NSAID **Dose:** 1–2 PO q4–6h PRN, w/ food/milk **Caution:** [C, M] ↓renal Fxn, gastritis/PUD, **Contra:** Component sensitivity; children w/chickenpox (Reye syndrome) **Supplied:** 5 mg hydrocodone/500 mg ASA/tab **SE:** GI upset, sedation, fatigue **Notes:** Monitor for GI bleed

Hydrocodone & Guaifenesin (Hycotuss Expectorant, others) [C-III] **Uses:** *Nonproductive cough* associated with resp Infxn **Action:** Expectorant w/ cough suppressant **Dose:** *Adults & Peds >12 y.* 5 mL q4h pc & hs. *Peds. < 2 y.* 0.3 mg/kg/d ÷ qid. *2–12 y.* 2.5 mL q4h pc & hs **Caution:** [C, M] **Contra:** Component sensitivity **Supplied:** Hydrocodone 5 mg/guaifenesin 100 mg/5 mL **SE:** GI upset, sedation, fatigue

Hydrocodone & Homatropine (Hycodan, Hydromet, others) [C-III] **Uses:** *Relief of cough* **Action:** Combo antitussive **Dose:** (Based on hydrocodone) *Adults.* 5–10 mg q4–6h. *Peds.* 0.6 mg/kg/d ÷ tid–qid **Caution:** [C, M] **Contra:** NA glaucoma, ↑ ICP, depressed ventilation **Supplied:** Syrup 5 mg hydrocodone/5 mL; tabs 5 mg hydrocodone **SE:** Sedation, fatigue, GI upset **Notes:** Do not give >q4h; see individual Rx monographs

Hydrocodone & Ibuprofen (Vicoprofen) [C-III] **Uses:** *Moderate–severe pain (<10 d)* **Action:** Narcotic w/ NSAID **Dose:** 1–2 tabs q4–6h PRN **Caution:** [C, M] Renal insuff; ↓ effect w/ ACE inhibitors & diuretics; ↑ effect w/ CNS depressants, EtOH, MAOI, aspirin, TCA, anticoagulants **Contra:** Component sensitivity **Supplied:** Tabs 7.5 mg hydrocodone/200 mg ibuprofen **SE:** Sedation, fatigue, GI upset

Hydrocodone & Pseudoephedrine (Detussin, Histussin-D, others) [C-III] **Uses:** *Cough & nasal congestion* **Action:** Narcotic cough suppressant with decongestant **Dose:** 5 mL qid, PRN **Caution:** [C, M] **Contra:** MAOIs **Supplied:** 5 mg hydrocodone/60 mg pseudoephedrine/5 mL **SE:** ↑ BP, GI upset, sedation, fatigue

Hydrocodone, Chlorpheniramine, Phenylephrine, Acetaminophen, & Caffeine (Hycomine Compound)[C-III] **Uses:** *Cough & Sxs of URI* **Action:** Narcotic cough suppressant w/ decongestants &

analgesic **Dose:** 1 tab PO q4h PRN **Caution:** [C, M] **Contra:** NA glaucoma **Supplied:** Hydrocodone 5 mg/chlorpheniramine 2 mg/phenylephrine 10 mg/APAP 250 mg/caffeine 30 mg/tab **SE:** ↑BP, GI upset, sedation, fatigue

Hydrocortisone, Rectal (Anusol-HC Suppository, Cortifoam Rectal, Proctocort, others) **Uses:** *Painful anorectal conditions,* radiation proctitis, management of ulcerative colitis **Action:** Antiinflammatory steroid **Dose:** *Adults. Ulcerative colitis:* 10–100 mg PR qd–bid for 2–3 wk **Caution:** [B, ?/–] **Contra:** Component sensitivity **Supplied:** *Hydrocortisone acetate:* Rectal aerosol 90 mg/applicator; supp 25 mg. *Hydrocortisone base:* Rectal 1%; rectal susp 100 mg/60 mL **SE:** Minimal systemic effect

Hydrocortisone, Topical & Systemic (Cortef, Solu-Cortef) See Steroids, page 169, & Tables 4 & 5, pages 206 & 207 **Caution:** [B, –] **Contra:** Viral, fungal, or tubercular skin lesions; serious Infxns (except septic shock or tuberculous meningitis) **SE:** Systemic forms: ↑ appetite, insomnia, hyperglycemia, bruising **Notes:** May cause HPA axis suppression

Hydromorphone (Dilaudid) [C–II] **Uses:** *Moderate/severe pain* **Action:** Narcotic analgesic **Dose:** 1–4 mg PO, IM, IV, or PR q4–6h PRN; 3 mg PR q6–8h PRN; ↓ w/ hepatic failure **Caution:** [B (D if prolonged use or high doses near term), ?] ↑ effects w/ CNS depressants, phenothiazines, TCA **Contra:** Component sensitivity **Supplied:** Tabs 1, 2, 3, 4, 8 mg; liq 5 mg/mL; inj 1, 2, 4, 10 mg/mL; supp 3 mg **SE:** Sedation, dizziness, GI upset **Notes:** Morphine 10 mg IM = hydromorphone 1.5 mg IM

Hydroxyurea (Hydrea, Droxia) **Uses:** *CML, head & neck, ovarian & colon CA, melanoma, acute leukemia, sickle cell anemia, polycythemia vera, HIV* **Action:** ↓ ribonucleotide reductase system **Dose:** *(per protocol) 50–75 mg/kg for WBC >100,000 cells/mL; 20–30 mg/kg in refractory CML. HIV:* 1000–1500 mg/d in single or ÷ doses; ↓ in renal insuff **Caution:** [D, –] ↑ effects w/ zidovudine, zalcitabine, didanosine, stavudine, fluorouracil **Contra:** Severe anemia, severe BM suppression, WBC <2500 or plt <100,000, PRG **Supplied:** Caps 200, 300, 400, 500 mg, tabs 1000 mg **SE:** Myelosuppression (primarily leukopenia), N/V, rashes, facial erythema, radiation recall Rxns, & renal dysfunction **Notes:** Capsules can be opened & emptied into H₂O

Hydroxyzine (Atarax, Vistaril) **Uses:** *Anxiety, sedation, itching* **Action:** Antihistamine, antianxiety **Dose:** *Adults. Anxiety or sedation:* 50–100 mg PO or IM qid or PRN (max 600 mg/d). *Itching:* 25–50 mg PO or IM tid–qid. *Peds.* 0.5–1.0 mg/kg/24 h PO or IM q6h; ↓ in hepatic failure **Caution:** [C, +/–] ↑ effects w/ CNS depressants, anticholinergics, EtOH **Contra:** Component sensitivity **Supplied:** Tabs 10, 25, 50, 100 mg; caps 25, 50, 100 mg; syrup 10 mg/5 mL; susp 25 mg/5 mL; inj 25, 50 mg/mL **SE:** Drowsiness & anticholinergic effects **Notes:** Useful to potentiate narcotics effects; not for IV/SQ (thrombosis & digital gangrene)

Hyoscyamine (Anaspaz, Cystospaz, Levsin, others) **Uses:** *Spasm associated w/ GI & bladder disorders* **Action:** Anticholinergic **Dose:**

Adults. 0.125–0.25 mg (1–2 tabs) SL/PO tid–qid, ac & hs; 1 SR cap q12h **Caution:** [C, +] ↑ effects w/ amantadine, antihistamines, antimuscarinics, haloperidol, phenothiazines, TCA, MAOI **Contra:** BOO, GI obstruction, glaucoma, MyG, paralytic ileus, severe ulcerative colitis, MI **Supplied:** (Cystospaz-M, Levsinex): cap timed release 0.375 mg; elixir (EtOH) soln 0.125 mg/5 mL; inj 0.5 mg/mL; tab 0.125 mg; tab (Cystospaz) 0.15 mg; XR tab (Levbid): 0.375 mg; SL (Levsin SL) 0.125 mg **SE:** Dry skin, xerostomia, constipation, anticholinergic SE, heat prostration may occur in hot weather **Notes:** Administer tabs before meals/food

Hyoscyamine, Atropine, Scopolamine, & Phenobarbital (Donnatal, others)
Uses: *Irritable bowel, spastic colitis, peptic ulcer, spastic bladder* **Action:** Anticholinergic, antispasmodic **Dose:** 0.125–0.25 mg (1–2 tabs) tid–qid, 1 cap q12h (SR), 5–10 mL elixir tid–qid or q8h **Contra:** [D, M] NA glaucoma **Supplied:** Many combos/manufacturers; *Cap* (Donnatal, others). Hyosc. 0.1037 mg/atropine 0.0194 mg/scop 0.0065 mg/phenobarbital 16.2 mg. *Tabs* (Donnatal, others): Hyosc. 0.1037 mg/atropine 0.0194 mg/scop 0.0065 mg/phenobarbital 16.2 mg. *Long-acting* (Donnatal): Hyosc. 0.311 mg/atropine 0.0582 mg/scop 0.0195 mg/phenobarbital 48.6 mg. *Elixirs* (Donnatal, others): Hyosc. 0.1037 mg/atropine 0.0194 mg/scop 0.0065 mg/phenobarbital 16.2 mg/5 mL **SE:** Sedation, xerostomia, constipation

Ibandronate (Boniva)
Uses: Rx & prevent osteoporosis in postmenopausal women **Action:** Bisphosphonate, ↓ osteoclast-mediated bone-resorption **Dose:** 2.5 mg PO qd or 150 mg once each month on the same day (do not lie down for 60 min after) **Caution:** [C, ?/–] avoid w/ CrCl < 30 mL/min **Contra:** Uncorrected ↓ Ca^{2+}; inability to stand/sit upright for 60 min **Supplied:** Tabs 2.5, 150 mg **SE:** N/D, HA, dizziness, asthenia, HTN, Infxn, dysphagia, esophagitis, esophageal/gastric ulcer, musculoskeletal pain, jaw osteonecrosis (avoid extensive dental procedures) **Notes:** Take 1st thing in AM w/ H_2O (6–8 oz) > 60 min before 1st food/beverage & any meds containing multivalent cations; adequate Ca^{2+} & vit D supls necessary

Ibuprofen (Motrin, Rufen, Advil, others) [OTC]
WARNING: May ↑ risk of cardiovascular events & GI bleeding **Uses:** *Arthritis, pain, fever* **Action:** NSAID **Dose:** *Adults.* 200–800 mg PO bid–qid (max 2.4 g/d); *Peds.* 30–40 mg/kg/d in 3–4 ÷ doses (max 40 mg/kg/d); w/ food **Caution:** [B, +] **Contra:** 3rd tri PRG severe hepatic impair, allergy & use w/ other NSAIDs, UGI bleed, ulcers **Supplied:** Tabs 100, 200, 400, 600, 800 mg; chew tabs 50, 100 mg; caps 200 mg; susp 100 mg/2.5 mL, 100 mg/5 mL, 40 mg/mL (200 mg is OTC preparation) **SE:** Dizziness, peptic ulcer, plt inhibition, worsening of renal insuff

Ibutilide (Corvert)
Uses: *Rapid conversion of AF/flutter* **Action:** Class III antiarrhythmic **Dose:** 0.01 mg/kg (max 1 mg) IV inf over 10 min; may repeat once **Caution:** [C, –] Do not use w/ class I or III antiarrhythmics or w/in 4 h of ibutilide **Contra:** QTc > 440 ms **Supplied:** Inj 0.1 mg/mL **SE:** Arrhythmias, HA **Notes:** Observe w/ continuous ECG monitoring

Idarubicin (Idamycin)
Uses: *Acute leukemias* (AML, ALL, ANLL), *CML in blast crisis, breast CA* **Action:** DNA intercalating agent; ↓ DNA topoi-

somerases I & II **Dose:** (per protocol) 10–12 mg/m²/d for 3–4 d; ↓ in renal/hepatic dysfunction **Caution:** [D, –] **Contra:** Bilirubin >5 mg/dL, PRG **Supplied:** Inj 1 mg/mL (5-, 10-, 20-mg vials) **SE:** Myelosuppression, cardiotox, N/V, mucositis, alopecia, & IV site Rxns, renal/hepatic Fxn **Notes:** Avoid extravasation—potent vesicant; only given IV

Ifosfamide (Ifex, Holoxan) **Uses:** Lung, breast, pancreatic & gastric CA, HL/NHL, soft tissue sarcoma **Action:** Alkylating agent **Dose:** (per protocol) 1.2 g/m²/d for 5 d by bolus or cont inf; 2.4 g/m²/d for 3 d; w/ mesna uroprotection; ↓ in renal/hepatic impair **Caution:** [D, M] ↑ effect w/ phenobarbital, carbamazepine, phenytoin; St. John's wort may ↓ levels **Contra:** ↓ BM Fxn, PRG **Supplied:** Inj 1, 3, g **SE:** Hemorrhagic cystitis, nephrotox, N/V, mild–moderate leukopenia, lethargy & confusion, alopecia, & ↑ hepatic enzyme **Notes:** Administer w/ mesna to prevent hemorrhagic cystitis

Iloprost (Ventavis) WARNING: Associated with syncope; may require dosage adjustment **Uses:** NYHA Class III/IV pulmonary arterial HTN * **Action:** Prostaglandin analog **Dose:** If initial 2.5 mcg tolerated, ↑ to 5 mcg inh 6–9 ×/d (at least 2 h apart) while awake **Caution:** [C, ?/–] Antiplatelet effects, ↑ bleeding risk w/anticoagulants; may have additive hypotensive effects **Contra:** SBP <85 mm Hg **Supplied:** In soln 10 mcg/mL **SE:** Syncope, ↓ BP, vasodilation, cough, HA, trismus **Notes:** Requires Pro-Dose AAD nebulizer; advise pt of syncope risk

Imatinib (Gleevec) **Uses:** *Rx of CML, blast crisis, gastrointestinal stromal tumors (GIST)* **Action:** ↓ BCL-ABL tyrosine kinase (signal transduction) **Dose:** *Chronic phase CML:* 400–600 mg PO qd. *Accelerated/blast crisis:* 600–800 mg PO qd. *GIST:* 400–600 mg PO qd **Caution:** [D, ?/–] w/CYP3A4 meds, warfarin, **Contra:** Component sensitivity **Supplied:** Caps 100 mg **SE:** GI upset, fluid retention, muscle cramps, musculoskeletal pain, arthralgia, rash, HA, neutropenia, thrombocytopenia **Notes:** Follow CBCs & LFTs baseline & monthly; administer w/ large glass of H₂O & food to ↓ GI irritation

Imipenem–Cilastatin (Primaxin) **Uses:** *Serious Infxns* caused by a wide variety of susceptible bacteria **Action:** Bactericidal; interferes with cell wall synthesis. **Spectrum:** Gram(+) (inactive against *S. aureus*, group A & B streptococci, gram(–) (not *Legionella*), anaerobes **Dose:** *Adults.* 250–1000 mg (imipenem) IV q6–8h. *Peds.* 60–100 mg/kg/24 h IV ÷ q6h; ↓ in renal Dz if calculated CrCl is <70 mL/min **Caution:** [C, +/–] Probenecid may ↑ tox **Contra:** Ped pts w/ CNS Infxn (↑ Sz risk) & <30 kg w/ renal impair **Supplied:** Inj (imipenem/cilastatin) 250/250 mg, 500/500 mg **SE:** Szs may occur if drug accumulates, GI upset, thrombocytopenia

Imipramine (Tofranil) **Uses:** *Depression, enuresis,* panic attack, chronic pain **Action:** TCA; ↑ synaptic conc of serotonin or norepinephrine in the CNS **Dose:** *Adults.* Hospitalized: Initial 100 mg/24 h PO in ÷ doses; can ↑ over several wks to max 300 mg/d. *Outpatient:* Maint 50–150 mg PO hs, 300 mg/24 h max. *Peds. Antidepressant:* 1.5–5 mg/kg/24 h ÷ qd–qid. *Enuresis:>6 y:* 10–25 mg PO qhs; ↑ by 10–25 mg at 1–2-wk intervals (max 50 mg for 6–12 y, 75 mg for >12 y);

treat for 2–3 mo, then taper **Caution:** [D, ?/–] **Contra:** Use with MAOIs, NA glaucoma, acute recovery phase of MI, PRG, CHF, angina, CVD, arrhythmias **Supplied:** Tabs 10, 25, 50 mg; caps 75, 100, 125, 150 mg **SE:** CV Sxs, dizziness, xerostomia, discolored urine **Notes:** Less sedation than with amitriptyline

Imiquimod Cream, 5% (Aldara) **Uses:** *Anogenital warts, HPV, condylomata acuminata* **Action:** Unknown; may induce cytokines **Dose:** Applied 3×/wk, leave on skin for 6–10 h & wash off with soap & water, continue therapy 16 wk max **Caution:** [B, ?] **Contra:** Component sensitivity **Supplied:** Single-dose packets 5% (250 mg cream) **SE:** Local skin reactions common **Notes:** Not a cure; may weaken condoms/vaginal diaphragms, wash hands before & after application

Immune Globulin, IV (Gamimune N, Sandoglobulin, Gammar IV) **Uses:** *IgG Ab deficiency Dz states, (eg, congenital agammaglobulinemia, CVH, & BMT), HIV, hepatitis A prophylaxis, ITP* **Action:** IgG supl **Dose:** *Adults & Peds.* *Immunodeficiency:* 100–200 mg/kg/mo IV at a rate of 0.01–0.04 mL/kg/min to a max of 400 mg/kg/dose. *ITP:* 400 mg/kg/dose IV qd × 5 d. *BMT:* 500 mg/kg/wk; ↓ in renal insuff **Caution:** [C, ?] Separate administration of live vaccines by 3 mo **Contra:** Isolated immunoglobulin A deficiency w/ Abs to IgA, severe thrombocytopenia or coagulation disorders **Supplied:** Inj **SE:** Adverse effects mostly with rate of inf, GI upset

Inamrinone [Amrinone] (Inocor) **Uses:** *Acute CHF, ischemic cardiomyopathy* **Action:** Positive inotrope w/ vasodilator **Dose:** IV bolus 0.75 mg/kg over 2–3 min. Maint 5–10 mcg/kg/min. 10 mg/kg/d max; ↓ if ClCr <10 mL/min **Caution:** [C, ?] **Contra:** Allergy to bisulfites **Supplied:** Inj 5 mg/mL **SE:** Monitor for fluid, electrolyte, & renal changes **Notes:** Incompatible w/ dextrose solns

Indapamide (Lozol) **Uses:** *HTN, edema, CHF* **Action:** Thiazide diuretic; ↑ Na, Cl, & H_2O excretion in the proximal segment of the distal tubule **Dose:** 1.25–5 mg/d PO **Caution:** [D, ?] ↑ effect w/ loop diuretics, ACE inhibitors, cyclosporine, digoxin, Li **Contra:** Anuria, thiazide/sulfonamide allergy, renal decompensation, PRG **Supplied:** Tabs 1.25, 2.5 mg **SE:** ↓ BP, dizziness, photosensitivity **Notes:** No additional effects on BP w/ doses >5 mg, take early to avoid nocturia; use sunscreen; OK w/ food/milk

Indinavir (Crixivan) **Uses:** *HIV Infxn* **Action:** Protease inhibitor; ↓ maturation of immature noninfectious virions to mature infectious virus **Dose:** 800 mg PO q8h; in combo w/ other antiretrovirals; on empty stomach; ↓ in hepatic impair **Caution:** [C, ?] Numerous drug interactions **Contra:** Concomitant use w/ triazolam, midazolam, pimozide, ergot alkaloids; not OK w/ simvastatin, lovastatin, sildenafil, St. John's wort **Supplied:** Caps 100, 200, 333, 400 mg **SE:** Nephrolithiasis, dyslipidemia, lipodystrophy, GI effects **Notes:** Drink six 8-oz glasses of H_2O/d

Indomethacin (Indocin) **WARNING:** May ↑ risk of cardiovascular events & GI bleeding **Uses:** *Arthritis; close ductus arteriosus; ankylosing spondylitis* **Action:** ↓ prostaglandins **Dose:** *Adults.* 25–50 mg PO bid–tid, max 200 mg/d. *Infants:* 0.2–0.25 mg/kg/dose IV; may repeat in 12–24 h up to 3 doses; w/ food

Caution: [B, +] **Contra:** ASA/NSAID sensitivity, peptic ulcer Dz/active GI bleed, precipitation of asthma/urticaria/rhinitis by NSAIDs/aspirin, premature neonates w/ NEC, ↓ renal Fxn, active bleeding, thrombocytopenia, 3rd tri PRG **Supplied:** Inj 1 mg/vial; caps 25, 50 mg; SR caps 75 mg; susp 25 mg/5 mL **SE:** GI bleeding or upset, dizziness, edema **Notes:** Monitor renal Fxn

Infliximab (Remicade) **WARNING:** TB, invasive fungal Infxns, & other opportunistic Infxns reported, some fatal; perform TB skin testing prior to therapy **Uses:** *Moderate–severe Crohn Dz; fistulizing Crohn Dz; RA (w/ MTX), ulcerative colitis* **Action:** IgG1K neutralizes TNFα (human & murine regions) **Dose:** *Crohn Dz: Induction:* 5 mg/kg IV inf, w/doses 2 & 6 wk after. *Maint:* 5 mg/kg IV inf q8wk. *RA:* 3 mg/kg IV inf at 0, 2, 6 wk, then q8wk **Caution:** [B, ?/–] Active Infxn, hepatic insult **Contra:** Murine allergy, moderate–severe CHF **Supplied:** Inj **SE:** Allergic Rxns; pts predisposed to Infxn (especially TB); HA, fatigue, GI upset, infusion Rxns; hepatotoxicity or reactivation hepatitis B, monitor LFTs, pneumonia, BM suppression, systemic vasculitis, pericardial effusion

Influenza Vaccine (Fluzone, FluShield, Fluvirin) **Uses:** *Prevent influenza*; all adults >50 y, children 6–23 mo, pregnant women (2nd/3rd tri during flu season), nursing home residents, chronic Dzs, health care workers & household contacts of high-risk pts, children < 9 y receiving vaccine for the first time **Action:** Active immunization **Dose:** *Adults.* 0.5 mL/dose IM. *Peds.* ≥ 3 y: 0.5 mL IM; 6–35 mo 0.25 mL IM; *6 mo to < 9 y* (first-time vaccination): 2 doses > 4 wk apart, 2nd dose before Dec if possible **Caution:** [C, +] **Contra:** Egg, gentamicin, or thimerosal allergy, Infxn at site; high risk of influenza complications, Hx of Guillain–Barré, asthma, children 5–17 y on aspirin **Supplied:** Based on specific manufacturer, 0.25- & 0.5-mL prefilled syringes **SE:** Soreness at site, fever, myalgia, malaise, Guillain–Barré syndrome (controversial) **Notes:** Optimal in U.S.: Oct–Nov, protection begins 1–2 wk after, lasts up to 6 mo; each yr, vaccines based on predictions of flu active in flu season (December–Spring in U.S.); whole or split virus for adults; Peds <13 y split virus or purified surface antigen to ↓ febrile Rxns

Influenza Virus Vaccine Live, Intranasal (FluMist) **Uses:** *Prevent influenza* **Action:** Live-attenuated vaccine **Dose:** *Adults 9–49 y.* 1 dose (0.5 mL)/season **Caution:** [C,?/–] **Contra:** Egg allergy, PRG, Hx Guillain–Barré syndrome, known/suspected immune deficiency, asthma or reactive airway Dz **Supplied:** Prefilled, single-use, intranasal sprayer **SE:** Runny nose, nasal congestion, HA, cough **Notes:** 0.25 mL into each nostril; do not administer concurrently w/ other vaccines; avoid contact w/ immunocompromised individuals for 21 days

Insulin **Uses:** *Type 1 or type 2 DM refractory to diet or PO hypoglycemic agents; acute life-threatening ↑ K+* **Action:** Insulin supl **Dose:** Based on serum glucose; usually SQ; can give IV (only regular)/IM; type 1 MTX usual start dose 0.5–1 units/kg/d; type 2 0.3–0.4 Units/kg/d; renal failure may ↓ insulin needs **Caution:** [B, +] **Contra:** Hypoglycemia **Supplied:** Table 6, (page 210) **SE:** Highly purified insulins ↑ free insulin; monitor for several wks when changing doses/agents

Interferon Alfa (Roferon-A, Intron A) Uses: *Hairy cell leukemia, Kaposi sarcoma, melanoma, CML, chronic hepatitis C, follicular NHL, condylomata acuminata,* multiple myeloma, renal cell carcinoma, & bladder CA **Action:** Antiproliferative against tumor cells; modulates host immune response **Dose:** Per protocols. *Adults.* Hairy cell leukemia: Alfa-2a (Roferon-A): 3 M units/d for 16–24 wk SQ/IM. Alfa-2b (Intron A): 2 M units/m² IM/ SQ 3×/wk for 2–6 mo *Peds. CML:* Alfa-2a (Roferon-A): 2.5–5 M units/m² IM qd. *Chronic hepatitis B:* Alfa-2b (Intron A): 3–10 M units/m² SQ 3×/wk **Contra:** Benzyl alcohol sensitivity, decompensated liver Dz, autoimmune Dz, rapidly progressing AIDS-related Kaposi sarcoma **Supplied:** Injectable forms **SE:** Flu-like Sxs; fatigue; anorexia in 20–30%; neurotox at high doses; neutralizing Ab in up to 40% of pts receiving prolonged systemic therapy

Interferon Alfa-2b & Ribavirin Combo (Rebetron) WARNING: Contraindicated in pregnant females & their male partners Uses: *Chronic hepatitis C in pts w/ compensated liver Dz who have relapsed following α-interferon therapy* **Action:** Combo antiviral agents **Dose:** 3 M units Intron A SQ 3×/wk w/ 1000–1200 mg of Rebetron PO ÷ bid dose for 24 wk. *Pts <75 kg:* 1000 mg of Rebetron/d **Caution:** [X, ?] **Contra:** PRG, males w/ PRG female partner, autoimmune hepatitis, creatinine clearance < 50 mL/min **Supplied:** *Pts <75 kg:* Combo packs: 6 vials Intron A (3 M units/0.5 mL) w/ 6 syringes & EtOH swabs, 70 Rebetron caps; one 18 M units multidose vial of Intron A inj (22.8 M units/3.8 mL; 3 M units/0.5 mL) & 6 syringes & swabs, 70 Rebetron caps; one 18 M units Intron A inj multidose pen (22.5 M units/1.5 mL; 3 M units/0.2 mL) w/ 6 needles & swabs, 70 Rebetron caps. *Pts <75 kg:* Identical except 84 Rebetron caps/pack **SE:** Flu-like syndrome, HA, anemia **Notes:** Negative PRG test required monthly; instruct pts in self-administration of SQ Intron A

Interferon Alfacon-1 (Infergen) Uses: *Chronic hepatitis C* **Action:** Biologic response modifier **Dose:** 9 mcg SQ 3×/wk × 24 wk **Caution:** [C, M] **Contra:** Allergy to E. coli-derived products **Supplied:** Inj 9, 15 mcg **SE:** Flu-like syndrome, depression, blood dyscrasias **Notes:** Allow > 48 h between inj

Interferon β-1b (Betaseron) Uses: *MS, relapsing-remitting & secondary progressive* **Action:** Biologic response modifier **Dose:** 0.25 mg SQ qod **Caution:** [C, ?] **Contra:** Allergy to human albumin products **Supplied:** Powder for inj 0.3 mg **SE:** Flu-like syndrome, depression, blood dyscrasias; monitor LFTs

Interferon γ-1b (Actimmune) Uses: *↓ Incidence of serious Infxns in chronic granulomatous Dz (CGD), osteopetrosis* **Action:** Biologic response modifier **Dose:** *Adults. CGD:* 50 mcg/m² SQ (1.5 million units/m²) BSA >0.5 m²; if BSA <0.5 m², give 1.5 mcg/kg/dose; given 3×/wk. *Peds.* BSA ≤ 0.5 m²: 1.5 mcg/kg SQ tid; BSA > 0.5 m²: 50 mcg/m² SQ tid **Caution:** [C, ?] **Contra:** Allergy to E. coli-derived products **Supplied:** Inj 100 mcg (2 million units) **SE:** Flu-like syndrome, depression, blood dyscrasias

Ipecac Syrup [OTC] Uses: *Drug OD, certain cases of poisoning* **NOTE:** Usage is falling out of favor & is no longer recommended by some groups **Action:**

Irritation of the GI mucosa; stimulation of the chemoreceptor trigger zone **Dose:** *Adults.* 15–30 mL PO, followed by 200–300 mL of H_2O; if no emesis in 20 min, repeat once. *Peds. 6–12 y:* 5–10 mL PO, followed by 10–20 mL/kg of H_2O; if no emesis in 20 min, repeat once. *1–12 y:* 15 mL PO followed by 10–20 mL/kg of H_2O; if no emesis in 20 min, repeat once **Caution:** [C, ?] **Contra:** Ingestion of petroleum distillates, strong acid, base, or other caustic agents; comatose/ unconscious **Supplied:** Syrup 15, 30 mL (OTC) **SE:** Lethargy, D, cardiotox, protracted vomiting **Notes:** Caution in CNS depressant OD; (www.clintox.org/ Pos_Statements/Ipecac.html)

Ipratropium (Atrovent) Uses: *Bronchospasm w/ COPD, rhinitis, rhinorrhea* **Action:** Synthetic anticholinergic similar to atropine **Dose:** *Adults & Peds >12 y.* 2–4 puffs qid. *Nasal:* 2 sprays/nostril bid–tid **Caution:** [B, +/–] **Contra:** Allergy to soya lecithin/related foods **Supplied:** Met-dose inhaler 18 mcg/dose; inhal soln 0.02%; nasal spray 0.03%, 0.06%; nasal inhaler 20 mcg/dose **SE:** Nervousness, dizziness, HA, cough, bitter taste, nasal dryness **Notes:** Not for acute bronchospasm

Irbesartan (Avapro) Uses: *HTN*, DN, CHF **Action:** Angiotensin II receptor antagonist **Dose:** 150 mg/d PO, may ↑ to 300 mg/d **Caution:** [C (1st tri; D 2nd/3rd), ?/–] **Supplied:** Tabs 75, 150, 300 mg **SE:** Fatigue, ↓ BP

Irinotecan (Camptosar) Uses: *Colorectal* & lung CA **Action:** Topoisomerase I inhibitor; ↓DNA synthesis **Dose:** Per protocol; 125–350 mg/m² qwk–q3wk (↓ hepatic dysfunction, as tolerated per tox) **Caution:** [D, –] **Contra:** Allergy to component **Supplied:** Inj 20 mg/mL **SE:** Myelosuppression, N/V/D, abdominal cramping, alopecia; D is dose-limiting; Rx acute D w/ atropine; Rx subacute D w/ loperamide **Notes:** D correlated to levels of metabolite SN-38

Iron Dextran (Dexferrum, INFeD) Uses: *Fe deficiency when cannot supplement PO* **Action:** Fe supl **Dose:** Estimate Fe deficiency, give IM/IV. A 0.5-mL test dose; total replacement dose (mL) = $0.0476 \times$ weight (kg) $\times$ [desired Hgb (g/dL) − measured Hgb (g/dL)] + 1 mL/5 kg weight (max 14 mL). *Adults. Max daily dose:* 100 mg Fe. *Peds.* Max daily dose: *<5 kg:* 25 mg Fe. *5–10 kg:* 50 mg Fe. *10–50 kg:* 100 mg Fe **Caution:** [C, M] **Contra:** Anemia w/o Fe deficiency. **Supplied:** Inj 50 mg (Fe)/mL **SE:** Anaphylaxis, flushing, dizziness, inj site & inf Rxns, metallic taste **Notes:** Give deep IM using "Z-track" technique; IV preferred

Iron Sucrose (Venofer) Uses: *Fe deficiency anemia w/chronic HD in those receiving erythropoietin* **Actions:** Fe replacement. **Dose:** 5 mL (100 mg) IV during dialysis, 1 mL (20 mg)/min max. **Caution:** [C, M] **Contra:** Anemia w/o Fe deficiency **Supplied:** 20 mg elemental Fe per mL, 5-mL vials. **SE:** Anaphylaxis, ↓ BP, cramps, N/V/D, HA **Notes:** Most pts require cumulative doses of 1000 mg; ensure administration at slow rate

Isoniazid (INH) Uses: *Rx & prophylaxis of TB* **Action:** Bactericidal; interferes w/ mycolic acid synthesis, disrupts cell wall **Dose:** *Adults. Active TB:* 5 mg/kg/24 h PO or IM (usually 300 mg/d). *Prophylaxis:* 300 mg/d PO for 6–12

mo. **Peds.** *Active TB:* 10–20 mg/kg/24 h PO or IM 300 mg/d max. *Prophylaxis:* 10 mg/kg/24 h PO; ↓ in hepatic/renal dysfunction **Caution:** [C, +] Liver Dz, dialysis; avoid EtOH **Contra:** Acute liver Dz, Hx INH hepatitis **Supplied:** Tabs 100, 300 mg; syrup 50 mg/5 mL; inj 100 mg/mL **SE:** Hepatitis, peripheral neuropathy, GI upset, anorexia, dizziness, skin Rxn **Notes:** Give w/ 2–3 other drugs for active TB, based on INH resistance patterns when TB acquired & sensitivity results; prophylaxis usually w/ INH alone. IM rarely used. ↓ Peripheral neuropathy w/ pyridoxine 50–100 mg/d. Check CDC guidelines (in MMWR) for current recommendations

Isoproterenol (Isuprel) Uses: *Shock, bronchospasm, cardiac arrest, AV nodal block* **Action:** β₁- & β₂-receptor stimulant **Dose:** *Adults.* 2–10 mcg/min IV inf; titrate to effect. *Inhal:* 1–2 inhal 4–6×/d. *Peds.* 0.2–2 mcg/kg/min IV inf; titrate to effect. *Inhal:* 1–2 inhal 4–6×/d **Caution:** [C, ?] **Contra:** Angina, tachyarrhythmias (digitalis-induced or others) **Supplied:** Met-inhaler; soln for neb 0.5%, 1%; inj 0.02 mg/mL, 0.2 mg/mL **SE:** Insomnia, arrhythmias, HA, trembling, dizziness **Notes:** Pulse > 130 bpm may induce arrhythmias

Isosorbide Dinitrate (Isordil, Sorbitrate, Dilatrate-SR) Uses: *Rx & prevent angina,* CHF (w/ hydralazine) **Action:** Relaxes vascular smooth muscle **Dose:** *Acute angina:* 5–10 mg PO (chew tabs) q2–3h or 2.5–10 mg SL PRN q5–10min; do not give >3 doses in a 15–30-min period. *Angina prophylaxis:* 5–40 mg PO q6h; do not give nitrates on a chronic q6h or qid basis >7–10 d; tolerance may develop; provide 10–12-h drug-free intervals **Caution:** [C, ?] **Contra:** Severe anemia, closed-angle glaucoma, postural ↓ BP, cerebral anemia, head trauma (can ↑ ICP), w/ sildenafil, tadalafil, vardenafil **Supplied:** Tabs 5, 10, 20, 30, 40 mg; SR tabs 40 mg; SL tabs 2.5, 5, 10 mg; chew tabs 5, 10 mg; SR caps 40 mg **SE:** HA, ↓ BP, flushing, tachycardia, dizziness **Notes:** Higher PO dose usually needed to achieve same results as SL forms

Isosorbide Mononitrate (Ismo, Imdur) Uses: *Prevention/Rx of angina pectoris* **Action:** Relaxes vascular smooth muscle **Dose:** 20 mg PO bid, w/ the 2 doses 7 h apart or XR (Imdur) 30–120 mg/d PO **Caution:** [C, ?] **Contra:** Head trauma/cerebral hemorrhage (can ↑ ICP), w/ sildenafil, tadalafil, vardenafil **Supplied:** Tabs 10, 20 mg; XR 30, 60, 120 mg **SE:** HA, dizziness, ↓ BP

Isotretinoin [13-*cis* Retinoic Acid] (Accutane, Amnesteem, Claravis, Sotret) WARNING: Must not be used by PRG females; can induce severe birth defects; pt must be capable of complying w/ mandatory contraceptive measures; prescribed according to product-specific risk management system. Because of teratogenicity, Accutane is approved for marketing only under a special restricted distribution FDA program called iPLEDGE Uses: *Refractory severe acne* **Action:** Retinoic acid derivative **Dose:** 0.5–2 mg/kg/d PO ÷ bid (↓ in hepatic Dz, take w/ food) **Caution:** [X, –] Avoid tetracyclines **Contra:** Retinoid sensitivity, PRG **Supplied:** Caps 10, 20, 40 mg **SE:** Rare: Depression, psychosis, suicidal thoughts; dermatologic sensitivity, xerostomia, photosensitivity, ↑ LFTs, ↑ triglycerides **Notes:** Risk management program requires 2 (–) PRG tests before Rx

& use of 2 forms of contraception 1 mo before, during, & 1 mo after therapy; to prescribe isotretinoin, the Prescriber must access the iPLEDGE system via the Internet (www.ipledgeprogram.com); monitor LFTs & lipids

Isradipine (DynaCirc) Uses: *HTN* Action: CCB Dose: *Adults.* 2.5–10 mg PO bid. *Peds.* 0.05–0.15 mg/kg PO tid–qid, up to 20 mg/d (do not crush or chew) Caution: [C, ?] Contra: Severe heart block, sinus bradycardia, CHF, dosing w/in several hours of IV β-blockers Supplied: Caps 2.5, 5 mg; tabs CR 5, 10 mg SE: HA, edema, flushing, fatigue, dizziness, palpitations

Itraconazole (Sporanox) WARNING: Potential for negative inotropic effects on the heart; if signs or Sxs of CHF occur during administration, continued use should be assessed Uses: *Fungal Infxns (aspergillosis, blastomycosis, histoplasmosis, candidiasis)* Action: ↓ Synthesis of ergosterol Dose: 200 mg PO or IV qd–bid (capsule w/ meals or cola/grapefruit juice); PO soln on empty stomach; avoid antacids Caution: [C, ?] Numerous drug interactions Contra: CrCl <30 mL/min, Hx of CHF or ventricular dysfunction, or w/ H_2-antagonist, omeprazole Supplied: Caps 100 mg; soln 10 mg/mL; inj 10 mg/mL SE: Nausea, rash, hepatitis, ↓ K^+, CHF Notes: PO soln & caps not interchangeable; useful in pts who cannot take amphotericin B; watch for s/Sxs of CHF w/ IV use

Kaolin-Pectin (Kaodene, Kao-Spen, Kapectolin, Parepectolin) [OTC] Uses: *Diarrhea* Action: Absorbent demulcent Dose: *Adults.* 60–120 mL PO after each loose stool or q3–4h PRN. *Peds. 3–6 y:* 15–30 mL/dose PO PRN. *6–12 y:* 30–60 mL/dose PO PRN Caution: [C, +] Contra: D secondary to pseudomembranous colitis Supplied: Multiple OTC forms; also available w/ opium (Parepectolin) SE: Constipation, dehydration

Ketoconazole (Nizoral, Nizoral AD Shampoo) [Shampoo–OTC] Uses: *Systemic fungal Infxns; topical for local fungal Infxns due to dermatophytes & yeast; shampoo for dandruff;* short term in CAP when rapid ↓ testosterone needed (ie, cord compression) Action: ↓ fungal cell wall synthesis Dose: *Adults. PO:* 200 mg PO qd; ↑ to 400 mg PO qd for serious Infxn; CAP 400 mg PO tid (short-term). *Topical:* Apply qd (cream/shampoo). *Peds >2 y.* 5–10 mg/kg/24 h PO ÷ q12–24h (↓ in hepatic Dz) Caution: [C, +/–] Any agent ↑ gastric pH decreases absorption; may enhance anticoagulants; w/ EtOH (disulfiram-like Rxn) numerous drug interactions Contra: CNS fungal Infxns (poor CNS penetration), concurrent astemizole, cisapride, PO triazolam Supplied: Tabs 200 mg; topical cream 2%; shampoo 2% SE: Monitor LFTs w/ systemic use; can cause nausea

Ketoprofen (Orudis, Oruvail) WARNING: May ↑ risk of cardiovascular events & GI bleeding Uses: *Arthritis, pain* Action: NSAID; ↓ prostaglandins Dose: 25–75 mg PO tid–qid, 300 mg/d/max; w/ food Caution [B (D 3rd tri), ?] Contra: NSAID/ASA sensitivity Supplied: Tabs 12.5 mg; caps 25, 50, 75 mg; caps, SR 100, 150, 200 mg SE: GI upset, peptic ulcers, dizziness, edema, rash

Ketorolac (Toradol) WARNING: Indicated for short term (≥ 5 d) Rx of moderate–severe acute pain that requires opioid analgesia levels Uses: *Pain* Action: NSAID; ↓ prostaglandins **Dose:** 15–30 mg IV/IM q6h or 10 mg PO qid; max IV/IM 120 mg/d, max PO 40 mg/d; do not use for > 5 d; ↓ for age & renal dysfunction **Caution:** [B (D 3rd tri), –] **Contra:** Peptic ulcer Dz, NSAID sensitivity, advanced renal Dz, CNS bleeding, anticipated major surgery, labor & delivery, nursing mothers **Supplied:** Tabs 10 mg; inj 15 mg/mL, 30 mg/mL **SE:** Bleeding, peptic ulcer Dz, renal failure, edema, dizziness, allergy **Notes:** PO only as continuation of IM/IV therapy

Ketorolac Ophthalmic (Acular) **Uses:** *Ocular itching w/ seasonal allergies* **Action:** NSAID **Dose:** 1 gt qid **Caution:** [C, +] **Supplied:** Soln 0.5% **SE:** Local irritation

Ketotifen (Zaditor) **Uses:** *Allergic conjunctivitis* **Action:** H₁-receptor antagonist, mast cell stabilizer **Dose:** *Adults & Peds.* 1 gt in eye(s) q8–12h **Caution:** [C,?/–] **Supplied:** Soln 0.025%/5 mL **SE:** Local irritation, HA, rhinitis

Labetalol (Trandate, Normodyne) **Uses:** *HTN* & hypertensive emergencies* **Action:** α- & β-Adrenergic blocking agent **Dose:** *Adults. HTN:* Initial, 100 mg PO bid, then 200–400 mg PO bid. *Hypertensive emergency:* 20–80 mg IV bolus, then 2 mg/min IV inf, titrate. *Peds. PO:* 3–20 mg/kg/d in ÷ doses. *Hypertensive emergency:* 0.4–1.5 mg/kg/h IV cont inf **Caution:** [C (D in 2nd or 3rd tri), +] **Contra:** Asthma/COPD, cardiogenic shock, uncompensated CHF, heart block **Supplied:** Tabs 100, 200, 300 mg; inj 5 mg/mL **SE:** Dizziness, nausea, ↓ BP, fatigue, CV effects

Lactic Acid & Ammonium Hydroxide [Ammonium Lactate] (Lac-Hydrin) **Uses:** *Severe xerosis & ichthyosis* **Action:** Emollient moisturizer **Dose:** Apply bid **Caution:** [B, ?] **Supplied:** Lactic acid 12% w/ ammonium hydroxide **SE:** Local irritation

Lactobacillus (Lactinex Granules) [OTC] **Uses:** Control of D, especially after antibiotic therapy **Action:** Replaces nl intestinal flora **Dose:** *Adults & Peds >3 y.* 1 packet, 2 caps, or 4 tabs PO tid–qid (w/ meals or liq) **Caution:** [A, +] **Contra:** Milk/lactose allergy **Supplied:** Tabs; caps; EC caps; powder in packets (all OTC) **SE:** Flatulence

Lactulose (Chronulac, Cephulac, Enulose) **Uses:** *Hepatic encephalopathy; constipation* **Action:** Acidifies the colon, allows ammonia to diffuse into colon **Dose:** *Acute hepatic encephalopathy:* 30–45 mL PO q1h until soft stools, then tid–qid. *Chronic laxative therapy:* 30–45 mL PO tid–qid; adjust q1–2d to produce 2–3 soft stools/d. *Rectally:* 200 g in 700 mL of H₂O PR. *Peds. Infants:* 2.5–10 mL/24 h ÷ tid–qid. *Peds:* 40–90 mL/24 h ÷ tid–qid **Caution:** [B, ?] **Contra:** Galactosemia **Supplied:** Syrup 10 g/15 mL, soln 10 g/15 mL, 10 g/packet **SE:** Severe D, flatulence; life-threatening electrolyte disturbances

Lamivudine (Epivir, Epivir-HBV) **WARNING:** Lactic acidosis & severe hepatomegaly w/ steatosis reported w/ nucleoside analogs **Uses:** *HIV Infxn, chronic hepatitis B* **Action:** ↓ HIV RT & hepatitis B viral polymerase, resulting in viral DNA chain termination **Dose:** *HIV: Adults & Peds >12 y.* 150 mg PO bid.

Peds <12 y. 4 mg/kg PO bid. *HBV: Adults.* 100 mg/d PO. *Peds 2–17 y.* 3 mg/kg/d PO, 100 mg max; ↓ in renal impair **Caution:** [C, ?] **Contra:** Component hypersensitivity **Supplied:** Tabs 100, 150 mg (HBV); soln 5 mg/mL, 10 mg/mL **SE:** HA, pancreatitis, anemia, GI upset, lactic acidosis

Lamotrigine (Lamictal)   WARNING: Serious rashes requiring hospitalization & D/C of Rx reported; rash less frequent in adults

Uses: *Partial Szs, bipolar disorder, Lennox–Gastaut syndrome* **Action:** Phenyltriazine antiepileptic **Dose: *Adults.*** *Szs:* Initial 50 mg/d PO, then 50 mg PO bid for 2 wk, then maint 300–500 mg/d in 2 ÷ doses. *Bipolar:* Initial 25 mg/d PO, then 50 mg PO qd for 2 wk, then 100 mg PO qd for 1 wk; Maint 200 mg/d. *Peds.* 0.15 mg/kg in 1–2 ÷ doses for wk 1 & 2, then 0.3 mg/kg for wk 3 & 4, then Maint 1 mg/kg/d in 1–2 ÷ (↓ in hepatic Dz or if w/ enzyme inducers or valproic acid) **Caution:** [C, –] Interactions w/ other antiepileptics **Supplied:** Tabs 25, 100, 150, 200 mg; chew tabs 5, 25 mg **SE:** Photosensitivity; HA, GI upset, dizziness, ataxia, rash (potentially life-threatening in children > adults) **Notes:** Value of therapeutic monitoring not established

Lansoprazole (Prevacid, Prevacid IV)   Uses: *Duodenal ulcers, prevent & Rx NSAID gastric ulcers, IV alternative for ≤ 7 d /w erosive esophagitis.* *H. pylori* Infxn, erosive esophagitis, & hypersecretory conditions **Action:** Proton pump inhibitor **Dose:** 15–30 mg/d PO; NSAID ulcer prevention 15 mg/d PO ≤ 12 wk, NSAID ulcers 30 mg/d PO, ×8 wk; 30 mg IV qd ≤ 7 d change to PO for 6–8 wk; ↓ in severe hepatic impair **Caution:** [B, ?/–] **Supplied:** Caps 15, 30 mg; inj set w/ filter **SE:** HA, fatigue **Notes:** For IV provided in-line filter must be used

Lanthanum Carbonate (Fosrenol)   Uses: Hyperphosphatemia in renal disease * **Action:** Phosphate binder **Dose:** 750–1500 mg PO qd ÷ doses, w/ or immed after meal; titrate every 2–3 wk based on PO_4^{-2} levels **Caution:** [C, ?/–], no data in GI disease **Supplied:** Chew tabs 250, 500 mg **SE:** N/V, graft occlusion **Notes:** Chew tabs before swallowing; separate from meds that interact with antacids by 2 h

Latanoprost (Xalatan)   Uses: *Refractory glaucoma* **Action:** Prostaglandin **Dose:** 1 gt eye(s) hs **Caution:** [C, ?] **Supplied:** 0.005% soln **SE:** May darken light irides; blurred vision, ocular stinging, & itching

Leflunomide (Arava)   WARNING: PRG must be excluded prior to start of Rx

Uses: *Active RA* **Action:** ↓ Pyrimidine synthesis **Dose:** Initial 100 mg/d PO for 3 d, then 10–20 mg/d **Caution:** [X, –] **Contra:** PRG **Supplied:** Tabs 10, 20, 100 mg **SE:** Monitor LFTs during initial therapy; D, Infxn, HTN, alopecia, rash, nausea, joint pain, hepatitis

Lepirudin (Refludan)   Uses: *HIT* **Action:** Direct thrombin inhibitor **Dose:** Bolus 0.4 mg/kg IV, then 0.15 mg/kg inf (↓ dose & inf rate if CrCl <60 mL/min) **Caution:** [B, ?/–] Hemorrhagic event or severe HTN **Contra:** Active bleeding **Supplied:** Inj 50 mg **SE:** Bleeding, anemia, hematoma **Notes:** Adjust dose based on aPTT ratio, maintain aPTT ratio of 1.5–2.0

Letrozole (Femara) Uses: *Advanced breast CA* **Action:** Nonsteroidal aromatase inhibitor **Dose:** 2.5 mg/d PO **Caution:** [D, ?] **Contra:** PRG **Supplied:** Tabs 2.5 mg **SE:** Requires periodic CBC, thyroid Fxn, electrolyte, LFT, & renal monitoring; anemia, nausea, hot flashes, arthralgia

Leucovorin (Wellcovorin) Uses: *OD of folic acid antagonist; augmentation of 5-FU, impaired MTX elimination* **Action:** Reduced folate source; circumvents action of folate reductase inhibitors (eg, MTX) **Dose:** *Adults & Peds. MTX rescue:* 10 mg/m²/dose IV or PO q6h for 72 h until MTX level <10⁻⁸. *5-FU:* 200 mg/m²/d IV 1–5 d during daily 5-FU Rx or 500 mg/m²/wk w/ weekly 5-FU therapy. *Adjunct to antimicrobials:* 5–15 mg/d PO **Caution:** [C, ?/–] **Contra:** Pernicious anemia **Supplied:** Tabs 5, 15, 25 mg; inj **SE:** Allergic Rxn, N/V/D, fatigue **Notes:** Many dosing schedules for leucovorin rescue following MTX therapy; do not use intrathecally/intraventrically

Leuprolide (Lupron, Lupron DEPOT, Lupron DEPOT-Ped, Viadur, Eligard) Uses: *Advanced CAP (all products), endometriosis (Lupron), uterine fibroids (Lupron), & CPP (Lupron-Ped)* **Action:** LHRH agonist; paradoxically ↓ release of gonadotropin, resulting in ↓ pituitary gonadotropins (↓ LH) in men ↓ testosterone **Dose:** *Adults. CAP:* 7.5 mg IM q28d or 22.5 mg IM q3mo or 30 mg IM q4mo of depot; 45 mg SQ 6 mo (Eligard) Viadur implant (CAP only); insert in inner upper arm using local anesthesia, replace q12mo. *Endometriosis (Lupron DEPOT):* 3.75 mg IM qmo ×6. *Fibroids:* 3.75 mg IM qmo ×3. *Peds. CPP (Lupron-Ped):* 50 mcg/kg/d SQ inj; ↑ by 10 mcg/kg/d until total down-regulation achieved. *DEPOT: <25 kg:* 7.5 mg IM q4wk. *>25–37.5 kg:* 11.25 mg IM q4wk. *>37.5 kg:* 15 mg IM q4wk **Caution:** [X, ?] PRG **Caution:** Undiagnosed vaginal bleeding, implant dosage form in women & peds; PRG **Supplied:** Inj 5 mg/mL; Lupron DEPOT 3.75 (1 mo for fibroids, endometriosis); Lupron DEPOT for CAP: 7.5 mg (1 mo), 22.5 (3 mo), 30 mg (4 mo); Eligard depot for CAP: 7.5 mg (1 mo); 45 mg (6 mo); Viadur 12-mo SQ implant, Lupron-Ped 7.5, 11.25, 15 mg **SE:** Hot flashes, gynecomastia, N/V, alopecia, anorexia, dizziness, HA, insomnia, paresthesias, depression exacerbation, peripheral edema, & bone pain (transient "flare Rxn" at 7–14 d after the 1st dose [LH/testosterone surge before suppression]) **Notes:** Nonsteroidal antiandrogen can block flare

Levalbuterol (Xopenex) Uses: *Asthma (Rx & prevention of bronchospasm)* **Action:** Sympathomimetic bronchodilator **Dose:** 0.63 mg neb q6–8h **Caution:** [C, ?] **Supplied:** Soln for inhal 0.63, 1.25 mg/3 mL **SE:** Tachycardia, nervousness, trembling, flu syndrome **Notes:** *R*-isomer of albuterol; potential for lower incidence of CV side effects compared with albuterol

Levamisole (Ergamisol) Uses: *Adjuvant therapy of Dukes C colon CA (in combo w/ 5-FU)* **Action:** Immunostimulatory **Dose:** 50 mg PO q8h for 3 d q14d during 5-FU; ↓ in hepatic dysfunction **Caution:** [C, ?/–] **Supplied:** Tabs 50 mg **SE:** N/V/D, abdominal pain, taste disturbance, anorexia, hyperbilirubinemia, disulfiram-like Rxn on EtOH ingestion, minimal BM supression, fatigue, fever, conjunctivitis

Levetiracetam (Keppra) Uses: *Partial onset Szs* **Action:** Unknown **Dose:** *Adults.* 500 mg PO bid, may ↑ 3000 mg/d max; *Peds. 4–16 y:* 10–20 mg/kg/d ÷ in 2 doses, 60 mg/kg/d max (↓ in renal insuff) **Caution:** [C, ?/–] **Contra:** Component allergy **Supplied:** Tabs 250, 500, 750 mg **SE:** Dizziness & somnolence; impaired coordination

Levobunolol (A-K Beta, Betagan) Uses:* Glaucoma* **Action:** β-Adrenergic blocker **Dose:** 1–2 gtt/d 0.5% or 1–2 gtt 0.25% bid **Caution:** [C, ?] **Supplied:** Soln 0.25, 0.5% **SE:** Ocular stinging or burning **Notes:** Possible systemic effects if absorbed

Levocabastine (Livostin) Uses: *Allergic seasonal conjunctivitis* **Action:** Antihistamine **Dose:** 1 gt in eye(s) qid ≤ 4 wk **Caution:** [C, +/–] **Supplied:** 0.05% gtt **SE:** Ocular discomfort

Levofloxacin (Levaquin, Quixin & Iquix Ophthalmic) Uses: *Lower resp tract Infxns, sinusitis, UTI; topical for bacterial conjunctivitis, skin Infxns* **Action:** Quinolone antibiotic, ↓ DNA gyrase. *Spectrum:* Excellent gram(+) except MRSA & *E. faecium;* excellent gram(–) except *S. maltophilia* & *Acinetobacter* sp; poor anaerobic **Dose:** 250–500 mg PO or IV; community acquired pneumonia 750 mg/day for 5 d; ophth 1–2 gtt in eye(s) q2h while awake for 2 d, then q4h while awake for 5 d; ↓ in renal insuff, avoid antacids if PO **Caution:** [C, –] Interactions w/ cation-containing products (eg, antacids) **Contra:** Quinolone sensitivity **Supplied:** Tabs 250, 500 mg; premixed IV 250, 500 mg; Leva-Pak 750 mg × 5 d; ophth soln 0.5% (Quixin), 1.5% (Iquix) **SE:** N/D, dizziness, rash, GI upset, photosensitivity

Levonorgestrel (Plan B) Uses: *Emergency contraceptive ("morning-after pill")*; prevents PRG if taken < 72 h after unprotected sex/contraceptive fails **Action:** Progestin **Dose:** 1 pill q12h × 2 **Caution:** [X, M] **Contra:** Known/suspected PRG, abnormal uterine bleeding **Supplied:** Tab, 0.75 mg, 2 blister pack **SE:** N/V, abdominal pain, fatigue, HA, menstrual changes. **Notes:** Will not induce abortion; ↑ risk of ectopic PRG

Levonorgestrel Implant (Norplant) Uses: * Contraceptive* **Action:** Progestin **Dose:** Implant 6 caps in midforearm **Caution:** [X, +/–] **Contra:** Undiagnosed abnormal uterine bleeding, Hepatic Dz, thromboembolism, Hx of intracranial HTN, breast CA, renal impair **Supplied:** Kits containing 6 implantable caps, (36 mg each) **SE:** Uterine bleeding, HA, acne, nausea **Notes:** Prevents PRG for up to 5 y; remove if PRG desired

Levorphanol (Levo-Dromoran) [C-II] Uses: * Moderate–severe pain; chronic pain* **Action:** Narcotic analgesic **Dose:** 2 mg PO or SQ PRN q6–8h (↓ in hepatic failure) **Caution:** [B/D (prolonged use or high doses at term), ?] **Contra:** Component allergy **Supplied:** Tabs 2 mg; inj 2 mg/mL **SE:** Tachycardia, ↓ BP, drowsiness, GI upset, constipation, resp depression, pruritus

Levothyroxine (Synthroid, Levoxyl, others) Uses: * Hypothyroidism, myxedema coma* **Action:** Supplement L-thyroxine **Dose:** *Adults.* Initial,

25–50 mcg/d PO or IV; ↑ by 25–50 mcg/d every mo; usual 100–200 mcg/d. **Peds.** *0–1 y:* 8–10 mcg/kg/24 h PO or IV. *1–5 y:* 4–6 mcg/kg/24 h PO or IV. *>5 y:* 3–4 mcg/kg/24 h PO or IV; titrate based on response & thyroid tests; dose can ↑ rapidly in young/middle-aged **Caution:** [A, +] **Contra:** Recent MI, uncorrected adrenal insuff **Supplied:** Tabs 25, 50, 75, 88, 100, 112, 125, 137, 150, 175, 200, 300 mcg; inj 200, 500 mcg **SE:** Insomnia, weight loss, alopecia, arrhythmia **Notes:** Take w/full glass of water (prevents choking)

Lidocaine (Anestacon Topical, Xylocaine, others) Uses: Local anesthetic; Rx cardiac arrhythmias **Action:** Anesthetic; class IB antiarrhythmic **Dose:** *Adults. Antiarrhythmic, ET:* 5 mcg/kg; follow w/ 0.5 mg/kg in 10 min if effective. *IV load:* 1 mg/kg/dose bolus over 2–3 min; repeat in 5–10 min; 200–300 mg/h max; cont inf 20–50 mcg/kg/min or 1–4 mg/min. **Peds.** *Antiarrhythmic, ET, load:* 1 mg/kg; repeat in 10–15 min 5 mg/kg max total, then IV inf 20–50 mcg/kg/min. *Topical:* Apply max 3 mg/kg/dose. *Local inj anesthetic:* Max 4.5 mg/kg (Table 3, page 205) **Caution:** [C, +] **Contra:** Do not use lidocaine w/ epi on digits, ears, or nose (risk of vasoconstriction & necrosis); heart block **Supplied:** *Inj local:* 0.5, 1, 1.5, 2, 4, 10, 20%. *Inj IV:* 1% (10 mg/mL), 2% (20 mg/mL); admixture 4, 10, 20%. *IV inf:* 0.2%, 0.4%; cream 2%; gel 2, 2.5%; oint 2.5, 5%; liq 2.5%; soln 2, 4%; viscous 2% **SE:** Dizziness, paresthesias, & convulsions associated w/ tox **Notes:** 2nd line to amiodarone in ECC; dilute ET dose 1–2 mL w/ NS; epi may be added for local anesthesia to ↑ effect & ↓ bleeding; for IV forms, ↓ w/ liver Dz or CHF; see Table 2 (page 200) for systemic levels

Lidocaine/Prilocaine (EMLA, LMX) Uses: *Topical anesthetic*; adjunct to phlebotomy or dermal procedures **Action:** Topical anesthetic **Dose:** *Adults.* EMLA cream, anesthetic disc (1 g/10 cm²): Thick layer 2–2.5 g to intact skin, cover w/ occlusive dressing (eg, Tegaderm) for at least 1 h. *Anesthetic disc:* 1 g/10 cm² for at least 1 h. **Peds.** *Max dose:* <3 mo or <5 kg: 1 g/10 cm² for 1 h. *3–12 mo & >5 kg:* 2 g/20 cm² for 4 h. *1–6 y & >10 kg:* 10 g/100 cm² for 4 h. *7–12 y & >20 kg:* 20 g/200 cm² for 4 h **Caution:** [B, +] Methemoglobinemia **Contra:** Use on mucous membranes, broken skin, eyes; allergy to amide-type anesthetics **Supplied:** Cream 2.5% lidocaine/2.5% prilocaine; anesthetic disc (1 g) **SE:** Burning, stinging, methemoglobinemia **Notes:** Longer contact time ↑ effect

Lindane (Kwell) [OTC] Uses: * Head lice, crab lice, scabies* **Action:** Ectoparasiticide & ovicide **Dose:** *Adults & Peds.* Cream or lotion: Thin layer after bathing, leave for 8–12 h, pour on laundry. Shampoo: Apply 30 mL, develop a lather w/ warm water for 4 min, comb out nits **Caution:** [C, +/–] **Contra:** Open wounds, Sz disorder **Supplied:** Lotion 1%; shampoo 1% **SE:** Arrhythmias, Szs, local irritation, GI upset **Notes:** Caution w/ overuse (may be absorbed); may repeat Rx in 7 days

Linezolid (Zyvox) Uses: *Infxns caused by gram(+) bacteria (including vancomycin-resistant enterococcus, VRE), pneumonia, skin Infxns* **Action:** Unique, binds ribosomal bacterial RNA; bactericidal for strep, bacteriostatic for enterococci & staph. *Spectrum:* Excellent gram(+) activity including VRE & MRSA

Dose: *Adults.* 400–600 mg IV or PO q12h. *Peds.* 10 mg/kg IV or PO q8h (q12h in preterm neonates) **Caution:** [C, ?/–] W/ reversible MAOI, avoid foods w/ tyramine & cough/cold products w/pseudoephedrine; w/myelosuppression **Supplied:** Inj 2 mg/mL; tabs 400, 600 mg; susp 100 mg/5 mL **SE:** HTN, N/D, HA, insomnia, GI upset, myelosuppression, tongue discoloration **Notes:** Follow weekly CBC

Liothyronine (Cytomel) **Uses:** *Hypothyroidism, goiter, myxedema coma, thyroid suppression therapy* **Action:** T_3 replacement **Dose:** *Adults.* Initial 25 mcg/24 h, titrate q1–2wk to response & TFT; maint of 25–100 mcg/d PO. *Myxedema coma:* 25–50 mcg IV. *Peds.* Initial 5 mcg/24 h, titrate by 5-mcg/24 h increments at 1–2-wk intervals; Maint 25–75 mcg/24 h PO qd; ↓ in elderly **Caution:** [A, +] **Contra:** Recent MI, uncorrected adrenal insuff, uncontrolled HTN **Supplied:** Tabs 5, 12.5, 25, 50 mcg; inj 10 mcg/mL **SE:** Alopecia, arrhythmias, CP, HA, sweating **Notes:** Monitor TFT

Lisinopril (Prinivil, Zestril) **Uses:** *HTN, CHF, prevent DN & AMI* **Action:** ACE inhibitor **Dose:** 5–40 mg/24 h PO qd–bid. *AMI:* 5 mg w/in 24 h of MI, then 5 mg after 24 h, 10 mg after 48 h, then 10 mg/d; ↓ in renal insuff **Caution:** [D, –] **Contra:** ACE inhibitor sensitivity **Supplied:** Tabs 2.5, 5, 10, 20, 30, 40 mg **SE:** Dizziness, HA, cough, ↓ BP, angioedema, ↑ K+ **Notes:** To prevent DN, start when urinary microalbuminemia begins

Lithium Carbonate (Eskalith, Lithobid, others) **Uses:** *Manic episodes of bipolar Dz* **Action:** Effects shift toward intraneuronal metabolism of catecholamines **Dose:** *Adults. Acute mania:* 600 mg PO tid or 900 mg SR bid. *Maint:* 300 mg PO tid–qid *Peds 6–12 y.* 15–60 mg/kg/d in 3–4 + doses; must titrate; follow serum levels; ↓ in renal insuff, elderly **Caution:** [D, –] Many drug interactions **Contra:** Severe renal impair or CV Dz, lactation **Supplied:** Caps 150, 300, 600 mg; tabs 300 mg; SR tabs 300, 450 mg; syrup 300 mg/5 mL **SE:** Polyuria, polydipsia, nephrogenic DI, tremor; Na retention or diuretic use may ↑tox; arrhythmias, dizziness **Notes:** See Table 2 (page 200) for drug levels

Lodoxamide (Alomide) **Uses:** *Seasonal allergic conjunctivitis* **Action:** Stabilizes mast cells **Dose:** *Adults & Peds >2 y.* 1–2 gtt in eye(s) qid ≤ 3 mon **Caution:** [B, ?] **Supplied:** Soln 0.1% **SE:** Ocular burning, stinging, HA

Lomefloxacin (Maxaquin) **Uses:** *UTI, acute exacerbation of chronic bronchitis; prophylaxis in transurethral procedures* **Action:** Quinolone antibiotic; ↓ DNA gyrase. *Spectrum:* Good gram(–) activity including *H. influenzae* except *Stenotrophomonas maltophilia, Acinetobacter* sp, & some *P. aeruginosa* **Dose:** 400 mg/d PO; ↓ in renal insuff, avoid antacids **Caution:** [C, –] Interactions w/ cation-containing products **Contra:** Allergy to other quinolones, children < 18 y **Supplied:** Tabs 400 mg **SE:** Photosensitivity, Szs, HA, dizziness

Loperamide (Imodium) [OTC] **Uses:** *Diarrhea* **Action:** Slows intestinal motility **Dose:** *Adults.* Initial 4 mg PO, then 2 mg after each loose stool, up to 16 mg/d. *Peds.* 2–5 y, 13–20 kg: 1 mg PO tid. 6–8 y, 20–30 kg: 2 mg PO bid. 8–12 y, >30 kg: 2 mg PO tid **Caution:** [B, +] Not for acute diarrhea caused by *Salmo-*

nella, Shigella, or *C. difficile* **Contra:** Pseudomembranous colitis, bloody diarrhea **Supplied:** Caps 2 mg; tabs 2 mg; liq 1 mg/5 mL (OTC) **SE:** Constipation, sedation, dizziness

Lopinavir/Ritonavir (Kaletra)

Uses: *HIV Infxn* **Action:** Protease inhibitor **Dose:** *Adults.* 3 caps or 5 mL PO bid. *Peds. 7–15 kg:* 12/3 mg/kg PO bid. *15–40 kg:* 10/2.5 mg/kg PO bid. *>40 kg:* Adult dose (w/ food) **Caution:** [C, ?/–] Numerous drug interactions **Contra:** Concomitant drugs dependent on CYP3A or CYP2D6 **Supplied:** Caps 133.3 mg/33.3 mg (lopinavir/ritonavir); soln 400 mg/100 mg/5 mL **SE:** Soln has EtOH, avoid disulfiram, metronidazole; GI upset, asthenia, ↑ cholesterol/triglycerides, pancreatitis; protease metabolic syndrome

Loracarbef (Lorabid)

Uses: *Upper & lower resp tract, skin, bone, urinary tract, abdomen, & gynecologic system bacterial Infxns* **Action:** 2nd-gen cephalosporin; ↓ cell wall synthesis. *Spectrum:* Weaker than 1st-gen against gram(+), enhanced gram(–) **Dose:** *Adults.* 200–400 mg PO bid. *Peds.* 7.5–15 mg/kg/d PO ÷ bid; on empty stomach; ↓ in severe renal insuff **Caution:** [B, +] **Supplied:** Caps 200, 400 mg; susp 125, 250 mg/5 mL **SE:** D

Loratadine (Claritin, Alavert)

Uses: *Allergic rhinitis, chronic idiopathic urticaria* **Action:** Nonsedating antihistamine **Dose:** *Adults.* 10 mg/d PO *Peds. 2–5 y:* 5 mg PO qd. *>6 y:* Adult dose; on empty stomach; ↓ in hepatic insuff **Caution:** [B, +/–] **Contra:** Component allergy **Supplied:** Tabs 10 mg (OTC); rapidly disintegrating Reditabs 10 mg; syrup 1 mg/mL **SE:** HA, somnolence, xerostomia

Lorazepam (Ativan, others) [C-IV]

Uses: *Anxiety & anxiety w/ depression; preop sedation; control status epilepticus*; EtOH withdrawal; antiemetic **Action:** Benzodiazepine; antianxiety agent **Dose:** *Adults. Anxiety:* 1–10 mg/d PO in 2–3 ÷ doses. *Preop:* 0.05 mg/kg to 4 mg max IM 2 h before surgery. *Insomnia:* 2–4 mg PO hs. *Status epilepticus:* 4 mg/dose IV PRN q10–15 min; usual total dose 8 mg. *Antiemetic:* 0.5–2 mg IV or PO q4–6h PRN. *EtOH withdrawal:* 2–5 mg IV or 1–2 mg PO initial depending on severity; titrate based on response *Peds. Status epilepticus:* 0.05 mg/kg/dose IV, repeat at 1–20 min intervals × 2 PRN. *Antiemetic, 2–15 y:* 0.05 mg/kg (to 2 mg/dose) pre chemo; ↓ in elderly; do not administer IV >2 mg/min or 0.05 mg/kg/min **Caution:** [D, ?/–] **Contra:** Severe pain, severe ↓ BP, sleep apnea, NA glaucoma, allergy to propylene glycol or benzyl alcohol **Supplied:** Tabs 0.5, 1, 2 mg; soln, PO conc 2 mg/mL; inj 2, 4 mg/mL **SE:** Sedation, ataxia, tachycardia, constipation, resp depression **Notes:** ≤10 min for effect if IV

Losartan (Cozaar)

Uses: *HTN,* *CHF, DN* **Action:** Angiotensin II antagonist **Dose:** 25–50 mg PO qd–bid; ↓ in elderly/hepatic impair **Caution:** [C (1st tri, D 2nd & 3rd tri), ?/–] **Supplied:** Tabs 25, 50, 100 mg **SE:** ↓ BP in pts on diuretics; GI upset, angioedema

Lovastatin (Mevacor, Altocor)

Uses: *Hypercholesterolemia* **Action:** HMG-CoA reductase inhibitor **Dose:** 20 mg/d PO w/ PM meal; may ↑ at 4-wk intervals to 80 mg/d max; take w/ meals **Caution:** [X, –] Avoid w/ grapefruit juice, gemfibrozil. **Contra:** Active liver Dz **Supplied:** Tabs 10, 20, 40 mg **SE:** HA & GI intolerance common; promptly report any unexplained muscle pain, tenderness, or weakness (myopathy) **Notes:** Maintain cholesterol-lowering diet; monitor LFT q12wk × 1 y, then q6mo

Lutropin Alfa (Luveris) **Uses:** *Infertility* **Action:** Recombinant LH **Dose:** 75 units SC with 75–150 units FSH, 2 separate injs **Caution:** [X, ?/M] **Contra:** Primary ovarian failure, uncontrolled thyroid/adrenal dysfunction, intracranial lesion, abnormal uterine bleeding, hormone-dependent GU tumor, ovarian cyst, PRG **Supplied:** Inj 75 units **SE:** HA, N, ovarian hyperstimulation syndrome, breast pain, ovarian cysts; ↑ risk of multiple births **Notes:** Rotate inj sites; do not exceed 14 d duration unless signs of imminent follicular development

Lymphocyte Immune Globulin [Antithymocyte Globulin, ATG] (Atgam) **Uses:** *Allograft rejection in transplant pts; aplastic anemia if not candidates for BMT* **Action:** ↓ circulating T lymphocytes **Dose:** *Adults. Prevent rejection:* 15 mg/kg/day IV ×14 d, then qod ×7; initial w/in 24 h before/after transplant. *Rx rejection:* Same except use 10–15 mg/kg/d. *Peds.* 5–25 mg/kg/d IV. **Caution:** [C, ?] **Contra:** Hx Rxn to other equine γ-globulin preparation, leukopenia, thrombocytopenia **Supplied:** Inj 50 mg/mL **SE:** D/C w/ severe thrombocytopenia/leukopenia; rash, fever, chills, ↓ BP, HA, ↑ K+ **Notes:** *Test dose:* 0.1 mL 1:1000 dilution in NS

Magaldrate (Riopan, Lowsium) [OTC] **Uses:** *Hyperacidity associated w/ peptic ulcer, gastritis, & hiatal hernia* **Action:** Low-Na antacid **Dose:** 5–10 mL PO between meals & hs **Caution:** [B, ?] **Contra:** Ulcerative colitis, diverticulitis, ileostomy/colostomy, renal insuff (Mg content) **Supplied:** Susp (OTC) **SE:** GI upset **Notes:** <0.3 mg Na/tab or tsp

Magnesium Citrate (various) [OTC] **Uses:** *Vigorous bowel preparation*; constipation **Action:** Cathartic laxative **Dose:** *Adults.* 120–240 mL PO PRN. *Peds.* 0.5 mL/kg/dose, to 200 mL PO max; w/ a beverage **Caution:** [B, +] **Contra:** Severe renal Dz, heart block, N/V, rectal bleeding **Supplied:** Effervescent soln (OTC) **SE:** Abdominal cramps, gas

Magnesium Hydroxide (Milk of Magnesia) [OTC] **Uses:** *Constipation* **Action:** NS laxative **Dose:** *Adults.* 15–30 mL PO PRN. *Peds.* 0.5 mL/kg/dose PO PRN (follow dose w/ 8 oz of H2O) **Caution:** [B, +] **Contra:** Renal insuff or intestinal obstruction, ileostomy/colostomy **Supplied:** Tabs 311 mg; liq 400, 800 mg/5 mL (OTC) **SE:** D, abdominal cramps

Magnesium Oxide (Mag-Ox 400, others) [OTC] **Uses:** *Replacement for low Mg levels* **Action:** Mg supl **Dose:** 400–800 mg/d ÷ qd–qid w/ full glass of H2O **Caution:** [B, +] **Contra:** Ulcerative colitis, diverticulitis, ileostomy/ colostomy, heart block, renal insuff **Supplied:** Caps 140 mg; tabs 400 mg (OTC) **SE:** D, nausea

Magnesium Sulfate (various) **Uses:** * Replacement for low Mg levels; preeclampsia & premature labor*; refractory ↓ K+ & ↓ Ca2+ **Action:** Mg supl

Dose: *Adults.* Supl: 1–2 g IM or IV; repeat PRN. *Preeclampsia/premature labor:* 4 g load then 1–4 g/h IV inf. *Peds.* 25–50 mg/kg/dose IM or IV q4–6h for 3–4 doses; repeat PRN; ↓ dose w/ low urine output or renal insuff **Caution:** [B, +] **Contra:** Heart block, renal failure **Supplied:** Inj 100, 125, 250, 500 mg/mL; PO soln 500 mg/mL; granules 40 mEq/5 g **SE:** CNS depression, D, flushing, heart block

Mannitol (various)
Uses: *Cerebral edema, ↑ intraocular pressure, renal impair, poisonings* **Action:** Osmotic diuretic **Dose:** *Diuresis: Adults.* 0.2 g/kg/dose IV over 3–5 min; if no diuresis w/in 2 h, D/C. *Peds.* 0.75 g/kg/dose IV over 3–5 min; if no diuresis w/in 2 h, D/C. *Cerebral edema: Adults & Peds.* 0.25 g/kg/dose IV push, repeated at 5-min intervals PRN; ↑ slowly to 1 g/kg/dose PRN for ↑ ICP **Caution:** [C, ?] w/ CHF or volume overload **Contra:** Anuria, dehydration, heart failure, PE **Supplied:** Inj 5, 10, 15, 20, 25% **SE:** Initial volume ↑ may exacerbate CHF; monitor for volume depletion, N/V/D

Measles, Mumps, Rubella and Varicella Virus Vaccine Live (Proquad)
Uses: *Simultaneous vaccination against measles, mumps, rubella, & varicella in peds 12 mo–12 y or second dose of MMR* **Action:** Active immunization, live attenuated virus **Dose:** 1 vial IM inj **Caution:** [N/A] Hx of cerebral injury or Szs (febrile reaction) **Contra:** Hx anaphylaxis to neomycin, blood dyscrasia, lymphoma, leukemia, immunosuppressive steroids, febrile illness, untreated TB **Supplied:** Inj **SE:** Fever, inj site Rxn, rash **Notes:** Allow 1 mo between inj & any other measles-containing vaccine

Mechlorethamine (Mustargen)
WARNING: Highly toxic, handle w/ care **Uses:** *Hodgkin Dz & NHL, cutaneous T-cell lymphoma (mycosis fungoides), lung CA, CML, malignant pleural effusions,* & CLL **Action:** Alkylating agent (bifunctional) **Dose:** 0.4 mg/kg single dose or 0.1 mg/kg/d for 4 d; 6 mg/m² 1–2 ×/mo **Caution:** [D, ?] **Contra:** Known infectious Dz **Supplied:** Inj 10 mg **SE:** Myelosuppression, thrombosis, or thrombophlebitis at site; tissue damage w/ extravasation (Na thiosulfate used topically to treat); N/V, skin rash, amenorrhea, sterility (especially in men), secondary leukemia if treated for Hodgkin Dz **Notes:** Highly volatile; administer w/in 30–60 min of prep

Meclizine (Antivert)
Uses: *Motion sickness; vertigo* **Action:** Antiemetic, anticholinergic, & antihistaminic properties **Dose:** *Adults & Peds >12 y.* 25 mg PO tid–qid PRN **Caution:** [B, ?] **Supplied:** Tabs 12.5, 25, 50 mg; chew tabs 25 mg; caps 25, 30 mg (OTC) **SE:** Drowsiness, xerostomia, & blurred vision common

Medroxyprogesterone (Provera, Depo-Provera)
WARNING: May cause loss of bone density; associated w/ duration of use **Uses:** *Contraception; secondary amenorrhea, abnormal uterine bleeding (AUB) caused by hormonal imbalance; endometrial CA* **Action:** Progestin supl **Dose:** *Contraception:* 150 mg IM q3mo or 450 mg IM q6mo. *Secondary amenorrhea:* 5–10 mg/d PO for 5–10 d. *AUB:* 5–10 mg/d PO for 5–10 d beginning on the 16th or 21st d of menstrual cycle. *Endometrial CA:* 400–1000 mg/wk IM; ↓ in hepatic insuff **Caution:**

[X, +] **Contra:** Hx of thromboembolic disorders, hepatic Dz, PRG **Supplied:** Tabs 2.5, 5, 10 mg; depot inj 100, 150, 400 mg/mL **SE:** Breakthrough bleeding, spotting, altered menstrual flow, anorexia, edema, thromboembolic complications, depression, weight gain **Notes:** Perform breast exam & Pap smear before contraceptive therapy; obtain PRG test if last inj > 3 mo

Megestrol Acetate (Megace) **Uses:** * Breast/endometrial CAs; appetite stimulant in cachexia (CA & HIV)* **Action:** Hormone; progesterone analog **Dose:** *CA:* 40–320 mg/d PO in ÷ doses. *Appetite:* 800 mg/d PO ÷ **Caution:** [X, –] Thromboembolism **Contra:** PRG **Supplied:** Tabs 20, 40 mg; soln 40 mg/mL **SE:** May induce DVT; do not D/C abruptly; edema, menstrual bleeding; photosensitivity, insomnia, rash, myelosuppression

Meloxicam (Mobic) **WARNING:** May ↑ risk of cardiovascular events & GI bleeding **Uses:** *Osteoarthritis* **Action:** NSAID w/ ↑ COX-2 activity **Dose:** 7.5–15 mg/d PO; ↓ in renal insuff; take w/food **Caution:** [C, ?/–] Peptic ulcer, NSAID, or ASA sensitivity **Supplied:** Tabs 7.5 mg **SE:** HA, dizziness, GI upset, GI bleeding, edema

Melphalan [L-PAM] (Alkeran) **WARNING:** Severe BM depression, leukemogenic, & mutagenic **Uses:** *Multiple myeloma, ovarian CAs,* breast, testicular CAs, melanoma; allogenic & ABMT (high dose) **Action:** Alkylating agent (bifunctional) **Dose:** (Per protocol) 6 mg/d or 0.25 mg/kg/d for 4–7 d, repeat 4–6-wk intervals, or 1-mg/kg/d ×1 q4–6wk; 0.15 mg/kg/d for 5 d q6wk. *High-dose high-risk multiple myeloma:* Single dose 140 mg/m². *ABMT:* 140–240 mg/m² IV; ↓ in renal insuff **Caution:** [D, ?] Allergy or resistance **Supplied:** Tabs 2 mg; inj 50, 100 mg **SE:** ↓ BM, secondary leukemia, alopecia, dermatitis, stomatitis, & pulmonary fibrosis; rare allergic Rxns **Notes:** Take PO on empty stomach

Memantine (Namenda) **Uses:** Moderate/severe Alzheimer Dz **Action:** *N*-methyl-D-aspartate receptor antagonist **Dose:** Target 20 mg/d, start 5 mg/d, ↑ 5 mg/d to 20 mg/d, wait > 1 wk before ↑ dose; use ÷ doses >5 mg/d **Caution:** [B, ?/–] Hepatic/mild–moderate renal impair **Supplied:** Tabs 5, 10 mg **SE:** Dizziness **Notes:** Renal clearance ↓ by alkaline urine (↓ 80% @ pH 8)

Meningococcal Polysaccharide Vaccine (Menomune) **Uses:** *Immunize against N. meningitidis (meningococcus)* **Action:** OK in some complement deficiency, asplenia, lab workers w/ exposure; college students by some professional groups **Action:** Live vaccine, active immunization **Dose:** *Adults & Peds >2 y.* 0.5 mL SQ (not indradermal or IV); keep epi (1:1000) available for anaphylactic/allergic Rxns **Caution:** [C, ?/–] **Contra:** Thimerosal sensitivity **Supplied:** Inj **SE:** Local inj site Rxns, HA **Notes:** Active against meningococcal serotypes A, C, Y, & W-135; not group B

Meperidine (Demerol) [C–II] **Uses:** * Moderate–severe pain* **Action:** Narcotic analgesic **Dose:** *Adults.* 50–150 mg PO or IM q3–4h PRN. *Peds.* 1–1.5 mg/kg/dose PO or IM q3–4h PRN, up to 100 mg/dose; ↓ in elderly/renal impair **Caution:** [C/D (prolonged use or high dose at term), +] ↓ Sz threshold **Contra:**

Recent/concomitant MAOIs, renal failure **Supplied:** Tabs 50, 100 mg; syrup 50 mg/mL; inj 10, 25, 50, 75, 100 mg/mL **SE:** Resp depression, Szs, sedation, constipation **Notes:** Analgesic effects potentiated w/ use of hydroxyzine; 75 mg IM = 10 mg morphine IM

Meprobamate (Equinil, Miltown) [C-IV]
Uses: *Short-term relief of anxiety* **Action:** Mild tranquilizer; antianxiety **Dose:** *Adults.* 400 mg PO tid–qid up to 2400 mg/d; SR 400–800 mg PO bid. *Peds 6–12 y.* 100–200 mg bid–tid; SR 200 mg bid; ↓ in renal/liver insuff **Caution:** [D, +/–] **Contra:** NA glaucoma, porphyria, PRG **Supplied:** Tabs 200, 400, 600 mg; SR caps 200, 400 mg **SE:** May cause drowsiness, syncope, tachycardia, edema

Mercaptopurine [6-MP] (Purinethol)
Uses: *Acute leukemias,* 2nd-line Rx of CML & NHL, maint ALL in children, immunosuppressant w/ autoimmune Dzs (Crohn Dz) **Action:** Antimetabolite, mimics hypoxanthine **Dose:** 80–100 mg/m²/d or 2.5–5 mg/kg/d; maint 1.5–2.5 mg/kg/d; w/ allopurinol requires a 67–75% ↓ dose of 6-MP (interference w/ xanthine oxidase metabolism); ↓ in renal/hepatic insuff; take on empty stomach **Caution:** [D, ?] **Contra:** Severe hepatic Dz, BM suppression, PRG **Supplied:** Tabs 50 mg **SE:** Mild hematotox; uncommon GI tox, except mucositis, stomatitis, & D; rash, fever, eosinophilia, jaundice, hepatitis **Notes:** Handle properly; ensure adequate hydration

Meropenem (Merrem)
Uses: * Intraabdominal Infxns, bacterial meningitis* **Action:** Carbapenem; ↓ cell wall synthesis, a β-lactam. *Spectrum:* Excellent gram(+) (except MRSA & E. faecium); excellent gram(–) including extended-spectrum β-lactamase producers; good anaerobic **Dose:** *Adults.* 1 g IV q8h. *Peds.* 20–40 mg/kg IV q 8h; ↓ in renal insuff **Caution:** [B, ?] **Contra:** β-Lactam sensitivity **Supplied:** Inj 1 g/30 mL, 500 mg/20 mL **SE:** Less Sz potential than imipenem; D, thrombocytopenia **Notes:** Overuse can ↑ bacterial resistance

Mesalamine (Rowasa, Asacol, Pentasa)
Uses: * Mild–moderate distal ulcerative colitis, proctosigmoiditis, proctitis* **Action:** Unknown; may inhibit prostaglandins **Dose:** *Retention enema:* qd hs or 1 supp bid. *PO:* 800–1000 mg PO tid–qid; ↓ initial dose in elderly **Caution:** [B, M] May discolor urine yellow-brown **Contra:** Salicylate sensitivity **Supplied:** Tabs 400 mg; caps 250 mg; supp 500 mg; rectal susp 4 g/60 mL **SE:** HA, malaise, abdominal pain, flatulence, rash, pancreatitis, pericarditis

Mesna (Mesnex)
Uses: *↓ ifosamide- & cyclophosphamide-induced hemorrhagic cystitis* **Action:** Antidote **Dose:** 20% of ifosfamide dose (±) or cyclophosphamide dose IV 15 min prior to & 4 & 8 h after chemo **Caution:** [B; ?/–] **Contra:** Thiol sensitivity **Supplied:** Inj 100 mg/mL; tablets 400 mg **SE:** ↓ BP, allergic Rxns, HA, GI upset, taste perversion **Notes:** Hydration helps ↓ hemorrhagic cystitis

Mesoridazine (Serentil)
WARNING: Can prolong QT interval in dose-related fashion; torsades de pointes reported **Uses:** *Schizophrenia,* acute & chronic alcoholism, chronic brain syndrome **Action:** Phenothiazine antipsychotic **Dose:** Initial, 25–50 mg PO or IV tid; ↑ to 300–400 mg/d max **Caution:** [C, ?/–]

Contra: Phenothiazine sensitivity, coadministration w/ drugs that cause QT_c prolongation, CNS depression **Supplied:** Tabs 10, 25, 50, 100 mg; PO conc 25 mg/mL; inj 25 mg/mL **SE:** Low incidence of EPS; ↓ BP, xerostomia, constipation, skin discoloration, tachycardia, lowered Sz threshold, blood dyscrasias, pigmentary retinopathy at high doses

Metaproterenol (Alupent, Metaprel)
Uses: * Asthma & reversible bronchospasm* **Action:** Sympathomimetic bronchodilator **Dose:** *Adults. Inhal:* 1–3 inhal q3–4h, 12 inhal max/24 h; wait 2 min between inhal. *PO:* 20 mg q6–8h. *Peds. Inhal:* 0.5 mg/kg/dose, 15 mg/dose max inhaled q4–6h by neb or 1–2 puffs q4–6h. *PO:* 0.3–0.5 mg/kg/dose q6–8h **Caution:** [C, ?/–] **Contra:** Tachycardia, other arrhythmias **Supplied:** Aerosol 0.65 mg/inhal; soln for inhal 0.4, 0.6, 5%; tabs 10, 20 mg; syrup 10 mg/5 mL **SE:** Fewer β_1 effects than isoproterenol & longer acting; nervousness, tremor, tachycardia, HTN

Metaxalone (Skelaxin)
Uses: * Painful musculoskeletal conditions* **Action:** Centrally acting skeletal muscle relaxant **Dose:** 800 mg PO tid–qid **Caution:** [C, ?/–] anemia **Contra:** Severe hepatic/renal impair **Supplied:** Tabs 400 mg **SE:** N/V, HA, drowsiness, hepatitis

Metformin (Glucophage, Glucophage XR)
WARNING: Associated w/ lactic acidosis **Uses:** *Type 2 DM* **Action:** ↓ Hepatic glucose production & intestinal absorption of glucose; ↑ insulin sensitivity **Dose:** *Adults.* Initial: 500 mg PO bid; may ↑ to 2550 mg/d max (w/ AM & PM meals; can convert total daily dose to qd dose of XR form). *Peds 10–16 y.* 500 mg PO bid, ↑ 500 mg/wk to 2000 mg/d max in ÷ doses; do not use XR formulation in peds **Caution:** [B, +/–] **Contra:** SCr >1.4 in females or >1.5 in males; contra in hypoxemic conditions, including acute CHF/sepsis; avoid EtOH; hold dose before & 48 h after ionic contrast **Supplied:** Tabs 500, 850, 1000 mg; XR tabs 500 mg **SE:** Anorexia, N/V, rash, lactic acidosis (rare, but serious)

Methadone (Dolophine) [C-II]
Uses: * Severe pain; detox, maint of narcotic addiction* **Action:** Narcotic analgesic **Dose:** *Adults.* 2.5–10 mg IM q3–8h or 5–15 mg PO q8h; titrate as needed *Peds.* 0.7 mg/kg/24 h PO or IM ÷ q8h; ↑ slowly to avoid resp depression; ↓ in renal Dz **Caution:** [B/D (prolonged use or high doses at term), + (w/ doses = 20 mg/24 h)], severe liver Dz **Supplied:** Tabs 5, 10, 40 mg; PO soln 5, 10 mg/5 mL; PO conc 10 mg/mL; inj 10 mg/mL **SE:** Resp depression, sedation, constipation, urinary retention, ventricular arrhythmias **Notes:** Equianalgesic w/ parenteral morphine; longer half-life; prolongs QT interval

Methenamine (Hiprex, Urex, others)
Uses: *Suppress/eliminate bacteriuria associated w/ chronic/ recurrent UTI* **Action:** Converted to formaldehyde & ammonia in acidic urine; nonspecific bactericidal action **Dose:** *Adults.* Hippurate: 1 g bid. *Mandelate:* 1 g qid PO pc & hs *Peds 6–12 y. Hippurate:* 25–50 mg/kg/d PO ÷ bid. *Mandelate:* 50–75 mg/kg/d PO ÷ qid (take w/ food, ascorbic acid w/ adequate hydration) **Caution:** [C, +] **Contra:** Renal insuff, severe hepatic Dz, & severe dehydration; sulfonamide allergy **Supplied:** *Methenamine hippurate*

(Hiprex, Urex): Tabs 1g. *Methenamine mandelate:* 500mg, 1g EC tabs **SE:** Rash, GI upset, dysuria, ↑ LFTs

Methimazole (Tapazole) Uses: *Hyperthyroidism, thyrotoxicosis,* prep for thyroid surgery or radiation **Action:** Blocks T_3 & T_4 formation **Dose:** *Adults. Initial:* 15–60 mg/d PO ÷ tid. *Maint:* 5–15 mg PO qd. *Peds. Initial:* 0.4–0.7 mg/kg/24 h PO ÷ tid. *Maint:* ½–⅔ of initial dose PO qd; w/ food **Caution:** [D, +/–] **Contra:** Breast-feeding **Supplied:** Tabs 5, 10 mg **SE:** GI upset, dizziness, blood dyscrasias **Notes:** Follow clinically & w/ TFT

Methocarbamol (Robaxin) Uses: *Relief of discomfort associated w/ painful musculoskeletal conditions* **Action:** Centrally acting skeletal muscle relaxant **Dose:** *Adults.* 1.5 g PO qid for 2–3 d, then 1-g PO qid maint therapy; IV form rarely indicated. *Peds.* 15 mg/kg/dose, may repeat PRN (OK for tetanus only) **Caution:** Sz disorders [C, +] **Contra:** MyG, renal impair **Supplied:** Tabs 325, 500, 750 mg; inj 100 mg/mL **SE:** Can discolor urine; drowsiness, GI upset

Methotrexate (Folex, Rheumatrex) Uses: *ALL & AML (including leukemic meningitis), trophoblastic tumors (chorioepithelioma, choriocarcinoma, chorioadenoma destruens, hydatidiform mole), breast CA, Burkitt lymphoma, mycosis fungoides, osteosarcoma, head & neck CA, Hodgkin Dz & NHL, lung CA; psoriasis; RA* **Action:** ↓ Dihydrofolate reductase-mediated gen. of tetrahydrofolate **Dose:** *CA:* Per protocol. *RA:* 7.5 mg/wk PO ×1 or 2.5 mg q12h PO for 3 doses/wk; "high dose" Rx requires leucovorin rescue (↓ hematologic/mucosal tox); ↓ in renal/hepatic impair **Caution:** [D, –] **Contra:** Severe renal/hepatic impair, PRG/lactation **Supplied:** Tabs 2.5, 5, 7.5, 10, 15 mg; inj 2.5, 25 mg/mL; preservative-free inj 25 mg/mL **SE:** Myelosuppression, N/V/D, anorexia, mucositis, hepatotox (transient & reversible; may progress to atrophy, necrosis, fibrosis, cirrhosis), rashes, dizziness, malaise, blurred vision, alopecia, photosensitivity, renal failure, pneumonitis; rarely, pulmonary fibrosis; chemical arachnoiditis & HA w/ IT delivery **Notes:** Monitor CBC, LFTs, Cr MTX levels & CXR

Methyldopa (Aldomet) Uses: *HTN* **Action:** Centrally acting antihypertensive **Dose:** *Adults.* 250–500 mg PO bid–tid (max ~2–3 g/d) or 250 mg–1 g IV q6–8h. *Peds.* 10 mg/kg/24 h PO in 2–3 ÷ doses (max 40 mg/kg/24 h ÷ q6–12h) or 5–10 mg/kg/dose IV q6–8h to total dose of 20–40 mg/kg/24 h; ↓ in renal insuff/elderly **Caution:** [B (PO), C (IV), +] **Contra:** Liver Dz; MAOIs **Supplied:** Tabs 125, 250, 500 mg; PO susp 50 mg/mL; inj 50 mg/mL **SE:** Can discolor urine; initial transient sedation or drowsiness frequent; edema, hemolytic anemia; hepatic disorders

Methylergonovine (Methergine) Uses: *Postpartum bleeding (uterine subinvolution)* **Action:** Ergotamine derivative **Dose:** 0.2 mg IM after placental delivery, may repeat 2–4-h intervals or 0.2–0.4 mg PO q6–12h for 2–7 d **Caution:** [C, ?] **Contra:** HTN, PRG **Supplied:** Injectable forms; tabs 0.2 mg **SE:** HTN, N/V **Notes:** Give IV doses over a period of >1 min w/ frequent BP monitoring

Methylprednisolone (Solu-Medrol) [See Steroids, Table 4, page 206]

Metoclopramide (Reglan, Clopra, Octamide) Uses: *Relief of diabetic gastroparesis, symptomatic GERD; chemo-induced N/V, facilitate small-bowel intubation & radiologic evaluation of the upper GI tract,* stimulate gut in prolonged postop ileus **Action:** Stimulates upper GI tract motility; blocks dopamine in chemoreceptor trigger zone **Dose:** *Adults.* Diabetic gastroparesis: 10 mg PO 30 min ac & hs for 2–8 wk PRN, or same dose given IV for 10 d, then PO. Reflux: 10–15 mg PO 30 min ac & hs. Antiemetic: 1–3 mg/kg/dose IV 30 min before chemo, then q2h ×2 doses, then q3h ×3 doses. *Peds.* Reflux: 0.1 mg/kg/dose PO qid. Antiemetic: 1–2 mg/kg/dose IV as adults **Caution:** [B, –] Drugs w/ extrapyramidal ADRs **Contra:** Sz disorders, GI obstruction **Supplied:** Tabs 5, 10 mg; syrup 5 mg/5 mL; soln 10 mg/mL; inj 5 mg/mL **SE:** Dystonic Rxns common w/ high doses, (Rx w/ IV diphenhydramine); restlessness, drowsiness, D

Metolazone (Mykrox, Zaroxolyn) Uses: *Mild–moderate essential HTN & edema of renal Dz or cardiac failure* **Action:** Thiazide-like diuretic; ↓ distal tubule Na reabsorption **Dose:** HTN: 2.5–5 mg/d PO. Edema: 5–20 mg/d PO. *Peds.* 0.2–0.4 mg/kg/d PO ÷ q12h–qd **Caution:** [D, +] **Contra:** Thiazide/sulfonamide sensitivity, anuria **Supplied:** *Tabs:* Mykrox (rapid acting) 0.5 mg, Zaroxolyn 2.5, 5, 10 mg **SE:** Monitor fluid/electrolytes; dizziness, ↓ BP, tachycardia, CP, photosensitivity **Notes:** Mykrox & Zaroxolyn not bioequivalent

Metoprolol (Lopressor, Toprol XL) **WARNING:** Do not acutely stop therapy as marked worsening of angina can result Uses: *HTN, angina, AMI, CHF* **Action:** β-Adrenergic receptor blocker **Dose:** Angina: 50–100 mg PO bid. HTN: 100–450 mg/d PO. AMI: 5 mg IV ×3 doses, then 50 mg PO q6h ×48 h, then 100 mg PO bid. CHF: 12–25 mg/d PO ×2 wk, ↑ at 2-wk intervals to 200 mg/max, use low dose in pts w/ greatest severity; ↓ in hepatic failure **Caution:** [C, +] Uncompensated CHF, bradycardia, heart block **Contra:** Arrhythmia w/ tachycardia **Supplied:** Tabs 50, 100 mg; ER tabs 50, 100, 200 mg; inj 1 mg/mL **SE:** Drowsiness, insomnia, ED, bradycardia, bronchospasm

Metronidazole (Flagyl, MetroGel) Uses: *Bone/joint, endocarditis, intraabdominal, meningitis, & skin Infxns; amebiasis; trichomoniasis; bacterial vaginosis* **Action:** Interferes w/ DNA synthesis. *Spectrum:* Excellent anaerobic coverage *C. difficile,* also *H. pylori* in combo therapy **Dose:** *Adults.* Anaerobic Infxns: 500 mg IV q6–8h. Amebic dysentery: 750 mg/d PO for 5–10 d. Trichomoniasis: 250 mg PO tid for 7 d or 2 g PO ×1. *C. difficile* Infxn: 500 mg PO or IV q8h for 7–10 d (PO preferred; IV only if pt NPO). Vaginosis: 1 applicatorful intravag bid or 500 mg PO bid for 7 d. Acne rosacea/skin: Apply bid. *Peds.* Anaerobic Infxns: 15 mg/kg/24 h PO or IV ÷ q6h. Amebic dysentery: 35–50 mg/kg/24 h PO in 3 ÷ doses for 5–10 d; ↓ in hepatic failure **Caution:** [B, M] Avoid EtOH **Contra:** First tri of PRG **Supplied:** Tabs 250, 500 mg; XR tabs 750 mg; caps 375 mg; topical lotion & gel 0.75%; intravag gel 0.75% (5 g/applicator 37.5 mg in 70-g tube), cream 1% **SE:** Disulfiram-like Rxn; dizziness, HA, GI upset, anorexia, urine discoloration **Notes:** For Trichomoniasis, Rx pt's partner; no aerobic bacteria activity; use in combo w/ serious mixed Infxns

Mexiletine (Mexitil) Uses: *Suppression of symptomatic ventricular arrhythmias*; diabetic neuropathy **Action:** Class IB antiarrhythmic **Dose:** *Adults.* 200–300 mg PO q8h; 1200 mg/d max. *Peds.* 2.5–5 mg/kg PO q 8h; drug interactions w/ hepatic enzyme inducers & suppressors requiring dosage changes; w/ food or antacids **Caution:** [C, +] May worsen severe arrhythmias **Contra:** Cardiogenic shock or 2nd-/3rd-degree AV block w/o pacemaker **Supplied:** Caps 150, 200, 250 mg **SE:** Monitor LFTs; lightheadedness, dizziness, anxiety, incoordination, GI upset, ataxia, hepatic damage, blood dyscrasias

Mezlocillin (Mezlin) Uses: *Infxns caused by susceptible gram(–) bacteria (skin, bone, resp tract, urinary tract, abdomen, septicemia)* **Action:** Bactericidal; ↓ cell wall synthesis. *Spectrum:* Gram(–) *Klebsiella, Proteus, E. coli, Enterobacter, P. aeruginosa,* & *Serratia* **Dose:** *Adults.* 3 g IV q4–6h. *Peds.* 200–300 mg/kg/d ÷ q4–6h; ↓ in renal/hepatic insuff **Caution:** [B, M] **Contra:** PCN sensitivity **Supplied:** Inj **SE:** GI upset, agranulocytosis, thrombocytopenia **Notes:** Often used w/ aminoglycoside

Miconazole (Monistat, others) Uses: *Candidal Infxns, dermatomycoses (various tinea forms)* **Action:** Fungicide; alters permeability of fungal membrane **Dose:** Apply to area bid for 2–4 wk. *Intravag:* 1 applicatorful or supp hs for 3 (4% or 200 mg) or 7 d (2% or 100 mg) **Caution:** [C, ?] Azole sensitivity **Supplied:** Topical cream 2%; lotion 2%; powder 2%; spray 2%; vaginal supp 100, 200 mg; vaginal cream 2%, 4% [OTC] **SE:** Vaginal burning, may ↑ warfarin **Notes:** Antagonistic to amphotericin B in vivo

Midazolam (Versed) [C-IV] Uses: *Preop sedation, conscious sedation for short procedures & mechanically ventilated pts, induction of general anesthesia* **Action:** Short-acting benzodiazepine **Dose:** *Adults.* 1–5 mg IV or IM; titrate to effect. *Peds. Preop:* 0.25–1 mg/kg, 20 mg max PO. *Conscious sedation:* 0.08 mg/kg IM × 1. *General anesthesia:* 0.15 mg/kg IV, then 0.05 mg/kg/dose q2min for 1–3 doses PRN to induce anesthesia (↓ in elderly, w/ narcotics or CNS depressants) **Caution:** [D, +/–] CYP3A4 substrate, several drug interactions **Contra:** NA glaucoma; use of amprenavir, nelfinavir, ritonavir **Supplied:** Inj 1, 5 mg/mL; syrup 2 mg/mL **SE:** Monitor for resp depression; ↓ BP in conscious sedation, nausea **Notes:** Reversal w/ flumazenil

Mifepristone [RU 486] (Mifeprex) **WARNING:** Pt counseling & information required; associated w/ fatal infections & bleeding Uses: *Termination of intrauterine pregnancies of <49 d* **Action:** Antiprogestin; ↑ prostaglandins, results in uterine contraction **Dose:** Administered w/ 3 office visits: day 1, three 200-mg tabs PO; day 3 if no abortion, two 200-mg misoprostol PO; on or about day 14, verify termination of PRG **Caution:** [X, –] **Contra:** Anticoagulation therapy, bleeding disorders **Supplied:** Tabs 200 mg **SE:** Abdominal pain & 1–2 wk of uterine bleeding **Notes:** Give under physician's supervision

Miglitol (Glyset) Uses: *Type 2 DM* **Action:** α-Glucosidase inhibitor; delays digestion of ingested carbohydrates **Dose:** Initial 25 mg PO tid; maint 50–100

mg tid (w/ 1st bite of each meal) **Caution:** [B, –] **Contra:** Obstructive or inflammatory GI disorders; SCr >2 **Supplied:** Tabs 25, 50, 100 mg **SE:** Used alone or in combo w/ sulfonylureas; flatulence, D, abdominal pain

Milrinone (Primacor) **Uses:** *CHF* **Action:** Positive inotrope & vasodilator; little chronotropic activity **Dose:** 50 mcg/kg, then 0.375–0.75 mcg/kg/min inf; ↓ in renal impair **Caution:** [C, ?] **Contra:** Allergy to drug or amrinone **Supplied:** Inj 1 mcg/mL **SE:** Arrhythmias, ↓ BP, HA **Notes:** Monitor fluid/electrolyte status & BP/HR

Mineral Oil [OTC] **Uses:** *Constipation* **Action:** Emollient laxative **Dose:** *Adults.* 5–45 mL PO PRN. *Peds >6 y.* 5–20 mL PO bid **Caution:** [C, ?] N/V, difficulty swallowing, bedridden pts **Contra:** Appendicitis, diverticulitis, ulcerative colitis **Supplied:** Liq [OTC] **SE:** Lipid pneumonia, anal incontinence, impaired vitamin absorption

Minoxidil (Loniten, Rogaine) **Uses:** *Severe HTN; male & female pattern baldness* **Action:** Peripheral vasodilator; stimulates vertex hair growth **Dose:** *Adults. PO:* 2.5–10 mg PO bid–qid. *Topical:* Apply bid to affected area. *Peds.* 0.2–1 mg/kg/24 h ÷ PO q12–24h; ↓ PO dose in elderly **Caution:** [C, +] **Contra:** Pheochromocytoma, allergy to components **Supplied:** Tabs 2.5, 5, 10 mg; topical soln (Rogaine) 2% **SE:** Pericardial effusion & volume overload may occur w/ PO use; hypertrichosis after chronic use; edema, ECG changes, weight gain

Mirtazapine (Remeron) **WARNING:** Closely monitor for worsening depression or emergence of suicidality, particularly in ped pts **Uses:** *Depression* **Action:** Tetracyclic antidepressant **Dose:** 15 mg PO hs, up to 45 mg/d hs **Caution:** [C, ?] **Contra:** MAOIs w/in 14 d **Supplied:** Tabs 15, 30, 45 mg **SE:** Somnolence, ↑ cholesterol, constipation, xerostomia, weight gain, agranulocytosis **Notes:** Do not ↑ dose at intervals of less than 1–2 wk

Misoprostol (Cytotec) **Uses:** * Prevent NSAID-induced gastric ulcers*; induction of labor, incomplete & therapeutic abortion **Action:** Prostaglandin w/ both antisecretory & mucosal protective properties **Dose:** *Ulcer prevention:* 200 mcg PO qid w/ meals; in females, start on 2nd or 3rd day of next nl menstrual period; 25–50 mcg for induction of labor (term); 400 mcg on day 3 of mifepristone for PRG termination (take w/ food) **Caution:** [X, –] **Contra:** PRG, component allergy **Supplied:** Tabs 100, 200 mcg **SE:** Can cause miscarriage w/ potentially dangerous bleeding; HA, GI Sxs common (D, abdominal pain, constipation)

Mitomycin (Mutamycin) **Uses:** *Stomach, pancreas,* breast, colon CA*; squamous cell carcinoma of the anus; non-small-cell lung, head & neck, cervical, & breast CA; bladder CA (intravesically) **Action:** Alkylating agent; may generate oxygen free radicals, w/ DNA strand breaks **Dose:** 20 mg/m² q6–8wk or 10 mg/m² in combo w/ other myelosuppressive drugs; bladder CA 20–40 mg in 40 mL NS via a urethral catheter once/wk for 8 wk, followed by monthly treatments for 1 y; ↓ in renal/hepatic impair **Caution:** [D, –] **Contra:** Thrombocytopenia, leukopenia, coagulation disorders, SCr >1.7 mg/dL **Supplied:** Inj **SE:** Myelosuppression (may persist up to 3–8 wk after dose, may be cumulative; minimize by a lifetime dose <50–60 mg/m²), N/V, anorexia, stomatitis, & renal tox; microangiopathic hemolytic anemia (similar to hemolytic–uremic syndrome) w/ progressive renal failure; venoocclusive Dz of the liver, interstitial pneumonia, alopecia (rare); extravasation Rxns

Mitoxantrone (Novantrone) Uses: *AML (w/ cytarabine), ALL, CML, CAP, MS,* breast CA, & NHL Action: DNA-intercalating agent; ↓ DNA topoisomerase II Dose: Per protocol; ↓ in hepatic failure, leukopenia, thrombocytopenia; maintain hydration Caution: [D, –] reports of secondary AML (monitor CBC) Contra: PRG Supplied: Inj 2 mg/mL SE: Myelosuppression, N/V, stomatitis, alopecia (infrequent), cardiotox; urine discoloration; cardiac monitoring prior to each dose

Modafinil (Provigil) Uses: * Improve wakefulness in pts w/ narcolepsy & excessive daytime sleepiness* Action: May alter dopamine & norepinephrine release, ↓ GABA-mediated neurotransmission Dose: 200 mg PO q morning Caution: [C, ?/–] ↑ effects of warfarin, diazepam, phenytoin; ↓ effects of oral contraceptives, cyclosporine, theophylline Contra: Component allergy Supplied: Tablets 100 mg, 200 mg SE: HA, N, D, paresthesias, rhinitis, agitation Notes: Lower dose in elderly pts ↓ by 50% in pts w/ hepatic impair; use w/ caution in pts w/ CV Dz

Moexipril (Univasc) Uses: *HTN, post-MI,* DN Action: ACE inhibitor Dose: 7.5–30 mg in 1–2 ÷ doses 1 h ac Caution: [C (1st tri, D 2nd & 3rd tri), ?] Contra: ACE inhibitor sensitivity Supplied: Tabs 7.5, 15 mg; ↓ in renal impair SE: ↓ BP, edema, angioedema, HA, dizziness, cough

Molindone (Moban) Uses: *Psychotic disorders* Action: Piperazine phenothiazine Dose: Adults. 50–75 mg/d, ↑ to 225 mg/d if necessary. Peds. 3–5 y: 1–2.5 mg/d in 4 ÷ doses. 5–12 y: 0.5–1.0 mg/kg/d in 4 ÷ doses Caution: [C, ?] NA glaucoma Contra: Drug or EtOH-induced CNS depression Supplied: Tabs 5, 10, 25, 50, 100 mg; conc 20 mg/mL SE: ↓ BP, tachycardia, arrhythmias, EPS, Szs, constipation, xerostomia, blurred vision

Montelukast (Singulair) Uses: *Prophylaxis & Rx of chronic asthma, seasonal allergic rhinitis* Action: Leukotriene receptor antagonist Dose: Asthma: Adults & Peds > 15y. 10 mg/d PO taken in PM. Peds. 2–5 y: 4 mg/d PO taken in PM. 6–14 y: 5 mg/d PO in PM. Rhinitis: Adults & Peds > 15y. 10 mg qd Peds. 2–5 y: 4 mg qd. 6–14 y: 5 mg qd Caution: [B, M] Contra: Component allergy Supplied: Tabs 10 mg; chew tabs 4, 5 mg SE: HA, dizziness, fatigue, rash, GI upset, Churg–Strauss syndrome Notes: Not for acute asthma attacks

Morphine (Avinza XR, Duramorph, Infumorph, MS Contin, Kadian SR, Oramorph SR, Palladone, Roxanol) [C-II] Uses: *Relief of severe pain* Action: Narcotic analgesic Dose: Adults. PO: 5–30 mg q4h PRN; SR tabs 30–60 mg q8–12h (do not chew/crush). IV/IM: 2.5–15 mg q2–6h; supp 10–30 mg q4h. IT: (Duramorph, Infumorph): Per protocol Peds. 0.1–0.2 mg/kg/dose IM/IV q2–4h PRN to 15 mg/dose max Caution: [B (D if prolonged use or high doses at term), +/−] **Contra:** Severe asthma, resp depression, GI obstruction **Supplied:** Immediate-release tabs 10, 14, 20 mg; MS Contin CR tabs 15, 30, 60, 100, 200 mg; Oramorph SR CR tabs 15, 30, 60, 100 mg; Kadian SR caps 20 30 50, 60, 100 mg; Palladone ER caps 12, 16, 24, 32 mg; Avinza XR caps 30, 60, 90, 120 mg; soln 10, 20, 100 mg/mL; supp 5, 10, 20 mg; inj 2, 4, 5, 8, 10, 15 mg/mL; Duramorph/Infumorph 0.5, 1 mg/mL; supp 5, 10, 20, 30 mg **SE:** Narcotic SE (resp depression, sedation, constipation, N/V, pruritus), granulomas w/ IT **Notes:** May require scheduled dosing to relieve severe chronic pain; do not crush/chew SR/ER forms

Morphine liposomal (DepoDur)
Uses: *Long-lasting epidural analgesia* **Action:** ER morphine analgesia **Dose:** 10–20 mg lumbar epidural inj (c-section 10 mg after cord clamped) **Caution:** [C,+/−] elderly, biliary Dz (sphincter of Oddi spasm) **Contra:** paralytic ileus, resp depression, asthma, obstructed airway, suspected/or known head injury ↑ ICP, allergy to morphine. **Supplied:** Inj 10 mg/mL **SE:** Hypoxia, resp depression, ↓ BP, retention, N/V, constipation, flatulence, pruritus, pyrexia, anemia, HA, dizziness, tachycardia, insomnia, ileus **Notes:** Effect ≤ 48 h; not for IT/IV/IM use

Moxifloxacin (Avelox, Vigamox ophthalmic)
Uses: *Acute sinusitis, acute bronchitis, skin/soft tissue Infxns, conjunctivitis, & community-acquired pneumonia* **Action:** 4th-gen quinolone; ↓ DNA gyrase. *Spectrum:* Excellent gram(+) coverage except MRSA & *E. faecium*; good gram(−) coverage except *P. aeruginosa, S. maltophilia*, & *Acinetobacter* sp; good anaerobic coverage **Dose:** 400 mg/d PO (avoid cation products, antacids) /IV qd. *Ophth:* 1 gt tid ×7d **Caution:** [C, ?/−] Quinolone sensitivity; interactions w/ Mg-, Ca-, Al-, & Fe-containing products & class IA & III antiarrhythmic agents **Contra:** Quinolone or component sensitivity **Supplied:** Tabs 400 mg, inj, ophth 0.5% **SE:** Dizziness, nausea, QT prolongation, Szs, photosensitivity, tendon rupture **Notes:** Take 4 h before or 8 h after antacids

Mupirocin (Bactroban)
Uses: *Impetigo; eradication of MRSA in nasal carriers* **Action:** ↓ bacterial protein synthesis **Dose:** *Topical:* Apply small amount to affected area. *Nasal:* Apply bid in nostrils **Caution:** [B, ?] **Contra:** Do not use concurrently w/ other nasal products **Supplied:** Oint 2%; cream 2% **SE:** Local irritation, rash

Muromonab-CD3 (Orthoclone OKT3)
WARNING: Can cause anaphylaxis; monitor fluid status **Uses:** *Acute rejection following organ transplantation* **Action:** Blocks T-cell Fxn **Dose:** *Adults.* 5 mg/d IV for 10–14 d. *Peds.* 0.1 mg/kg/d for 10–14 d **Caution:** [C, ?/−] Murine sensitivity, fluid overload **Contra:** Heart failure/fluid overload, Hx of Szs, PRG, uncontrolled HTN **Supplied:** Inj 5 mg/5 mL **SE:** Murine Ab; fever & chills after the 1st dose (premedicate w/ steroid/APAP/antihistamine); monitor closely for anaphylaxis or pulmonary edema **Notes:** Use 0.22-mcm filter for administration

Mycophenolic Acid (Myfortic)
WARNING: ↑ Risk of Infxns, possible development of lymphoma **Uses:** *Prevent rejection after renal transplant* **Action:**

Cytostatic to lymphocytes **Dose:** *Adults.* 720 mg PO bid; *Peds.* BSA 400–720 mg/m²: 750 mg PO bid; ↓ in renal insuff/neutropenia (on empty stomach) **Caution:** [C, ?/–] **Contra:** Component allergy **Supplied:** DR tabs 180, 360 mg **SE:** N/V/D, pain, fever, HA, Infxn, HTN, anemia, leukopenia, edema

Mycophenolate Mofetil (CellCept) WARNING: ↑ Risk of Infxns, possible development of lymphoma **Uses:** *Prevent organ rejection after transplant* **Action:** ↓ immunologically mediated inflammatory responses **Dose:** *Adults.* 1 g PO bid; *Peds.* BSA 1.2–1.5 m²: 750 mg PO bid; *BSA >1.5 m²:* 1 g PO bid; may taper up to 600 mg/m² PO bid; used w/ steroids & cyclosporine; ↓ in renal insuff or neutropenia. *IV:* Infuse over at least 2 h. *PO:* Take on empty stomach, do not open capsules **Caution:** [C, ?/–] **Contra:** Component allergy; IV use in polysorbate 80 allergy **Supplied:** Caps 250, 500 mg; inj 500 mg **SE:** N/V/D, pain, fever, HA, Infxn, HTN, anemia, leukopenia, edema

Nabumetone (Relafen) WARNING: May ↑ risk of cardiovascular events & GI bleeding **Uses:** *Arthritis & pain* **Action:** NSAID; ↓ prostaglandins **Dose:** 1000–2000 mg/d ÷ qd–bid w/ food **Caution:** [C (D 3rd tri), +] **Contra:** Peptic ulcer, NSAID sensitivity, severe hepatic Dz **Supplied:** Tabs 500, 750 mg **SE:** Dizziness, rash, GI upset, edema, peptic ulcer

Nadolol (Corgard) **Uses:** *HTN & angina* **Action:** Competitively blocks β-adrenergic receptors, β₁, β₂ **Dose:** 40–80 mg/d; ↑ to 240 mg/d (angina) or 320 mg/d (HTN) may be needed; ↓ in renal insuff & elderly **Caution:** [C (1st tri; D if 2nd or 3rd tri), +] **Contra:** Uncompensated CHF, shock, heart block, asthma **Supplied:** Tabs 20, 40, 80, 120, 160 mg **SE:** Nightmares, paresthesias, ↓ BP, bradycardia, fatigue

Nafcillin (Nallpen) **Uses:** *Infxns caused by susceptible strains of Staphylococcus & Streptococcus* **Action:** Bactericidal; ↓ cell wall synthesis. *Spectrum:* Good gram(+) **Dose:** *Adults.* 1–2 g IV q4–6h. *Peds.* 50–200 mg/kg/d ÷ q4–6h **Caution:** [B, ?] PCN allergy **Supplied:** Inj **SE:** Interstitial nephritis, D, fever, nausea **Notes:** No adjustments for renal Fxn

Naftifine (Naftin) **Uses:** *Tinea pedis, cruris, & corporis* **Action:** Antifungal antibiotic **Dose:** Apply bid **Caution:** [B, ?] **Contra:** Component sensitivity **Supplied:** 1% cream; gel **SE:** Local irritation

Nalbuphine (Nubain) **Uses:** *Moderate–severe pain; preop & obstetric analgesia* **Action:** Narcotic agonist–antagonist; ↓ ascending pain pathways **Dose:** *Adults.* 10–20 mg IM or IV q4–6h PRN; max of 160 mg/d; single max dose, 20 mg. *Peds.* 0.2 mg/kg IV or IM to a max dose of 20 mg; ↓ in hepatic insuff **Caution:** [B (D if prolonged or high doses at term), ?] **Contra:** Sulfite sensitivity **Supplied:** Inj 10, 20 mg/mL **SE:** Causes CNS depression & drowsiness; caution in pts receiving opiates

Naloxone (Narcan) **Uses:** *Opioid addiction (diagnosis) & OD* **Action:** Competitive narcotic antagonist **Dose:** *Adults.* 0.4–2.0 mg IV, IM, or SQ q5min; max total dose, 10 mg. *Peds.* 0.01–1 mg/kg/dose IV, IM, or SQ; repeat IV q3min ×

3 doses PRN **Caution:** [B, ?] May precipitate acute withdrawal in addicts **Supplied:** Inj 0.4, 1.0 mg/mL; neonatal inj 0.02 mg/mL **SE:** ↓ BP, tachycardia, irritability, GI upset, pulmonary edema **Notes:** If no response after 10 mg, suspect nonnarcotic cause

Naltrexone (ReVia) Uses: *EtOH & narcotic addiction* **Action:** Competitively binds to opioid receptors **Dose:** 50 mg PO; do not give until opioid-free for 7–10 d **Caution:** [C, M] **Contra:** Acute hepatitis, liver failure; opioid use **Supplied:** Tabs 50 mg **SE:** May cause hepatotox; insomnia, GI upset, joint pain, HA, fatigue

Naphazoline & Antazoline (Albalon-A Ophthalmic, others), Naphazoline & Pheniramine Acetate (Naphcon A) Uses: *Relieve ocular redness & itching caused by allergy* **Action:** Vasoconstrictor & antihistamine **Dose:** 1–2 gtt up to qid **Caution:** [C, +] **Contra:** Glaucoma, children <6 y, & w/ contact lenses **Supplied:** Soln 15 mL **SE:** CV stimulation, dizziness, local irritation

Naproxen (Aleve [OTC], Naprosyn, Anaprox) WARNING: May ↑ risk of cardiovascular events & GI bleeding Uses: *Arthritis & pain* **Action:** NSAID; ↓ prostaglandins **Dose:** *Adults & Peds >12 y.* 200–500 mg bid–tid to 1500 mg/d max; ↓ in hepatic impair **Caution:** [B (D 3rd tri), +] **Contra:** NSAID sensitivity, peptic ulcer **Supplied:** Tabs 200, 220, 250, 375, 500 mg; DR (EC) tabs 375, 500 mg; susp 125 mg/5 mL **SE:** Dizziness, pruritus, GI upset, peptic ulcer, edema

Naratriptan (Amerge) [OTC] Uses: *Acute migraine attacks* **Action:** Serotonin 5-HT$_1$ receptor antagonist **Dose:** 1–2.5 mg PO once; repeat PRN in 4 h; ↓ in mild renal/hepatic insuff, take w/ fluids **Caution:** [C, M] **Contra:** Severe renal/hepatic impair, avoid in angina, ischemic heart Dz, uncontrolled HTN, cerebrovascular syndromes, & ergot use **Supplied:** Tabs 1, 2.5 mg **SE:** Dizziness, sedation, GI upset, paresthesias, ECG changes, coronary vasospasm, arrhythmias

Natalizumab (Tysabri) Uses: *Relapsing MS* Withdrawn due to safety concerns

Nateglinide (Starlix) Uses: * Type 2 DM* **Action:** ↑ Pancreatic release of insulin **Dose:** 120 mg PO tid 1–30 min pc; ↓ to 60 mg tid if near target HbA$_{1c}$ (take 1–30 min ac) **Caution:** [C, –]. Caution w/ drugs metabolized by CYP2C9/3A4 **Contra:** Diabetic ketoacidosis, type 1 DM **Supplied:** Tabs 60, 120 mg **SE:** Hypoglycemia, URI; salicylates, nonselective β-blockers may enhance hypoglycemia

Nedocromil (Tilade) Uses: *Mild–moderate asthma* **Action:** Antiinflammatory agent **Dose:** *Inhal:* 2 inhal qid **Caution:** [B, ?/–] **Contra:** Component allergy **Supplied:** Met-dose inhaler **SE:** Chest pain, dizziness, dysphonia, rash, GI upset, Infxn **Notes:** Not for acute asthma attacks

Nefazodone (Serzone) WARNING: Fatal hepatitis & liver failure possible, D/C if LFT >3× ULN, do not re-treat; closely monitor for worsening depression or emergence of suicidality, particularly in ped pts Uses: *Depression* **Action:** ↓ Neuronal uptake of serotonin & norepinephrine **Dose:** Initial 100 mg PO bid; usual 300–600 mg/d in 2 ÷ doses **Caution:** [C, ?] **Contra:** MAOIs, pimozide, cisapride, carbamazepine **Supplied:** Tabs 100, 150, 200, 250 mg **SE:** Postural ↓ BP & allergic Rxns; HA, drowsiness, xerostomia, constipation, GI upset, liver failure **Notes:** Monitor LFTs, HR/BP

Nelfinavir (Viracept)
Uses: *HIV Infxn* **Action:** Protease inhibitor; results in formation of immature, noninfectious virion **Dose:** *Adults.* 750 mg PO tid or 1250 mg PO bid. **Peds.** 20–30 mg/kg PO tid; take w/ food **Caution:** [B, ?] Many significant drug interactions **Contra:** Phenylketonuria, triazolam/midazolam use or any other drug highly dependent on CYP3A4 (page 220) **Supplied:** Tabs 250 mg; PO powder **SE:** Food ↑ absorption; interacts w/ St. John's wort; dyslipidemia, lipodystrophy, D, rash

Neomycin, Bacitracin, & Polymyxin B (Neosporin Ointment)
(See Bacitracin, Neomycin, & Polymyxin B Topical, page 421)

Neomycin, Colistin, & Hydrocortisone (Cortisporin-TC Otic Drops); Neomycin, Colistin, Hydrocortisone, & Thonzonium (Cortisporin-TC Otic Suspension)
Uses: *External otitis,* Infxns of mastoid/fenestration cavities **Action:** Antibiotic w/antiinflammatory **Dose:** *Adults.* 4–5 gtt in ear(s) tid–qid. **Peds.** 3–4 gtt in ear(s) tid–qid **Caution:** [C, ?] **Supplied:** Otic gtt & susp **SE:** Local irritation

Neomycin & Dexamethasone (AK-Neo-Dex Ophthalmic, NeoDecadron Ophthalmic)
Uses: *Steroid-responsive inflammatory conditions of the cornea, conjunctiva, lid, & anterior segment* **Action:** Antibiotic w/ antiinflammatory corticosteroid **Dose:** 1–2 gtt in eye(s) q3–4h or thin coat tid–qid until response, then ↓ to qd **Caution:** [C, ?] **Supplied:** Cream neomycin 0.5%/dexamethasone 0.1%; oint neomycin 0.35%/dexamethasone 0.05%; soln neomycin 0.35%/dexamethasone 0.1% **SE:** Local irritation **Notes:** Use under ophthalmologist's supervision

Neomycin & Polymyxin B (Neosporin Cream) [OTC]
Uses: *Infxn in minor cuts, scrapes, & burns* **Action:** Bactericidal **Dose:** Apply bid–qid **Caution:** [C, ?] **Contra:** Component allergy **Supplied:** Cream neomycin 3.5 mg/polymyxin B 10,000 Units/g **SE:** Local irritation **Notes:** Different from Neosporin oint

Neomycin, Polymyxin B, & Dexamethasone (Maxitrol)
Uses: *Steroid-responsive ocular conditions w/ bacterial Infxn* **Action:** Antibiotic w/ antiinflammatory corticosteroid **Dose:** 1–2 gtt in eye(s) q4–6h; apply oint in eye(s) tid–qid **Caution:** [C, ?] **Supplied:** Oint neomycin sulfate 3.5 mg/polymyxin B sulfate 10,000 Units/dexamethasone 0.1%/g; susp identical/5 mL **SE:** Local irritation **Notes:** Use under supervision of ophthalmologist

Neomycin-Polymyxin Bladder Irrigant [Neosporin GU Irrigant]
Uses: *Continuous irrigant for prophylaxis against bacteriuria & gram(−) bacteremia associated w/ indwelling catheter use* **Action:** Bactericide **Dose:** 1 mL irrigant in 1 L of 0.9% NaCl; cont bladder irrigation w/ 1 L of soln/24 h **Caution:**

[D] Contra: Component allergy **Supplied:** Soln neomycin sulfate 40 mg & polymyxin B 200,000 Units/mL; amp 1, 20 mL **SE:** Neomycin-induced ototoxic or nephrotox (rare) **Notes:** Potential for bacterial or fungal super Infxn; not for inj

Neomycin, Polymyxin, & Hydrocortisone (Cortisporin Ophthalmic & Otic)
Uses: *Ocular & otic bacterial Infxns* **Action:** Antibiotic & antiinflammatory **Dose:** *Otic:* 3–4 gtt in the ear(s) tid–qid. *Ophth:* Apply a thin layer to the eye(s) or 1 gt qd–qid **Caution:** [C, ?] **Supplied:** Otic susp; ophth soln; ophth oint **SE:** Local irritation

Neomycin, Polymyxin B, & Prednisolone (Poly-Pred Ophthalmic)
Uses: *Steroid-responsive ocular conditions w/ bacterial Infxn* **Action:** Antibiotic & antiinflammatory **Dose:** 1–2 gtt in eye(s) q4–6h; apply oint in eye(s) tid–qid **Caution:** [C, ?] **Supplied:** Susp neomycin 0.35%/polymyxin B 10,000 Units/prednisolone 0.5%/mL **SE:** Irritation **Notes:** Use under supervision of ophthalmologist

Neomycin Sulfate (Myciguent) [OTC]
Uses: *Hepatic coma, bowel prep* **Action:** Aminoglycoside, poorly absorbed PO; ↓ GI bacterial flora **Dose:** *Adults.* 3–12 g/24 h PO in 3–4 ÷ doses. *Peds.* 50–100 mg/kg/24 h PO in 3–4 ÷ doses **Caution:** [C, ?/–] Renal failure, neuromuscular disorders, hearing impair **Contra:** Intestinal obstruction **Supplied:** Tabs 500 mg; PO soln 125 mg/5 mL **SE:** Hearing loss w/ long-term use; rash, N/V **Notes:** Do not use parenterally (↑ tox); part of the Condon bowel prep

Nesiritide (Natrecor)
Uses: *Acutely decompensated CHF* **Action:** Human B-type natriuretic peptide **Dose:** 2 mcg/kg IV bolus, then 0.01 mcg/kg/min IV **Caution:** [C, ?/–] When vasodilators are not appropriate **Contra:** SBP <90, cardiogenic shock **Supplied:** Vials 1.5 mg **SE:** ↓ BP, HA, GI upset, arrhythmias, ↑ Cr **Notes:** Requires continuous BP monitoring; some studies indicate ↑ in mortality

Nevirapine (Viramune)
WARNING: Reports of fatal hepatotox even after short-term use; severe life-threatening skin reactions (Stevens–Johnson, toxic epidermal necrolysis, & allergic Rxns); monitor closely during 1st 8 wk of Rx **Uses:** *HIV Infxn* **Action:** Nonnucleoside RT inhibitor **Dose:** *Adults.* Initial 200 mg PO × 14 d, then 200 mg bid. *Peds.* <8 y: 4 mg/kg/d × 14 d, then 7 mg/kg bid. >8 y: 4 mg/kg/d × 14 d, then 4 mg/kg bid (w/o regard to food) **Caution:** [C, +/–] OCP **Supplied:** Tabs 200 mg; susp 50 mg/5 mL **SE:** Life-threatening rash; HA, fever, D, neutropenia, hepatitis. **Notes:** Give w/out regard to food; not recommended in women if CD_4 > 250 or men > 400 unless benefit >> risk of hepatotoxicity

Niacin (Niaspan)
Uses: * Adjunct in significant hyperlipidemia* **Action:** ↓ Lipolysis; ↓ esterification of triglycerides; ↑ lipoprotein lipase **Dose:** 1–6 g ÷ doses PO tid; 9 g/d max (w/ food) **Caution:** [A (C if doses >RDA), +] **Contra:** Liver Dz, peptic ulcer, arterial hemorrhage **Supplied:** SR caps 125, 250, 300, 400, 500 mg; tabs 25, 50, 100, 250, 500 mg; SR tabs 150, 250, 500, 750 mg; elixir 50 mg/5 mL **SE:** Upper body/facial flushing & warmth; GI upset, flatulence, exacer-

bate peptic ulcer; HA, paresthesias, liver damage, gout, or altered glucose control in DM. **Notes:** Flushing ↓ by taking aspirin or NSAID 30–60 min prior to dose

Nicardipine (Cardene) **Uses:** *Chronic stable angina & HTN*; prophylaxis of migraine **Action:** CCB **Dose:** *Adults.* *PO:* 20–40 mg PO tid. *SR:* 30–60 mg PO bid. *IV:* 5 mg/h IV cont inf; ↑ by 2.5 mg/h q15min to max 15 mg/h. *Peds.* *PO:* 20–30 mg PO q 8h. *IV:* 0.5–5 mcg/kg/min; ↓ in renal/hepatic impair **Caution:** [C, ?/–] Heart block, CAD **Contra:** Cardiogenic shock **Supplied:** Caps 20, 30 mg; SR caps 30, 45, 60 mg; inj 2.5 mg/mL **SE:** Flushing, tachycardia, ↓ BP, edema, HA **Notes:** *PO-to-IV conversion:* 20 mg tid = 0.5 mg/h, 30 mg tid = 1.2 mg/h, 40 mg tid = 2.2 mg/h; take w/ food (not high fat)

Nicotine Gum (Nicorette) [OTC] **Uses:** *Aid to smoking cessation for relief of nicotine withdrawal* **Action:** Systemic delivery of nicotine **Dose:** Chew 9–12 pieces/d PRN; max 30 pieces/d **Caution:** [C, ?] **Contra:** Life-threatening arrhythmias, unstable angina **Supplied:** 2 mg, 4 mg/piece; mint, orange, original flavors **SE:** Tachycardia, HA, GI upset, hiccups **Notes:** Must stop smoking & perform behavior modification for max effect

Nicotine Nasal Spray (Nicotrol NS) **Uses:** *Aid to smoking cessation for relief of nicotine withdrawal* **Action:** Systemic delivery of nicotine **Dose:** 0.5 mg/actuation; 1–2 sprays/h, 10 sprays/h max **Caution:** [D, M] **Contra:** Life-threatening arrhythmias, unstable angina **Supplied:** Nasal inhaler 10 mg/mL **SE:** Local irritation, tachycardia, HA, taste perversion **Notes:** Must stop smoking & perform behavior modification for max effect

Nicotine Transdermal (Habitrol, Nicoderm CQ [OTC], Nicotrol [OTC]) **Uses:** *Aid to smoking cessation; relief of nicotine withdrawal* **Action:** Systemic delivery of nicotine **Dose:** Individualized; 1 patch (14–22 mg/d), & taper over 6 wk **Caution:** [D, M] **Contra:** Life-threatening arrhythmias, unstable angina **Supplied:** Habitrol & Nicoderm CQ 7, 14, 21 mg of nicotine/24 h; Nicotrol 5, 10, 15 mg/24 h **SE:** Insomnia, pruritus, erythema, local site Rxn, tachycardia **Notes:** Nicotrol worn for 16 h to mimic smoking patterns; others worn for 24 h; must stop smoking & perform behavior modification for max effect

Nifedipine (Procardia, Procardia XL, Adalat, Adalat CC) **Uses:** *Vasospastic or chronic stable angina & HTN*; tocolytic **Action:** CCB **Dose:** *Adults.* SR tabs 30–90 mg/d. *Tocolysis:* 10–20 mg PO q4–6h. *Peds.* 0.6–0.9 mg/kg/24 h ÷ tid–qid **Caution:** [C, +] Heart block, aortic stenosis **Contra:** Immediate-release preparation for urgent or emergent HTN; acute MI **Supplied:** Caps 10, 20 mg; SR tabs 30, 60, 90 mg **SE:** HA common on initial Rx; reflex tachycardia may occur w/ regular release dosage forms; peripheral edema, ↓ BP, flushing, dizziness **Notes:** Adalat CC & Procardia XL not interchangeable; SL administration not OK

Nilutamide (Nilandron) **WARNING:** Interstitial pneumonitis possible; most cases in 1st 3 mo; follow CXR before Rx **Uses:** *Combo w/ surgical castration for metastatic CAP* **Action:** Nonsteroidal antiandrogen **Dose:** 300 mg/d PO in ÷ doses for 30 d, then 150 mg/d **Caution:** [N/A] **Contra:** Severe hepatic impair or resp insuff **Supplied:** Tabs 150 mg **SE:** Hot flashes, loss of libido, impotence, N/V/D, gynecomastia, hepatic dysfunction (follow LFTs), interstitial pneumonitis **Notes:** May cause Rxn when taken w/ EtOH

Nimodipine (Nimotop) **Uses:** *Prevent vasospasm following subarachnoid hemorrhage* **Action:** CCB **Dose:** 60 mg PO q4h for 21 d; ↓ in hepatic failure **Caution:** [C, ?] **Contra:** Component allergy **Supplied:** Caps 30 mg **SE:** ↓ BP, HA, constipation **Notes:** Administered via NG tube if caps cannot be swallowed whole

Nisoldipine (Sular) **Uses:** *HTN* **Action:** CCB **Dose:** 10–60 mg/d PO; do not take w/ grapefruit juice or high-fat meal; ↓ starting doses in elderly or hepatic impair **Caution:** [C, ?] **Supplied:** ER tabs 10, 20, 30, 40 mg **SE:** Edema, HA, flushing

Nitazoxanide (Alinia) **Uses:** *Cryptosporidium-* or *Giardia*-induced diarrhea in pts 1–11 y* **Action:** Antiprotozoal. *Spectrum: Cryptosporidium* or *Giardia* **Dose:** *Peds 12–47 mo.* 5 mL (100 mg) PO q 12h × 3 d. *4–11 y:* 10 mL (200 mg) PO q 12h × 3 d; take w/ food **Caution:** [B, ?] **Contra:** **Supplied:** 100 mg/5 mL PO susp **SE:** Abdominal pain **Notes:** Susp contains sucrose, interacts w/ highly protein-bound drugs

Nitrofurantoin (Macrodantin, Furadantin, Macrobid) **WARNING:** Pulmonary reactions possible **Uses:** *Prevention & Rx UTI* **Action:** Bacteriostatic; interferes w/ carbohydrate metabolism. *Spectrum:* Susceptible gram(–) & some gram(+) bacteria; *Pseudomonas, Serratia,* & most sp. *Proteus*-resistant **Dose:** *Adults.* Suppression: 50–100 mg/d PO. *Rx:* 50–100 mg PO qid. *Peds.* 4–7 mg/kg/24 h in 4 ÷ doses (w/ food/milk/antacid) **Caution:** [B, +] Avoid if CrCl <50 mL/min, pregnant at term **Contra:** Renal failure, infants < 1 mo **Supplied:** Caps/tabs 50, 100 mg; SR caps 100 mg; susp 25 mg/5 mL **SE:** GI side effects; dyspnea & a variety of acute/chronic pulmonary reactions, peripheral neuropathy **Notes:** Macrocrystals (Macrodantin) cause < nausea than other forms

Nitroglycerin (Nitrostat, Nitrolingual, Nitro-Bid Ointment, Nitro-Bid IV, Nitrodisc, Transderm-Nitro, others) **Uses:** *Angina pectoris, acute & prophylactic therapy, CHF, BP control* **Action:** Relaxation of vascular smooth muscle, dilates coronary arteries **Dose:** *Adults.* SL: 1 tab q5min SL PRN for 3 doses. *Translingual:* 1–2 met-doses sprayed onto PO mucosa q3–5min, max 3 doses. *PO:* 2.5–9 mg tid. *IV:* 5–20 mcg/min, titrated to effect. *Topical:* Apply ½ in. of oint to chest wall tid, wipe off at night. *TD:* 0.2–0.4 mg/h/patch qd. *Peds.* 1 mcg/kg/min IV, titrate. **Caution:** [B, ?] Restrictive cardiomyopathy **Contra:** *IV:* Pericardial tamponade, constrictive pericarditis. *PO:* Use w/ sildenafil, tadalafil, vardenfil, head trauma, closed-angle glaucoma **Supplied:** SL tabs 0.3, 0.4, 0.6 mg; translingual spray 0.4 mg/dose; SR caps 2.5, 6.5, 9, 13 mg; SR tabs 2.6, 6.5, 9.0 mg; inj 0.5, 5, 10 mg/mL; oint 2%; TD patches 0.1, 0.2, 0.4, 0.6 mg/h; buccal CR 2, 3 mg **SE:** HA, ↓ BP, lightheadedness, GI upset **Notes:** Nitrate tolerance w/ chronic use after 1–2 wk; minimize by providing nitrate-free period qd, using shorter-acting nitrates tid, & removing long-acting patches & oint before sleep to ↓ tolerance

Nitroprusside (Nipride, Nitropress)
Uses: *Hypertensive crisis, CHF, controlled ↓ BP periop (↓ bleeding),* aortic dissection, pulmonary edema **Action:** ↓ Systemic vascular resistance *Adult & Peds.* 0.5–10 mcg/kg/min IV inf, titrate; usual dose 3 mcg/kg/min **Caution:** [C, ?] ↓ cerebral perfusion **Contra:** High output failure, compensatory HTN **Supplied:** Inj 25 mg/mL **SE:** Excessive hypotensive effects, palpitations, HA **Notes:** Thiocyanate (metabolite w/renal excretion) w/ tox at 5–10 mg/dL, more likely if used for > 2–3 d; to Rx aortic dissection, use β-blocker concomitantly

Nizatidine (Axid, Axid AR [OTC])
Uses: *Duodenal ulcers, GERD, heartburn* **Action:** H$_2$-receptor antagonist **Dose:** *Adults. Active ulcer:* 150 mg PO bid or 300 mg PO hs; maint 150 mg PO hs. *Heartburn:* 75 mg PO bid. *Peds. GERD:* 10 mg/kg PO bid in ÷ doses, 150 mg bid max ↓ in renal impair **Caution:** [B, +] **Contra:** H$_2$-receptor antagonist sensitivity **Supplied:** Caps 75 [OTC], 150, 300 mg **SE:** Dizziness, HA, constipation, D

Norepinephrine (Levophed)
Uses: *Acute* ↓ BP, cardiac arrest (adjunct)* **Action:** Peripheral vasoconstrictor acts on arterial/venous beds **Dose:** *Adults.* 8–12 mcg/min IV, titrate. *Peds.* 0.05 – 0.1 mg/kg/min IV, titrate **Caution:** [C, ?] **Contra:** ↓ BP due to hypovolemia **Supplied:** Inj 1 mg/mL **SE:** Bradycardia, arrhythmia **Notes:** Correct volume depletion as much as possible before vasopressors; interaction w/ TCAs leads to severe HTN; infuse into large vein to avoid extravasation; phentolamine 5–10 mg/10 mL NS injected locally for extravasation

Norethindrone Acetate/Ethinyl Estradiol (FemHRT)
WARNING: Estrogens & progestins should not be used for the prevention of CV Dz; the WHI study reported ↑ risks of MI, breast CA, & DVT in postmenopausal women during 5 y of treatment with estrogens combined with medroxyprogesterone acetate relative to placebo **Uses:** *Rx of moderate–severe vasomotor Sxs associated w/ menopause; prevent osteoporosis*. **Action:** Hormone replacement **Dose:** 1 tablet qd **Caution:** [X, –] **Contra:** PRG; Hx breast CA; estrogen-dependent neoplasia; abnormal genital bleeding; Hx DVT, PE, or related disorders; recent (w/in past year) arterial thromboembolic Dz (CVA, MI) **Supplied:** 1 mg norethindrone/5 mcg ethinyl estradiol tablets **SE:** Thrombosis, dizziness, HA, libido changes **Notes:** Use in women w/ intact uterus

Norfloxacin (Noroxin, Chibroxin ophthal)
Uses: *Complicated & uncomplicated UTI due to gram(–) bacteria, prostatitis, gonorrhea,* & infectious D* **Action:** Quinolone, ↓ DNA gyrase. *Spectrum:* Susceptible *E. faecalis, E. coli, K. pneumoniae, P. mirabilis, P. aeruginosa, S. epidermidis, S. saprophyticus* **Dose:** 400 mg PO bid (↓ in renal impair). *Gonorrhea:* 800 mg single dose. *Prostatitis:* 400 mg PO bid *Adults, Peds > 1 y:* 1 gt each eye qid for 7 d **Caution:** [C, –] Tendinitis/tendon rupture, quinolone sensitivity, **Contra:** Hx of allergy or tendinitis w/ fluoroquinolones **Supplied:** Tabs 400 mg; ophth 3 mg/mL **SE:** Photosensitivity,

HA, GI; ocular burning w/ ophth **Notes:** Interactions w/ antacids, theophylline, caffeine; good conc in the kidney & urine, poor blood levels; do not use for urosepsis

Norgestrel (Ovrette) Uses: *PO Contraceptive* **Action:** Prevent follicular maturation & ovulation **Dose:** 1 tab/d; begin day 1 of menses **Caution:** [X, ?] **Contra:** Thromboembolic disorders, breast CA, PRG, severe hepatic Dz **Supplied:** Tabs 0.075 mg **SE:** Edema, breakthrough bleeding, thromboembolism **Notes:** Progestin-only products have ↑ risk of failure in prevention of PRG

Nortriptyline (Aventyl, Pamelor) Uses: *Endogenous depression* **Action:** TCA; ↑ synaptic CNS levels of serotonin &/or norepinephrine **Dose:** *Adults.* 25 mg PO tid–qid; >150 mg/d not OK. *Elderly.* 10–25 mg hs. *Peds. 6–7 y:* 10 mg/d. *8–11 y:* 10–20 mg/d. *>11 y:* 25–35 mg/d, ↓ w/ hepatic insuff **Caution:** [D, +/–] NA glaucoma, CV Dz **Contra:** TCA allergy, use w/ MAOI **Supplied:** Caps 10, 25, 50, 75 mg; soln 10 mg/5 mL **SE:** Anticholinergic (blurred vision, retention, xerostomia) **Notes:** Max effect seen after 2 wk

Nystatin (Mycostatin) Uses: *Mucocutaneous Candida* Infxns (oral, skin, vaginal)* **Action:** Alters membrane permeability. **Spectrum:** Susceptible *Candida* sp **Dose:** *Adults & children.* PO: 400,000–600,000 Units PO "swish & swallow" qid. *Vaginal:* 1 tab vaginally hs × 2 wk. *Topical:* Apply bid–tid to area. *Peds. Infants:* 200,000 Units PO q6h. **Caution:** [B (C PO), +] **Supplied:** PO susp 100,000 Units/mL; PO tabs 500,000 Units; troches 200,000 Units; vaginal tabs 100,000 U; topical cream/oint 100,000 Units/g **SE:** GI upset, Stevens–Johnson syndrome **Notes:** Not absorbed PO; not for systemic Infxns

Octreotide (Sandostatin, Sandostatin LAR) Uses: *Suppresses/↓ severe diarrhea associated w/ carcinoid & neuroendocrine GI tumors (eg, VIPoma, ZE syndrome)*; bleeding esophageal varices **Action:** Long-acting peptide; mimics natural hormone somatostatin **Dose:** *Adults.* 100–600 mcg/d SQ/IV in 2–4 ÷ doses; start 50 mcg q2–bid. *Sandostatin LAR (depot):* 10–30 mg IM q4wk **Peds.** 1–10 mcg/kg/24 h SQ in 2–4 ÷ doses. **Caution:** [B, +] Hepatic/renal impair **Supplied:** Inj 0.05, 0.1, 0.2, 0.5, 1 mg/mL; 10, 20, 30 mg/5 mL depot **SE:** N/V, abdominal discomfort, flushing, edema, fatigue, cholelithiasis, hyper-/hypoglycemia, hepatitis

Ofloxacin (Floxin, Ocuflox Ophthalmic) Uses: *Lower resp tract, skin & skin structure, & UTI, prostatitis, uncomplicated gonorrhea, & Chlamydia Infxns; topical (bacterial conjunctivitis; otitis externa; if perforated ear drum >12 y)* **Action:** ↓ DNA gyrase. **Spectrum:** S. pneumoniae, S. aureus, S. pyogenes, H. influenzae, P. mirabilis, N. gonorrhoeae, C. trachomatis, E. coli **Dose:** PO: *Adults.* 200–400 mg PO bid or IV q12h. *Ophth: Adults & Peds >1 y.* 1–2 gtt in eye(s) q2–4h for 2 d, then qid × 5 more d. *Otic: Adults & Peds >12 y.* 10 gtt in ear(s) bid for 10 d. *Peds 1–12 y.* 5 gtt in ear(s) bid for 10 d. ↓ in renal impair;(on empty stomach) **Caution:** [C, –] Interacts w/ antacids, sucralfate, Al-, Ca-, Mg-, Fe-, or Zn-containing drugs (↓ absorption) **Contra:** Quinolone allergy **Supplied:** Tabs 200, 300, 400 mg; inj 20, 40 mg/mL; ophth & otic 0.3% **SE:** N/V/D, photosensitivity, insomnia, & HA **Notes:** Use ophth form in ears

Olanzapine (Zyprexa, Zyprexa Zydis) **WARNING:** mortality in elderly w/ dementia-related psychosis **Uses:** *Bipolar mania, schizophrenia,* psychotic disorders, acute agitation in schizophrenia **Action:** Dopamine & serotonin antagonist **Dose:** *Bipolar/schizophrenia:* 5–10 mg/d, ↑ weekly PRN, 20 mg/d max *Agitation:* 10–20 mg IMq2–4h PRN, 40 mg day/max **Caution:** [C, –] **Supplied:** Tabs 2.5, 5, 7.5, 10, 15, 20 mg; PO disintegrating tabs 5, 10, 15, 20 mg **SE:** HA, somnolence, orthostatic ↓ BP, tachycardia, dystonia, xerostomia, constipation **Notes:** Takes weeks to titrate dose; smoking ↓ levels; may be confused w/ Zyrtec

Olopatadine (Patanol) **Uses:** *Allergic conjunctivitis* **Action:** H_1-receptor antagonist **Dose:** 1–2 gtt in eye(s) bid q6–8h **Caution:** [C, ?] **Supplied:** Soln 0.1% 5 mL **SE:** Local irritation, HA, rhinitis **Notes:** Do not instill w/ contacts in

Olsalazine (Dipentum) **Uses:** *Maint remission in ulcerative colitis* **Action:** Topical antiinflammatory **Dose:** 500 mg PO bid (w/ food) **Caution:** [C, M] Salicylate sensitivity **Supplied:** Caps 250 mg **SE:** D, HA, blood dyscrasias, hepatitis

Omalizumab (Xolair) **Uses:** *Moderate–severe asthma in ≥12 y w/ reactivity to an allergen & when Sxs inadequately controlled w/ inhaled steroids* **Action:** Anti-IgE Ab **Dose:** 150–375 mg SQ q2–4wk (dose/frequency based on serum IgE level & BW–see insert) **Caution:** [B,?/–] **Contra:** Component allergy **Supplied:** 150 mg single-use 5-mL vial **SE:** Site Rxn, sinusitis, HA, anaphylaxis reported in 3 pts **Notes:** Continue other asthma medications as indicated

Omeprazole (Prilosec, Zegerid) **Uses:** *Duodenal/gastric ulcers, ZE syndrome, GERD,* H. pylori Infxns **Action:** Proton-pump inhibitor **Dose:** 20–40 mg PO qd–bid Zegerid powder/hac; in small cup w/ 2 Tbsp H_2O (not food other liquids) refill and drink **Caution:** [C, –] **Supplied:** Caps 10, 20, 40 mg; Powder packets 20 mg; Zegerid PO Powder 20, 40 mg **SE:** HA, D **Notes:** Combo (ie, antibiotic) Rx for H. pylori

Ondansetron (Zofran) **Uses:** *Prevent chemo-associated & postop N/V* **Action:** Serotonin receptor antagonist **Dose:** *Chemo:* **Adults & Peds.** 0.15 mg/kg/dose IV prior to chemo, then 4 & 8 h after 1st dose or 4–8 mg PO tid; 1st dose 30 min prior to chemo & give on a schedule, not PRN. *Postop:* **Adults.** 4 mg IV immediately before anesthesia or postop. **Peds.** *<40 kg:* 0.1 mg/kg. *>40 kg:* 4 mg IV ↓ dose w/ hepatic impair **Caution:** [B, +/–] **Supplied:** Tabs 4, 8 mg; inj 2 mg/mL **SE:** D, HA, constipation, dizziness

Oprelvekin (Neumega) **Uses:** *Prevent severe thrombocytopenia w/ chemo* **Action:** ↑ Proliferation & maturation of megakaryocytes (interleukin-11) **Dose:** **Adults.** 50 mcg/kg/d SQ for 10–21 d. *Peds >12 y:* 75–100 mcg/kg/d SQ for 10–21 d. *<12 y:* Use only in clinical trials. **Caution:** [C, ?/–] **Supplied:** 5 mg powder for inj **SE:** Tachycardia, palpitations, arrhythmias, edema, HA, dizziness, insomnia, fatigue, fever, nausea, anemia, dyspnea

Oral Contraceptives, Biphasic, Monophasic, Triphasic, Progestin Only (Table 7, page 214) **Uses:** *Birth control & regulation of anovulatory bleeding* **Action:** *Birth control:* Suppresses LH surge, prevents ovulation; progestins thicken cervical mucus; ↓ fallopian tubule cilia, ↓ endometrial thickness to ↓ chances of fertilization. *Anovulatory bleeding:* Cyclic hormones mimic body's natural cycle & regulate endometrial lining, results in regular bleeding q28d; may also ↓ uterine bleeding & dysmenorrhea **Dose:** 28-d cycle pills take qd; 21-d cycle pills take qd, no pills during last 7 d of cycle (during menses); some available as transdermal patch **Caution:** [X, +] Migraine, HTN, DM, sickle cell Dz, gallbladder Dz **Contra:** Undiagnosed vaginal bleeding, PRG, estrogen-dependent malignancy, hypercoagulation disorders, liver Dz, hemiplegic migraine, smokers >35 y **Supplied:** 28-d cycle pills (21 active pills + 7 placebo/Fe supl); 21-d cycle pills (21 active pills) **SE:** Intramenstrual bleeding, oligomenorrhea, amenorrhea, ↑ appetite/weight gain, ↓ libido, fatigue, depression, mood swings, mastalgia, HA, melasma, ↑ vaginal discharge, acne/greasy skin, corneal edema, nausea **Notes:** Taken correctly, 99.9% effective for preventing PRG; no STDs prevention, use additional barrier contraceptive; long term, can ↓ risk of ectopic PRG, benign breast Dz, ovarian & uterine CA. *Rx for menstrual cycle control:* Start w/ monophasic; take for 3 mo before switching to another brand; if bleeding continues, change to pill w/ higher estrogen dose. *Rx for birth control:* Choose pill w/ lowest SE profile for particular pt; SEs numerous, due to Sxs of estrogen excess or progesterone deficiency; each pill's side effect profile is unique (see insert)

Orlistat (Xenical) **Uses:** *Manage obesity w/ BMI ≥ 30 kg/m² or ≥ 27 kg/m² w/ other risk factors; type 2 DM, dyslipidemia* **Action:** Reversible inhibitor of gastric & pancreatic lipases. **Dose:** 120 mg PO tid w/ a fat-containing meal **Caution:** [B, ?] May ↓ cyclosporine & ↓ warfarin dose requirements **Contra:** Cholestasis, malabsorption **Supplied:** Capsules 120 mg **SE:** Abdominal pain/discomfort, fatty/oily stools, fecal urgency **Notes:** Do not use if meal contains no fat; GI effects ↑ w/high-fat meals; supplement w/ fat-soluble vitamins

Orphenadrine (Norflex) **Uses:** *Muscle spasms* **Action:** Central atropine-like effects cause indirect skeletal muscle relaxation, euphoria, analgesia **Dose:** 100 mg PO bid, 60 mg IM/IV q12h **Caution:** [C, +] **Contra:** Glaucoma, GI obstruction, cardiospasm, MyG **Supplied:** Tabs 100 mg; SR tabs 100 mg; inj 30 mg/mL **SE:** Drowsiness, dizziness, blurred vision, flushing, tachycardia, constipation

Oseltamivir (Tamiflu) **Uses:** * Prevention & Rx influenza A & B* **Action:** ↓ viral neuraminidase **Dose:** *Adults.* 75 mg PO bid for 5 d. *Peds. PO* bid dosing: <14 kg: 30 mg. *16–23 kg:* 45 mg. *24–40 kg:* 60 mg; *>40 kg:* As adults; ↓ in renal impair **Caution:** [C, ?/–] **Contra:** Component allergy **Supplied:** Caps 75 mg, powder 12 mg/mL **SE:** N/V, insomnia **Notes:** Initiate w/in 48 h of Sx onset or exposure

Oxacillin (Bactocill, Prostaphlin) **Uses:** *Infxns due to susceptible S. aureus & Streptococcus* **Action:** Bactericidal; ↓ cell wall synthesis. *Spectrum:* Excellent gram(+), poor gram(–) **Dose:** *Adults.* 250–500 mg (1 g severe) IM/IV q4–6h. *Peds.* 150–200 mg/kg/d IV ÷ q4–6h; ↓ in significant renal Dz **Caution:** [B, M] **Contra:** PCN sensitivity **Supplied:** Inj; caps 250, 500 mg; soln 250 mg/5 mL **SE:** GI upset, interstitial nephritis, blood dyscrasias

Oxaliplatin (Eloxatin)   **WARNING:** Administer w/ supervision of physician experienced in chemo. Appropriate management is possible only w/ adequate diagnostic & Rx facilities. Anaphylactic-like Rxns reported. **Uses:** *Adjuvant Rx stage-III colon CA (primary resected) & metastatic colon CA in combo w/ 5-FU* **Action:** Metabolized to platinum derivatives, crosslinks DNA **Dose:** Per protocol; see insert. **Premedicate:** Antiemetics w/ or w/o dexamethasone **Caution:** [D, –] see Warning **Contra:** Allergy to components or platinum **Supplied:** Inj forms **SE:** Anaphylaxis, granulocytopenia, paresthesia, N/V/D, stomatitis, fatigue, neuropathy (common) hepatotox **Notes:** 5-FU & Luekovorin are given in combo; epi, corticosteroids, & antihistamines alleviate severe Rxns

Oxaprozin (Daypro)   **WARNING:** May ↑ risk of cardiovascular events & GI bleeding **Uses:** *Arthritis & pain* **Action:** NSAID; ↓ prostaglandins synthesis **Dose:** 600–1200 mg/d; ↓ in renal/hepatic impair **Caution:** [C (D in 3rd tri or near term), ?] ASA/NSAID sensitivity, peptic ulcer, bleeding disorders **Supplied:** Caps 600 mg **SE:** CNS inhibition, sleep disturbance, rash, GI upset, peptic ulcer, edema, renal failure

Oxazepam (Serax) [C-IV]   **Uses:** *Anxiety, acute EtOH withdrawal,* anxiety w/ depressive Sxs **Action:** Benzodiazepine **Dose:** *Adults.* 10–15 mg PO tid–qid; severe anxiety & EtOH withdrawal may require up to 30 mg qid. *Peds.* 1 mg/kg/d in ÷ doses **Caution:** [D, ?] **Supplied:** Caps 10, 15, 30 mg; tabs 15 mg **SE:** Sedation, ataxia, dizziness, rash, blood dyscrasias, dependence **Notes:** Avoid abrupt D/C; metabolite of diazepam (Valium)

Oxcarbazepine (Trileptal)   **Uses:** *Partial Szs,* bipolar disorders **Action:** Blocks voltage-sensitive Na⁺ channels, stabilization of hyperexcited neural membranes **Dose:** *Adults.* 300 mg PO bid, ↑ weekly to target maint 1200–2400 mg/d. *Peds.* 8–10 mg/kg bid, 500 mg/d max, ↑ weekly to target maint dose; ↓ in renal insuff **Caution:** [C, –] Cross-sensitivity to carbamazepine; reports of fatal skin and multiorgan hypersensitivity Rxns **Contra:** Components sensitivity **Supplied:** Tabs 150, 300, 600 mg **SE:** ↓ Na⁺, HA, dizziness, fatigue, somnolence, GI upset, diplopia, mental concentration difficulties **Notes:** Do not abruptly D/C, check Na⁺ if fatigue reported; advise about symptoms of Stevens-Johnson syndrome and topic epidermal necrolysis

Oxiconazole (Oxistat)   **Uses:** *Tinea pedis, cruris, & corporis* **Action:** Antifungal antibiotic. *Spectrum:* Most strains of *Epidermophyton floccosum, Trichophyton mentagrophytes, Trichophyton rubrum, Malassezia furfur* **Dose:** Apply bid **Caution:** [B, M] **Contra:** Component allergy **Supplied:** Cream 1%; lotion **SE:** Local irritation

Oxybutynin (Ditropan, Ditropan XL)   **Uses:** *Symptomatic relief of urgency, nocturia, & incontinence w/ neurogenic or reflex neurogenic bladder* **Action:** Direct smooth muscle antispasmodic; ↑ bladder capacity **Dose:** *Adults & Peds > 5 y.* 5 mg PO tid–qid; XL 5 mg PO qd; ↑ to 30 mg/d PO (5 & 10 mg/tab). *Peds 1–5 y.* 0.2 mg/kg/dose bid–qid (syrup 5 mg/5 mL); ↓ in elderly; periodic drug holidays

OK **Caution:** [B, ? (use w/ caution)] **Contra:** Glaucoma, MyG, GI or GU obstruction, ulcerative colitis, megacolon **Supplied:** Tabs 5 mg; XL tabs 5, 10, 15 mg; syrup 5 mg/5 mL **SE:** Anticholinergic (drowsiness, xerostomia, constipation, tachycardia)

Oxybutynin Transdermal System (Oxytrol)
Uses: *Rx OAB* **Action:** Smooth muscle antispasmodic; ↑ bladder capacity **Dose:** One 3.9 mg/d system apply 2×/wk to abdomen, hip, or buttock **Caution:** [B, ?/–] **Contra:** Urinary or gastric retention, uncontrolled NA glaucoma **Supplied:** 3.9 mg/d transdermal system **SE:** Anticholinergic effects, itching/redness at application site **Notes:** Avoid reapplication to the same site w/in 7 d

Oxycodone [Dihydrohydroxycodeinone] (OxyContin, OxyIR, Roxicodone) [C-II]
WARNING: Swallow whole, do not crush; high abuse potential **Uses:** *Moderate/severe pain, usually in combo w/ nonnarcotic analgesics* **Action:** Narcotic analgesic **Dose:** *Adults.* 5 mg PO q6h PRN. *Peds. 6–12 y:* 1.25 mg PO q6h PRN. *>12 y:* 2.5 mg q6h PRN. ↓ In severe liver Dz **Caution:** [B (D if prolonged use or near term), M] **Contra:** Allergy, resp depression **Supplied:** Immediate-release caps (OxyIR) 5 mg; tabs (Percolone) 5 mg; CR (OxyContin) 10, 20, 40, 80 mg; liq 5 mg/5 mL **SE:** ↓ BP, sedation, dizziness, GI upset, constipation, risk of abuse **Notes:** OxyContin for chronic CA pain; may be sought after as drug of abuse

Oxycodone & Acetaminophen (Percocet, Tylox) [C-II]
Uses: *Moderate–severe pain* **Action:** Narcotic analgesic **Dose:** *Adults.* 1–2 tabs/caps PO q4–6h PRN (acetaminophen max dose 4 g/d). *Peds.* Oxycodone 0.05–0.15 mg/kg/dose q 4–6h PRN, up to 5 mg/dose **Caution:** [B (D prolonged use or near term), M] **Contra:** Allergy, resp depression **Supplied:** Percocet tabs, mg oxycodone/mg APAP: 2.5/325, 5/325, 7.5/325, 10/325, 7.5/500, 10/650; Tylox caps 5 mg oxycodone, 500 mg APAP; soln 5 mg oxycodone & 325 mg APAP/5 mL **SE:** ↓ BP, sedation, dizziness, GI upset, constipation

Oxycodone & Aspirin (Percodan, Percodan-Demi) [C-II]
Uses: *Moderate–moderately severe pain* **Action:** Narcotic analgesic w/ NSAID **Dose:** *Adults.* 1–2 tabs/caps PO q4–6h PRN. *Peds.* Oxycodone 0.05–0.15 mg/kg/dose q 4–6h PRN, up to 5 mg/dose; ↓ in severe hepatic failure **Caution:** [B (D prolonged use or near term), M] Peptic ulcer **Contra:** Component allergy **Supplied:** Percodan 4.5 mg oxycodone hydrochloride, 0.38 mg oxycodone terephthalate, 325 mg ASA; Percodan-Demi 2.25 mg oxycodone hydrochloride, 0.19 mg oxycodone terephthalate, 325 mg ASA **SE:** Sedation, dizziness, GI upset, constipation

Oxycodone/Ibuprofen (Combunox) [C-II]
Uses: *Short term (not >7 d) management of acute moderate–severe pain* **Action:** Narcotic w/NSAID **Dose:** Initial Caution: [C, –] w/ impaired renal/hepatic Fxn; COPD, CNS depression **Contra:** Paralytic ileus, 3rd tri PRG, allergy to ASA or NSAIDs, where opioids are contraindicated PRG **Supplied:** Tabs 5 mg oxycodone /400 mg ibuprofen **SE:** N/V, somnolence, dizziness, sweating, flatulence, ↑ LFTs **Notes:** Monitor renal Fxn; abuse potential w/ oxycodone

Oxymorphone (Numorphan) [C-II] Uses: *Moderate/severe pain, sedative* Action: Narcotic analgesic Dose: 0.5 mg IM, SQ, IV initial, 1–1.5 mg q4–6h PRN. *PR:* 5 mg q4–6h PRN Caution: [B, ?] Contra: ↑ ICP, resp severe depression Supplied: Inj 1, 1.5 mg/mL; supp 5 mg SE: ↓ BP, sedation, GI upset, constipation, histamine release Notes: Chemically related to hydromorphone

Oxytocin (Pitocin) Uses: *Induce labor, control postpartum hemorrhage*; promote milk letdown in lactating women Action: Stimulate muscular contractions of the uterus & milk flow during nursing Dose: 0.001–0.002 Units/min IV inf; titrate 0.02 Units/min max. *Breast-feeding:* 1 spray in both nostrils 2–3 min before feeding Caution: [Uncategorized, no anomalies expected, +/–] Contra: Where vaginal delivery not favorable, fetal distress Supplied: Inj 10 Units/mL; nasal soln 40 Units/mL SE: Uterine rupture, fetal death; arrhythmias, anaphylaxis, H_2O intox Notes: Monitor vital signs; nasal form for breast-feeding only

Paclitaxel (Taxol, Abraxane) Uses: *Ovarian & breast CA* CAP Action: Mitotic spindle poison promotes microtubule assembly & stabilization against depolymerization Dose: Per protocols; use glass or polyolefin containers (eg, nitroglycerin tubing set); PVC sets result in plasticizer leaching; ↓ in hepatic failure; maintain hydration Caution: [D, –] Contra: Neutropenia <1500 WBC/mm³; solid tumors Supplied: Inj 6 mg/mL, 5 mg/mL albumin bound (Abraxane) SE: Myelosuppression, peripheral neuropathy, transient ileus, myalgia, bradycardia, ↓ BP, mucositis, N/V/D, fever, rash, HA, & phlebitis; hematologic tox schedule-dependent; leukopenia dose-limiting by 24-h inf; neurotox dose-limiting by short (1–3 h) inf Notes: Allergy Rxns (dyspnea, ↓ BP, urticaria, rash) usually w/in 10 min of inf; minimize w/ corticosteroid, antihistamine pretreatment.

Palivizumab (Synagis) Uses: *Prevent RSV Infxn* Action: MoAb Dose: *Peds.* 15 mg/kg IM monthly, typically Nov–Apr Caution: [C, ?] Renal/hepatic dysfunction Contra: Component allergy Supplied: Vials 50, 100 mg SE: URI, rhinitis, cough, ↑ LFT, local irritation

Palifermin (Kepivance) Uses: Oral mucositis w/ BMT * Action: Synthetic keratinocyte GF Dose: *Phase 1:* 60 mcg/kg IV qd ×3, 3rd dose 24–48 h before chemo *Phase 2:* 60 mcg/kg IV qd ×3, immediately after stem cell infusion Caution: [C, ?/-] Contra: N/A Supplied: Inj 6.25 mg SE: Unusual mouth sensations, tongue thickening, rash,↑ amylase & lipase Notes: *E coli*-derived; separate phases by 4 d; safety unknown w/ nonhematologic malignancies

Palonosetron (Aloxi) WARNING: May ↑ QT_c interval Uses: *Prevention acute & delayed N/V w/ emetogenic chemo* Action: 5HT3-receptor antagonist Dose: 0.25 mg IV 30 min prior to chemo; do not repeat w/in 7 d Caution: [B, ?] Contra: Component allergy Supplied: 0.25 mg/5 mL vial SE: HA, constipation, dizziness, abdominal pain, anxiety

Pamidronate (Aredia) Uses: *↑ Ca^{2+} of malignancy, Paget Dz, palliate symptomatic bone metastases* Action: ↓ Nl & abnormal bone resorption Dose: *↑ Ca^{2+}:* 60 mg IV over 4 h or 90 mg IV over 24 h. *Paget Dz:* 30 mg/d IV slow inf for

3 d **Caution:** [C, ?/–] Avoid invasive dental procedures in CA patients **Contra:** PRG **Supplied:** Powder for inj 30, 60, 90 mg **SE:** Fever, inj site Rxn, uveitis, fluid overload, HTN, abdominal pain, N/V, constipation, UTI, bone pain,↓ K⁺, ↓Ca^{2+},↓Mg^{2+}, hypophosphatemia; jaw osteonecrosis in CA patients, dental exam pre-therapy

Pancrelipase (Pancrease, Cotazym, Creon, Ultrase)
Uses: *Exocrine pancreatic secretion deficiency (eg, CF, chronic pancreatitis, pancreatic insuff), steatorrhea of malabsorption* **Action:** Pancreatic enzyme supl **Dose:** 1–3 caps (tabs) w/ meals & snacks; ↑ to 8 caps (tabs); do not crush or chew EC products; dose-dependent on digestive requirements of pt; avoid antacids **Caution:** [C, ?/–] **Contra:** Pork product allergy **Supplied:** Caps, tabs **SE:** N/V, abdominal cramps **Notes:** Individualize therapy

Pancuronium (Pavulon)
Uses: *Paralysis w/ mechanical ventilation* **Action:** Nondepolarizing neuromuscular blocker **Dose:** *Adults.* 2–4 mg IV q2–4h PRN. *Peds.* 0.02–0.1 mg/kg/dose q2–4h PRN; ↓ in renal/hepatic impair; intubate pt & keep on controlled ventilation; use adequate sedation or analgesia **Caution:** [C, ?/–] **Contra:** Component or bromide sensitivity **Supplied:** Inj 1, 2 mg/mL **SE:** Tachycardia, HTN, pruritus, other histamine reactions

Pantoprazole (Protonix)
Uses: *GERD, erosive gastritis,* ZE syndrome, PUD **Action:** Proton-pump inhibitor **Dose:** 40 mg/d PO; do not crush/chew tabs; 40 mg IV/d (not >3 mg/min, use Protonix filter) **Caution:** [B, ?/–] **Supplied:** Tabs 40 mg; inj **SE:** Chest pain, anxiety, GI upset, ↑ LFTs

Paregoric [Camphorated Tincture of Opium] [C-III]
Uses: *Diarrhea,* pain, & neonatal opiate withdrawal syndrome **Action:** Narcotic **Dose:** *Adults.* 5–10 mL PO qd–qid PRN. *Peds.* 0.25–0.5 mL/kg qd–qid. *Neonatal withdrawal syndrome:* 3–6 gtt PO q3–6 h PRN to relieve Sxs for 3–5 d, then taper over 2–4 wk **Caution:** [B (D w/ prolonged use/high dose near term, +] **Contra:** Tincture (children); convulsive disorder **Supplied:** Liq 2 mg morphine = 20 mg opium/5 mL **SE:** ↓ BP, sedation, constipation **Notes:** Contains anhydrous morphine from opium; short-term use only

Paroxetine (Paxil, Paxil CR)
WARNING: Closely monitor for worsening depression or emergence of suicidality, particularly in ped pts **Uses:** *Depression, OCD, panic disorder, social anxiety disorder,* PMDD **Action:** SSRI **Dose:** 10–60 mg PO single daily dose in AM; CR 25 mg/d PO; ↑ 12.5 mg/wk (max range 26–62.5 mg/d) **Caution:** [B, ?/] **Contra:** MAOI **Supplied:** Tabs 10, 20, 30, 40 mg; susp 10 mg/5 mL; CR 12.5, 25 mg **SE:** Sexual dysfunction, HA, somnolence, dizziness, GI upset, D, xerostomia, tachycardia

Pegfilgrastim (Neulasta)
Uses: *↓ Frequency of Infxn in pts w/ nonmyeloid malignancies receiving myelosuppressive anti-CA drugs that cause febrile neutropenia* **Action:** Colony-stimulating factor **Dose:** *Adults.* 6 mg SQ × 1/chemo cycle. *Peds.* 100 mcg/kg SQ × 1/chemo cycle **Caution:** [C, M] in sickle cell **Contra:** Drug allergy to treat *E. coli* or to filgrastim **Supplied:** *Syringes:* 6 mg/0.6 mL

SE: HA, fever, weakness, fatigue, dizziness, insomnia, edema, N/V/D, stomatitis, anorexia, constipation, taste perversion, dyspepsia, abdominal pain, granulocytopenia, neutropenic fever, ↑ LFT & uric acid, arthralgia, myalgia, bone pain, ARDS, alopecia, splenic rupture, aggravation of sickle cell Dz **Notes:** Never give between 14 d before & 24 h after dose of cytotoxic chemo

Peg Interferon Alfa-2a (Pegasys) Uses: *Chronic hepatitis C w/ compensated liver Dz* **Action:** Biologic response modifier **Dose:** 180 mcg (1 mL) SQ qwk × 48 wk; ↓ in renal impair **Caution:** [C, ?/–] **Contra:** Autoimmune hepatitis, decompensated liver Dz **Supplied:** 180 mcg/mL inj **SE:** Depression, insomnia, suicidal behavior, GI upset, neutropenia & thrombocytopenia, alopecia, pruritus **Notes:** May aggravate neuropsychiatric, autoimmune, ischemic, & infectious disorders

Peg Interferon Alfa-2b (PEG-Intron) Uses: *Rx hepatitis C* **Action:** Immune modulation **Dose:** 1 mcg/kg/wk SQ; 1.5 mcg/kg/wk combined w/ribavirin **Caution:** [C, ?/–] w/psychiatric Hx **Contra:** Autoimmune hepatitis, decompensated liver Dz, hemoglobinopathy **Supplied:** Vials 50, 80, 120, 150 mcg/0.5 mL **SE:** Depression, insomnia, suicidal behavior, GI upset, neutropenia, thrombocytopenia, alopecia, pruritus **Notes:** Give hs to ↓ flu-like Sxs by giving hs or w/APAP; monitor CBC/platelets

Pemetrexed (Alimta) Uses: *W/ cisplatin in nonresectable mesothelioma* NSCLC **Action:** Antifolate antineoplastic **Dose:** 500 mg/m² IV over 10 min every 3 wk; hold if CrCl <45 mL/min; give w/ vitamin B₁₂ (1000 mcg IM every 9 wk) & folic acid (350–1000 mcg PO qd); start 1 wk before; dexamethasone 4 mg PO bid × 3 start 1 d before each Rx **Caution:** [D, –] Renal/hepatic/BM impair **Contra:** Component sensitivity **Supplied:** 500-mg vial **SE:** Neutropenia, thombocytopenia, N/V/D, anorexia, stomatitis, renal failure, neuropathy, fever, fatigue, mood changes, dyspnea, anaphylactic reactions **Notes:** Avoid NSAIDs, follow CBC/platelets

Pemirolast (Alamast) Uses: *Allergic conjunctivitis* **Action:** Mast cell stabilizer **Dose:** 1–2 gtt in each eye qid **Caution:** [C, ?/–] **Supplied:** 1 mg/mL **SE:** HA, rhinitis, cold/flu symptoms, local irritation **Notes:** Wait 10 min before inserting contacts

Penbutolol (Levatol) Uses: *HTN* **Action:** β-adrenergic receptor blocker, β₁, β₂ **Dose:** 20–40 mg/d; ↓ in hepatic insuff **Caution:** [C (1st tri; D if 2nd/3rd tri), M] **Contra:** Asthma, cardiogenic shock, cardiac failure, heart block, bradycardia **Supplied:** Tabs 20 mg **SE:** Flushing, ↓ BP, fatigue, hyperglycemia, GI upset, sexual dysfunction, bronchospasm

Penciclovir (Denavir) Uses: *Herpes simplex (herpes labialis/cold sores)* **Action:** Competitive inhibitor of DNA polymerase **Dose:** Apply at 1st sign of lesions, then q2h for 4 d **Caution:** [B, ?/–] **Contra:** Allergy **Supplied:** Cream 1% [OTC] **SE:** Erythema, HA **Notes:** Do not apply to mucous membranes

Penicillin G, Aqueous (Potassium or Sodium) (Pfizerpen, Pentids) Uses: *Bacteremia, endocarditis, pericarditis, resp tract Infxns, meningitis, neurosyphilis, skin/skin structure Infxns* **Action:** Bactericide; ↓ cell wall synthesis. *Spectrum:* Most gram(+) (not staphylococci), streptococci, *N. meningitidis,* syphilis, clostridia, & anaerobes (not *Bacteroides*) **Dose: Adults.** 400,000–800,000 Units PO qid; IV doses vary depending on indications; range 0.6–24 MU/d in ÷ doses q4h. *Peds. Newborns <1 wk:* 25,000–50,000 Units/ kg/dose IV q12h. *Infants 1 wk–<1 mo:* 25,000–50,000 Units/kg/dose IV q8h. *Children:* 100,000–300,000 Units/kg/24h IV ÷ q4h; ↓ in renal impair **Caution:** [B, M] **Contra:** Allergy **Supplied:** Tabs 200,000, 250,000, 400,000, 800,000 Units; susp 200,000, 400,000 Units/5 mL; powder for inj **SE:** Allergic Rxns; interstitial nephritis, D, Szs **Notes:** Contains 1.7 mEq of K+/MU

Penicillin G Benzathine (Bicillin) Uses: *Single-dose regimen for streptococcal pharyngitis, rheumatic fever, glomerulonephritis prophylaxis, & syphilis* **Action:** Bactericide; ↓ cell wall synthesis. *Spectrum:* See Penicillin G **Dose: Adults.** 1.2–2.4 million units deep IM inj q2–4wk. *Peds.* 50,000 Units/kg/dose, 2.4 million units/dose max; deep IM inj q2–4 wk **Caution:** [B, M] **Contra:** Allergy **Supplied:** Inj 300,000, 600,000 Units/mL; Bicillin L-A benzathine salt only; Bicillin C-R combo of benzathine & procaine (300,000 Units procaine w/ 300,000 Units benzathine/mL or 900,000 Units benzathine w/ 300,000 Units procaine/2 mL) **SE:** Inj site pain, acute interstitial nephritis, anaphylaxis **Notes:** Sustained action, detectable levels up to 4 wk; drug of choice for noncongenital syphilis

Penicillin G Procaine (Wycillin, others) Uses: *Infxns of respir tract, skin/soft tissue, scarlet fever, syphilis* **Action:** Bactericidal; ↓ cell wall synthesis. *Spectrum:* PCN G-sensitive organisms that respond to low, persistent serum levels **Dose: Adults.** 0.6–4.8 million units/d in ÷ doses q12–24h; give probenecid at least 30 min prior to PCN to prolong action. *Peds.* 25,000–50,000 Units/kg/d IM ÷ qd–bid **Caution:** [B, M] **Contra:** Allergy **Supplied:** Inj 300,000, 500,000, 600,000 Units/mL **SE:** Pain at inj site, interstitial nephritis, anaphylaxis **Notes:** Long-acting parenteral PCN; levels up to 15 h

Penicillin V (Pen-Vee K, Veetids, others) Uses: Susceptible streptococci Infxns, otitis media, URIs, skin/soft tissue Infxns (PCN-sensitive staph) **Action:** Bactericidal; ↓ cell wall synthesis. *Spectrum:* Most gram(+), including strep **Dose: Adults.** 250–500 mg PO qid/6h, q8h, q12h. *Peds.* 25–50 mg/kg/24h PO in 4 doses; ↓ in renal Dz; on empty stomach **Caution:** [B, M] **Contra:** Allergy **Supplied:** Tabs 125, 250, 500 mg; susp 125, 250 mg/5 mL **SE:** GI upset, interstitial nephritis, anaphylaxis, convulsions **Notes:** Well-tolerated PO PCN; 250 mg = 400,000 Units of PCN G

Pentamidine (Pentam 300, NebuPent) Uses: *Rx & prevention of PCP* **Action:** ↓ DNA, RNA, phospholipid, & protein synthesis **Dose: Rx: Adults & Peds.** 4 mg/kg/24 h IV qd for 14–21 d. *Prevention: Adults & Peds >5 y.* 300 mg once q4wk, give via Respigard II neb; IV requires ↓ in renal impair **Caution:** [C, ?] **Contra:** Component allergy **Supplied:** Inj 300 mg/vial; aerosol 300 mg **SE:** Associated w/ pancreatic cell necrosis w/ hyperglycemia; pancreatitis, CP, fatigue, dizziness, rash, GI upset, renal impair, blood dyscrasias (leukopenia & thrombocytopenia)

Notes: Follow CBC, glucose, pancreatic Fxn monthly for the 1st 3 mo; monitor for ↓ BP following IV administration

Pentazocine (Talwin) [C-IV] **Uses:** *Moderate–severe pain* **Action:** Partial narcotic agonist–antagonist **Dose:** *Adults.* 30 mg IM or IV; 50–100 mg PO q3–4h PRN. *Peds. 5–8 y:* 15 mg IM q4h PRN. *8–14 y:* 30 mg IM q4h PRN; ↓ in renal/hepatic impair **Caution:** [C (1st tri, D w/ prolonged use/high dose near term), +/–] **Contra:** Allergy **Supplied:** Tabs 50 mg (+ naloxone 0.5 mg); inj 30 mg/mL **SE:** Considerable dysphoria; drowsiness, GI upset, xerostomia, Szs **Notes:** 30–60 mg IM = 10 mg of morphine IM

Pentobarbital (Nembutal, others) [C-II] **Uses:** *Insomnia, convulsions,* induced coma following severe head injury **Action:** Barbiturate **Dose:** *Adults. Sedative:* 20–40 mg PO or PR q6–12h. *Hypnotic:* 100–200 mg PO or PR hs PRN. *Induced coma:* Load 5–10 mg/kg IV, then maint 1–3 mg/kg/h IV inf (keep serum level 20–50 mg/mL). *Peds. Hypnotic:* 2–6 mg/kg/dose PO hs PRN. *Induced coma:* As adult **Caution:** [D, +/–] Severe hepatic impair **Contra:** Allergy **Supplied:** Caps 50, 100 mg; elixir 18.2 mg/5 mL (= 20 mg pentobarbital); supp 30, 60, 120, 200 mg; inj 50 mg/mL **SE:** Resp depression, ↓ BP w/ aggressive IV use for cerebral edema; bradycardia, ↓ BP, sedation, lethargy, hangover, rash, Stevens–Johnson syndrome, blood dyscrasias, resp depression **Notes:** Tolerance to sedative–hypnotic effect w/in 1–2 wk

Pentosan Polysulfate Sodium (Elmiron) **Uses:** * Relief of pain/discomfort associated w/ interstitial cystitis* **Action:** Bladder wall buffer **Dose:** 100 mg PO tid on empty stomach w/ H$_2$O 1 h ac or 2 h pc **Caution:** [B, ?/–] **Contra:** Allergy **Supplied:** Caps 100 mg **SE:** Alopecia, N/D, HA, ↑ LFTs, anticoagulant effects, thrombocytopenia **Notes:** Reassess after 3 mo

Pentoxifylline (Trental) **Uses:** *Symptomatic management of peripheral vascular Dz* **Action:** ↓ Blood cell viscosity by restoring erythrocyte flexibility **Dose:** *Adults.* 400 mg PO tid pc; Rx for at least 8 wk for full effect; ↓ to bid w/ GI/CNS SEs **Caution:** [C, +/–] **Contra:** Cerebral/retinal hemorrhage **Supplied:** Tabs 400 mg **SE:** Dizziness, HA, GI upset

Pergolide (Permax) **Uses:** *Parkinson Dz* **Action:** Centrally active dopamine receptor agonist **Dose:** Initial, 0.05 mg PO tid, titrated q2–3d to effect; maint 2–3 mg/d in ÷ doses **Caution:** [B, ?/–] **Contra:** Ergot sensitivity **Supplied:** Tabs 0.05, 0.25, 1.0 mg **SE:** Dizziness, somnolence, confusion, nausea, constipation, dyskinesia, rhinitis, MI **Notes:** May cause ↓ BP during initiation of therapy

Perindopril Erbumine (Aceon) **Uses:** *HTN,* CHF, DN, post-MI **Action:** ACE inhibitor **Dose:** 4–8 mg/d; avoid w/ food; ↓ in elderly/renal impair **Caution:** [C (1st tri, D 2nd & 3rd tri), ?/–] ACE-inhibitor–induced angioedema **Contra:** Bilateral renal artery stenosis, primary hyperaldosteronism **Supplied:** Tabs 2, 4, 8 mg **SE:** HA, ↓ BP, dizziness, GI upset, cough **Notes:** OK w/ diuretics

Permethrin (Nix, Elimite) [OTC] **Uses:** *Eradication of lice/scabies* **Action:** Pediculicide **Dose:** *Adults & Peds.* Saturate hair & scalp; allow 10 min before rinsing **Caution:** [B, ?/–] **Contra:** Allergy **Supplied:** Topical liq 1%; cream 5% **SE:** Local irritation **Notes:** Disinfect clothing, bedding, combs & brushes

Perphenazine (Trilafon) **Uses:** *Psychotic disorders, severe nausea,* intractable hiccups **Action:** Phenothiazine; blocks brain dopaminergic receptors **Dose:** *Antipsychotic:* 4–16 mg PO tid; max 64 mg/d. *Hiccups:* 5 mg IM q6h PRN or 1 mg IV at intervals not <1–2 mg/min, 5 mg max. *Peds. 1–6 y:* 4–6 mg/d PO in ÷ doses. *6–12 y:* 6 mg/d PO in ÷ doses. *>12 y:* 4–16 mg PO bid–qid; ↓ in hepatic insuff **Caution:** [C, ?/–] NA glaucoma, severe hyper-/↓ BP **Contra:** Phenothiazine sensitivity, BM depression, severe liver or cardiac Dz **Supplied:** Tabs 2, 4, 8, 16 mg; PO conc 16 mg/5 mL; inj 5 mg/mL **SE:** ↓ BP, tachycardia, bradycardia, EPS, drowsiness, Szs, photosensitivity, skin discoloration, blood dyscrasias, constipation

Phenazopyridine (Pyridium, others) **Uses:** *Lower urinary tract irritation* **Action:** Local anesthetic on urinary tract mucosa **Dose:** *Adults.* 100–200 mg PO tid. *Peds 6–12 y.* 12 mg/kg/24 h PO in 3 ÷ doses; ↓ in renal insuff **Caution:** [B, ?] Hepatic Dz **Contra:** Renal failure **Supplied:** Tabs 100, 200 mg; some available OTC **SE:** GI disturbances; red-orange urine color (can stain clothing); HA, dizziness, acute renal failure, methemoglobinemia

Phenelzine (Nardil) **Uses:** *Depression* **Action:** MAOI **Dose:** 15 mg PO tid. *Elderly:* 15–60 mg/d ÷ doses **Caution:** [C, –] Interacts w/ SSRI, ergots, triptans **Contra:** CHF, Hx liver Dz **Supplied:** Tabs 15 mg **SE:** Postural ↓ BP; edema, dizziness, sedation, rash, sexual dysfunction, xerostomia, constipation, urinary retention **Notes:** May take 2–4 wk for effect; avoid tyramine-containing foods (eg, cheeses)

Phenobarbital [C-IV] **Uses:** *Sz disorders,* insomnia, anxiety **Action:** Barbiturate **Dose:** *Adults. Sedative–hypnotic:* 30–120 mg/d PO or IM PRN. *Anticonvulsant:* Load 10–12 mg/kg in 3 ÷ doses, then 1–3 mg/kg/24 h PO, IM, or IV. *Peds. Sedative–hypnotic:* 2–3 mg/kg/24 h PO or IM hs PRN. *Anticonvulsant:* Load 15–20 mg/kg ÷ in 2 equal doses 4 h apart, then 3–5 mg/kg/24h PO ÷ in 2–3 doses. **Caution:** [D, M] **Contra:** Porphyria, liver dysfunction **Supplied:** Tabs 8, 15, 16, 30, 32, 60, 65, 100 mg; elixir 15, 20 mg/5 mL; inj 30, 60, 65, 130 mg/mL **SE:** Bradycardia, ↓ BP, hangover, Stevens–Johnson syndrome, blood dyscrasias, resp depression **Notes:** Tolerance develops to sedation; paradox hyperactivity seen in ped pts; long half-life allows single daily dosing (Table 2, page 200)

Phenylephrine (Neo-Synephrine) **Uses:** *Vascular failure in shock,* allergy, or drug-induced ↓ BP; *nasal congestion*; *mydriatic* **Action:** α-Adrenergic agonist **Dose:** *Adults. Mild–moderate ↓ BP:* 2–5 mg IM or SQ ↑ BP for 2 h; 0.1–0.5 mg IV elevates BP for 15 min. *Severe ↓ BP/shock:* Cont inf at 100–180 mg/min; after BP stabilized, maint 40–60 mg/min. *Nasal congestion:* 1–2 sprays/nostril PRN. *Ophth:* 1 gtt 15–30 min before exam. *Peds. ↓ BP:* 5–20 mcg/kg/dose IV q10–15 min or 0.1–0.5 mg/kg/min IV inf, titrate to effect. *Nasal congestion:* 1 spray/nostril q3–4h PRN **Caution:** [C, +/–] HTN, acute pancreatitis, hepatitis, coronary Dz, NA glaucoma, hyperthyroidism **Contra:** Bradycardia, arrhythmias **Supplied:** Inj 10 mg/mL; nasal soln 0.125, 0.16, 0.25, 0.5, 1%; ophth soln 0.12, 2.5, 10% **SE:** Arrhythmias,

HTN, peripheral vasoconstriction activity potentiated by oxytocin, MAOIs, & TCAs; HA, weakness, necrosis, ↓ renal perfusion **Notes:** Promptly restore blood volume if loss has occurred; use large veins for inf to avoid extravasation; phentolamine 10 mg in 10–15 mL of NS for local inj as antidote for extravasation

Phenytoin (Dilantin)   Uses: *Sz disorders* Action: ↓ Sz spread in the motor cortex **Dose:** *Load: Adults & Peds.* 15–20 mg/kg IV, 25 mg/min max or PO in 400-mg doses at 4-h intervals. *Maint: Adults.* Initial, 200 mg PO or IV bid or 300 mg hs; then follow levels. *Peds.* 4–7 mg/kg/24h PO or IV ÷ qd–bid; avoid PO susp (erratic absorption) **Caution:** [D, +] **Contra:** Heart block, sinus bradycardia **Supplied:** Caps 30, 100 mg; chew tabs 50 mg; PO susp 30, 125 mg/5 mL; inj 50 mg/mL **SE:** Nystagmus/ataxia early signs of tox; gum hyperplasia w/ long-term use. *IV:* ↓ BP, bradycardia, arrhythmias, phlebitis; peripheral neuropathy, rash, blood dyscrasias, Stevens–Johnson syndrome **Notes:** Follow levels (Table 2, page 200); phenytoin albumin bound & levels reflect bound & free phenytoin; w/↓ albumin & azotemia, low levels may be therapeutic (nl free levels); do not change dosage (↑ or ↓) at intervals <7–10 d

Physostigmine (Antilirium)   Uses: *Antidote for TCA, atropine, & scopolamine OD; glaucoma* **Action:** Reversible cholinesterase inhibitor **Dose:** *Adults.* 2 mg IV or IM q 20 min. *Peds.* 0.01–0.03 mg/kg/dose IV q15–30 min up to 2 mg total if needed **Caution:** [C, ?] **Contra:** GI/GU obstruction, CV Dz **Supplied:** Inj 1 mg/mL; ophth oint 0.25% **SE:** Rapid IV admin associated w/ convulsions; cholinergic side effects; sweating, salivation, lacrimation, GI upset, asystole, changes in heart rate **Notes:** Excessive readministration can result in cholinergic crisis; crisis reversed w/ atropine

Phytonadione [Vitamin K] (AquaMEPHYTON, others)   Uses: *Coagulation disorders due to faulty formation of factors II, VII, IX, X*; hyperalimentation **Action:** Cofactor for production of factors II, VII, IX, & X **Dose:** *Adults & Children. Anticoagulant-induced prothrombin deficiency:* 1–10 mg PO or IV slowly. *Hyperalimentation:* 10 mg IM or IV q wk. *Infants.* 0.5–1 mg/dose IM, SQ, or PO **Caution:** [C, +] **Contra:** Allergy **Supplied:** Tabs 5 mg; inj 2, 10 mg/mL **SE:** Anaphylaxis from IV dosage; give IV slowly; GI upset (PO), inj site Rxns **Notes:** W/ parenteral Rx, 1st change in PT usually seen in 12–24 h; use makes re-Coumadinization more difficult

Pimecrolimus (Elidel)   Uses: *Atopic dermatitis* refractory, severe perianal itching **Action:** Inhibits T-lymphocytes **Dose:** Apply bid; use at least 1 wk following resolution **Caution:** [C, ?/–] w/ local Infxn, lymphadenopathy; immunocompromise; avoid < 2 yrs of age **Contra:** Allergy **Supplied:** Oint 0.03%, 0.1%; 30-g, 60-g tubes **SE:** Phototox, local irritation/burning, flu-like Sxs, may ↑ malignancy **Notes:** Apply to dry skin only; wash hands after use; "?" ↑ cancer risk; second line/short term use only

Pindolol (Visken)   Uses: *HTN* **Action:** β-Adrenergic receptor blocker, β₁, β₂, ISA **Dose:** 5–10 mg bid, 60 mg/d max; ↓ in hepatic/renal failure **Caution:** [B (1st tri); D if 2nd or 3rd tri), +/–] **Contra:** Uncompensated CHF, cardiogenic shock, bradycardia, heart block, asthma, COPD **Supplied:** Tabs 5, 10 mg **SE:** Insomnia, dizziness, fatigue, edema, GI upset, dyspnea; fluid retention may exacerbate CHF

Pioglitazone/Metformin (ActoPlus Met)   WARNING: Can cause lactic acidosis which is fatal in 50% of cases. **Uses:** *Type 2 DM as adjunct to diet and exercise* **Action:** Combined ↑ insulin sensitivity w/ ↓ hepatic glucose release **Dose:** Initial 1 tab PO qd or bid, titrate; max daily pioglitazone 45 mg & metformin 2550 mg **Caution:** [C, –] stop w/ radiologic contrast agents **Contra:** Renal impair, acidosis **Supplied:** Tabs pioglitazone mg/metformin mg: 15/500, 15/850 **SE:** Lactic acidosis, hypoglycemia, edema, weight gain, URI, HA, GI upset, liver damage **Notes:** Follow LFTs

Pioglitazone (Actos) **Uses:** *Type 2 DM* **Action:** ↑ Insulin sensitivity **Dose:** 15–45 mg/d PO **Caution:** [C, –] **Contra:** Hepatic impair **Supplied:** Tabs 15, 30, 45 mg **SE:** Weight gain, URI, HA, hypoglycemia, edema

Piperacillin (Pipracil) **Uses:** *Infxns of skin, bone, resp &, urinary tract, abdomen, sepsis* **Action:** 4th-gen PCN; bactericidal; ↓ cell wall synthesis. *Spectrum:* Primarily gram(+), better *Enterococcus, H. influenza,* not staph; gram(–) *E. coli, Proteus, Shigella, Pseudomonas,* not β-lactamase-producing **Dose:** *Adults.* 3 g IV q4–6h. *Peds.* 200–300 mg/kg/d IV ÷ q4–6h; ↓ in renal failure **Caution:** [B, M] PCN sensitivity **Supplied:** Inj **SE:** ↓ Plt aggregation, interstitial nephritis, renal failure, anaphylaxis, hemolytic anemia **Notes:** Often used w/ aminoglycoside

Piperacillin–Tazobactam (Zosyn) **Uses:** *Infxns of skin, bone, resp & urinary tract, abdomen, sepsis* **Action:** PCN plus β-lactamase inhibitor; bactericidal; ↓ cell wall synthesis. *Spectrum:* Good gram(+), excellent gram(–); covers β-lactamase producers **Dose:** *Adults.* 3.375–4.5 g IV q6h; ↓ in renal failure **Caution:** [B, M] PCN or β-lactam sensitivity **Supplied:** Inj **SE:** D, HA, insomnia, GI upset, serum sickness-like reaction, pseudomembranous colitis **Notes:** Often used in combo w/ aminoglycoside

Pirbuterol (Maxair) **Uses:** *Prevention & Rx reversible bronchospasm* **Action:** β₂-Adrenergic agonist **Dose:** 2 inhal q4–6h; max 12 inhal/d **Caution:** [C, ?/–] **Supplied:** Aerosol 0.2 mg/actuation; Autohaler dry powder 0.2 mg/actuation **SE:** Nervousness, restlessness, trembling, HA, taste changes, tachycardia

Piroxicam (Feldene)   WARNING: May ↑ risk of cardiovascular events & GI bleeding **Uses:** *Arthritis & pain* **Action:** NSAID; ↓ prostaglandins **Dose:** 10–20 mg/d **Caution:** [B (1st tri; D if 3rd tri or near term), +] GI bleeding **Contra:** ASA or NSAID sensitivity **Supplied:** Caps 10, 20 mg **SE:** Dizziness, rash, GI upset, edema, acute renal failure, peptic ulcer

Plasma Protein Fraction (Plasmanate, others) **Uses:** *Shock & ↓ BP* **Action:** Plasma volume expander **Dose:** Initial, 250–500 mL IV (not >10 mL/min); subsequent inf based on response. *Peds.* 10–15 mL/kg/dose IV; subsequent inf based on response **Caution:** [C, +] **Contra:** Renal insuff, CHF **Supplied:** Inj 5% **SE:** ↓ BP associated w/ rapid inf; hypocoagulability, metabolic acidosis, PE **Notes:** 130–160 mEq Na/L; not substitute for RBC

Pneumococcal 7-Valent Conjugate Vaccine (Prevnar) Uses: *Immunization against pneumococcal Infxns in infants & children* Action: Active immunization Dose: 0.5 mL IM/dose; series of 3 doses; 1st dose 2 mo of age w/ subsequent doses q2mo Caution: [C, +] Thrombocytopenia Contra: Diphtheria toxoid sensitivity, febrile illness Supplied: Inj SE: Local reactions, arthralgia, fever, myalgia

Pneumococcal Vaccine, Polyvalent (Pneumovax-23) Uses: *Immunization against pneumococcal Infxns in pts at high risk (eg, all ≥65 y of age)* Action: Active immunization Dose: 0.5 mL IM. Caution: [C, ?] Contra: *Do not* vaccinate during immunosuppressive therapy Supplied: Inj 25 mg each of polysaccharide isolates per 0.5-mL dose SE: Fever, inj site Rxn, hemolytic anemia, thrombocytopenia, anaphylaxis

Podophyllin (Podocon-25, Condylox Gel 0.5%, Condylox) Uses: *Topical therapy of benign growths (genital & perianal warts [condylomata acuminata],* papillomas, fibromas) Action: Direct antimitotic effect; exact mechanism unknown Dose: *Condylox gel & Condylox:* Apply 3 consecutive d/wk for 4 wk. *Podocon-25:* Use sparingly on the lesion, leave on for 1–4 h, then thoroughly wash off Caution: [C, ?] Immunosuppression Contra: DM, bleeding lesions Supplied: Podocon-25 (w/ benzoin) 15-mL bottles; Condylox gel 0.5% 35 g clear gel; Condylox soln 0.5% 35 g clear SE: Local reactions, significant absorption; anemias, tachycardia, paresthesias, GI upset, renal/hepatic damage Notes: Podocon-25 applied only by the clinician; do not dispense directly to patient

Polyethylene Glycol [PEG]–Electrolyte Solution (GoLYTELY, CoLyte) Uses: *Bowel prep prior to examination or surgery* Action: Osmotic cathartic Dose: *Adults.* Following 3–4-h fast, drink 240 mL of soln q10min until 4 L consumed. *Peds.* 25–40 mL/kg/h for 4–10 h Caution: [C, ?] Contra: GI obstruction, bowel perforation, megacolon, ulcerative colitis Supplied: Powder for reconstitution to 4 L SE: Cramping or nausea, bloating Notes: 1st BM should occur in approximately 1 h

Polyethylene Glycol [PEG] 3350 (MiraLax) Uses: *Occasional constipation* Action: Osmotic laxative Dose: 17 g powder (1 heaping Tbsp) in 8 oz (1 cup) of H_2O & drink; max 14 d Caution: [C, ?] R/O bowel obstruction before use Contra: GI obstruction, allergy to PEG Supplied: Powder for reconstitution; bottle cap holds 17 g SE: Upset stomach, bloating, cramping, gas, severe D, hives Notes: Can add to H_2O, juice, soda, coffee, or tea

Polymyxin B & Hydrocortisone (Otobiotic Otic) Uses: *Superficial bacterial Infxns of external ear canal* Action: Antibiotic/antiinflammatory combo Dose: 4 gtt in ear(s) tid–qid Caution: [B, ?] Supplied: Soln polymyxin B 10,000 Units/hydrocortisone 0.5%/mL SE: Local irritation Notes: Useful in neomycin allergy

Potassium Citrate (Urocit-K) Uses: *Alkalinize urine, prevention of urinary stones (uric acid, calcium stones if hypocitraturic)* Action: Urinary alkalinizer Dose: 10–20 mEq PO tid w/ meals, max 100 mEq/d Caution: [A, +] Contra: Severe renal impair, dehydration, ↑ K⁺, peptic ulcer; use of K⁺-sparing diuretics or salt substitutes **Supplied:** 540-, 1080-mg tabs **SE:** GI upset, ↓ Ca²⁺, ↑ K⁺, metabolic alkalosis **Notes:** Tabs 540 mg = 5 mEq, 1080 mg = 10 mEq

Potassium Citrate & Citric Acid (Polycitra-K) Uses: *Alkalinize urine, prevent urinary stones (uric acid, Ca stones if hypocitraturic)* **Action:** Urinary alkalinizer **Dose:** 10–20 mEq PO tid w/ meals, max 100 mEq/d **Caution:** [A, +] **Contra:** Severe renal impair, dehydration, ↑ K⁺, peptic ulcer; use of K⁺-sparing diuretics or salt substitutes **Supplied:** Soln 10 mEq/5 mL; powder 30 mEq/packet **SE:** GI upset, ↓ Ca²⁺, ↑ K⁺, metabolic alkalosis

Potassium Iodide [Lugol Solution] (SSKI, Thyro-Block) Uses: *Thyroid storm,* ↓ vascularity before thyroid surgery, block thyroid uptake of radioactive iodine, thin bronchial secretions **Action:** Iodine supl **Dose:** *Adults & Peds >2 y.* Preop thyroidectomy: 50–250 mg PO tid (2–6 gtt strong iodine soln); give 10 d preop. *Peds 1 y. Thyroid crisis:* 300 mg (6 gtt SSKI q8h). *Peds <1 y:* ½ adult dose **Caution:** [D, +] ↑ K⁺, TB, PE, bronchitis, renal impair **Contra:** Iodine sensitivity **Supplied:** Tabs 130 mg; soln (SSKI) 1 g/mL; Lugol soln, strong iodine 100 mg/mL; syrup 325 mg/5 mL **SE:** Fever, HA, urticaria, angioedema, goiter, GI upset, eosinophilia

Potassium Supplements (Kaon, Kaochlor, K-Lor, Slow-K, Micro-K, Klorvess, others) Uses: *Prevention or Rx of ↓ K⁺* (eg, diuretic use) **Action:** K⁺ supl **Dose:** *Adults.* 20–100 mEq/d PO ÷ qd–bid; IV 10–20 mEq/h, max 40 mEq/d & 150 mEq/d (monitor K⁺ levels frequently w/ high-dose IV). *Peds.* Calculate K⁺ deficit; 1–3 mEq/kg/d PO ÷ qd–qid; IV max dose 0.5–1 mEq/kg/h **Caution:** [A, +] Renal insuff, use w/ NSAIDs & ACE inhibitors **Contra:** ↑ K⁺ **Supplied:** PO forms (Table 8, page 215); injectable forms **SE:** Can cause GI irritation; bradycardia, ↑ K⁺, heart block **Notes:** Mix powder & liq w/ beverage (unsalted tomato juice, etc); follow K⁺; Cl⁻ salt OK w/ alkalosis; w/ acidosis use acetate, bicarbonate, citrate, or gluconate salt

Pramipexole (Mirapex) Uses: *Parkinson Dz* **Action:** Dopamine agonist **Dose:** 1.5–4.5 mg/d PO, initial 0.375 mg/d in 3 ÷ doses; titrate slowly **Caution:** [C, ?/–] **Contra:** Component allergy **Supplied:** Tabs 0.125, 0.25, 1, 1.5 mg **SE:** Postural ↓ BP, asthenia, somnolence, abnormal dreams, GI upset, EPS

Pramoxine (Anusol Ointment, Proctofoam-NS, others) Uses: *Relief of pain & itching from hemorrhoids, anorectal surgery*; topical for burns & dermatosis **Action:** Topical anesthetic **Dose:** Apply freely to anal area q3h **Caution:** [C, ?] **Supplied:** [OTC] All 1%; foam (Proctofoam-NS), cream, oint, lotion, gel, pads, spray **SE:** Contact dermatitis, mucosal thinning w/ chronic use

Pramoxine + Hydrocortisone (Enzone, Proctofoam-HC) Uses: *Relief of pain & itching from hemorrhoids* **Action:** Topical anesthetic, antiinflammatory **Dose:** Apply freely to anal area tid–qid **Caution:** [C, ?/–] **Supplied:** Cream pramoxine 1% acetate 0.5/1%; foam pramoxine 1% hydrocortisone 1%; lotion pramoxine 1% hydrocortisone 0.25/1/2.5%, pramoxine 2.5% & hydrocortisone 1% **SE:** Contact dermatitis, mucosal thinning with chronic use

Pravastatin (Pravachol)   **Uses:** ↓ Cholesterol **Action:** HMG-CoA reductase inhibitor **Dose:** 10–40 mg PO hs; ↓ in significant renal/hepatic insuff **Caution:** [X, –] **Contra:** Liver Dz or persistent LFT ↑ **Supplied:** Tabs 10, 20, 40 mg **SE:** Use caution w/ concurrent gemfibrozil; HA, GI upset, hepatitis, myopathy, renal failure

Prazosin (Minipress)   **Uses:** * HTN* **Action:** Peripherally acting α-adrenergic blocker **Dose:** *Adults.* 1 mg PO tid; can ↑ to 20 mg/d max. *Peds.* 5–25 mcg/kg/dose q6h, to 25 mcg/kg/dose max **Caution:** [C, ?] **Contra:** Component allergy **Supplied:** Caps 1, 2, 5 mg **SE:** Dizziness, edema, palpitations, fatigue, GI upset **Notes:** Can cause orthostatic ↓ BP, take the 1st dose hs; tolerance develops to this effect; tachyphylaxis may result

Prednisolone   [See Table 4, page 206],
Prednisone   [See Table 4, page 206]

Pregabalin (Lyrica)   **Uses:** *DM peripheral neuropathy pain; postherpetic neuralgia; adjunct Rx adult partial onset seizures* **Action:** $α_2$–δ ligand; nerve transmission modulator **Dose:** *Neuropathic pain:* 50 mg PO tid, ↑ to 300 mg/d w/in 1 wk based on response (300 mg/d max) *Postherpetic neuralgia:* 75–150 mg bid, or 50–100 mg tid; start 75 mg bid or 50 mg tid; ↑to 300 mg/d w/in 1 wk based on response; if pt still has pain after 2–4 wk, ↑ to 600 mg/d; *Epilepsy:* Start 150 mg/d (75 mg bid or 50 mg tid) may ↑ to max 600 mg/d; ↓ w/ renal insuffic; w/ or w/o food **Caution:** [X, –] with significant renal impair, see insert for dosing **Contra:** PRG **Supplied:** Tabs 25, 50, 75, 100, 150, 200, 225, 300 mg **SE:** Dizziness, drowsiness, xerostomia, peripheral edema, blurred vision, weight gain, difficulty concentrating **Notes:** Related to gabapentin; w/ D/C, taper over at least 1 wk

Probenecid (Benemid, others)   **Uses:** *Prevent gout & hyperuricemia; prolongs levels of PCNs & cephalosporins* **Action:** Renal tubular blocking agent **Dose:** *Adults. Gout:* 250 mg bid × 1 wk, then 0.5 g PO bid; can ↑ by 500 mg/mo up to 2–3 g/d. *Antibiotic effect:* 1–2 g PO 30 min before dose. *Peds >2 y.* 25 mg/kg, then 40 mg/kg/d PO + qid **Caution:** [B, ?] **Contra:** High-dose ASA, moderate–severe renal impair, age <2 yr **Supplied:** Tabs 500 mg **SE:** HA, GI upset, rash, pruritus, dizziness, blood dyscrasias **Notes:** Do not use during acute gout attack

Procainamide (Pronestyl, Procan)   **Uses:** *Supraventricular/ventricular arrhythmias* **Action:** Class 1A antiarrhythmic **Dose:** *Adults. Recurrent VF/VT:* 20 mg/min IV (max total 17 mg/kg). *Maint:* 1–4 mg/min. *Stable wide-complex tachycardia of unknown origin, AF w/ rapid rate in WPW:* 20 mg/min IV until arrhythmia suppression, ↓ BP, QRS widens >50%, then 1–4 mg/min. *Chronic dosing:* 50 mg/kg/d PO in ÷ doses q4–6h. *Peds. Chronic maint:* 15–50 mg/kg/24 h PO ÷ q3–6h; ↓ in renal/hepatic impair **Caution:** [C, +] **Contra:** Complete heart block, 2nd- or 3rd-degree heart block w/o pacemaker, torsades de pointes, SLE **Supplied:** Tabs & caps 250, 375, 500 mg; SR tabs 250, 500, 750, 1000 mg; inj 100, 500 mg/mL **SE:** Can cause ↓ BP & a lupus-like syndrome; GI upset, taste perversion, arrhythmias, tachycardia, heart block, angioneurotic edema **Notes:** Follow levels (Table 2, page 200)

Procarbazine (Matulane) WARNING: Highly toxic; handle w/ care Uses: *Hodgkin Dz,* NHL, brain tumors **Action:** Alkylating agent; ↓ DNA & RNA synthesis **Dose:** Per protocol **Caution:** [D, ?] W/ EtOH ingestion **Contra:** Inadequate BM reserve **Supplied:** Caps 50 mg **SE:** Myelosuppression, hemolytic reactions (w/ G6PD deficiency), N/V/D; disulfiram-like Rxn; cutaneous & constitutional Sxs, myalgia, arthralgia, CNS effects, azoospermia, cessation of menses

Prochlorperazine (Compazine) Uses: *N/V, agitation, & psychotic disorders* **Action:** Phenothiazine; blocks postsynaptic dopaminergic CNS receptors **Dose:** *Adults. Antiemetic:* 5–10 mg PO tid–qid or 25 mg PR bid or 5–10 mg deep IM q4–6h. *Antipsychotic:* 10–20 mg IM acutely or 5–10 mg PO tid–qid for maint; ↑ doses may be required for antipsychotic effect. *Peds.* 0.1–0.15 mg/kg/dose IM q4–6h or 0.4 mg/kg/24 h PO ÷ tid–qid **Caution:** [C, +/–] NA glaucoma, severe liver/cardiac Dz **Contra:** Phenothiazine sensitivity, BM suppression **Supplied:** Tabs 5, 10, 25 mg; SR caps 10, 15, 30 mg; syrup 5 mg/5 mL; supp 2.5, 5, 25 mg; inj 5 mg/mL **SE:** EPS common; Rx w/ diphenhydramine

Promethazine (Phenergan) Uses: *N/V, motion sickness* **Action:** Phenothiazine; blocks postsynaptic mesolimbic dopaminergic receptors **Dose:** *Adults.* 12.5–50 mg PO, PR, or IM bid–qid PRN. *Peds.* 0.1–0.5 mg/kg/dose PO or IM q2–6h PRN **Caution:** [C, +/–] use w/ agents w/ respiratory depressant effects **Contra:** Component allergy, NA glaucoma, age < 2 yrs **Supplied:** Tabs 12.5, 25, 50 mg; syrup 6.25 mg/5 mL, 25 mg/5 mL; supp 12.5, 25, 50 mg; inj 25, 50 mg/mL **SE:** Drowsiness, tardive dyskinesia, EPS, lowered Sz threshold, ↓ BP, GI upset, blood dyscrasias, photosensitivity, respiratory depression in children

Propafenone (Rythmol) Uses: *Life-threatening ventricular arrhythmias, AF* **Action:** Class IC antiarrhythmic; **Dose:** *Adults.* 150–300 mg PO q8h. *Peds.* 8–10 mg/kg/d ÷ in 3–4 doses; may ↑ 2 mg/kg/d, to max of 20 mg/kg/d **Caution:** [C, ?] w/ amprenavir, ritonavir **Contra:** Uncontrolled CHF, bronchospasm, cardiogenic shock, conduction disorders **Supplied:** Tabs 150, 225, 300 mg **SE:** Dizziness, unusual taste, 1st-degree heart block, arrhythmias, prolongs QRS & QT intervals; fatigue, GI upset, blood dyscrasias

Propantheline (Pro-Banthine) Uses: *PUD,* symptomatic Rx of small intestine hypermotility, spastic colon, ureteral spasm, bladder spasm, pylorospasm **Action:** Antimuscarinic **Dose:** *Adults.* 15 mg PO ac & 30 mg PO hs; ↓ in elderly. *Peds.* 2–3 mg/kg/24h PO ÷ tid–qid **Caution:** [C, ?] **Contra:** NA glaucoma, ulcerative colitis, toxic megacolon, GI/GU obstruction **Supplied:** Tabs 7.5, 15 mg **SE:** Anticholinergic (eg, xerostomia, blurred vision)

Propofol (Diprivan) Uses: *Induction & maint of anesthesia; sedation in intubated pts* **Action:** Sedative–hypnotic; mechanism unknown **Dose:** *Adults. Anesthesia:* 2–2.5 mg/kg induction, then 0.1–0.2 mg/kg/min inf *ICU sedation:* 5–50 mcg/kg/min cont inf; ↓ in elderly, debilitated, ASA II/IV pts *Peds. Anesthesia:* 2.5–3.5 mg/kg induction; then 125–300 mcg/kg/min **Caution:** [B, +] **Contra:** If general anesthesia contraindicated **Supplied:** Inj 10 mg/mL **SE:** May ↑ triglycerides w/ extended dosing; ↓ BP, pain at site, apnea, anaphylaxis **Notes:** 1 mL of propofol has 0.1 g fat

Propoxyphene (Darvon); Propoxyphene & Acetaminophen (Darvocet); & Propoxyphene & Aspirin (Darvon Compound-65, Darvon-N + Aspirin) [C-IV] **Uses:** *Mild–moderate pain* **Action:** Narcotic analgesic **Dose:** 1–2 PO q4h PRN; ↓ in hepatic impair, elderly **Caution:** [C (D if prolonged use), M] Hepatic impair (APAP), peptic ulcer (ASA); severe renal impair **Contra:** Allergy **Supplied:** *Darvon:* Propoxyphene HCl caps 65 mg. *Darvon-N:* Propoxyphene napsylate 100-mg tabs. *Darvocet-N:* Propoxyphene napsylate 50 mg/APAP 325 mg. *Darvocet-N 100:* Propoxyphene napsylate 100 mg/APAP 650 mg. *Darvon Compound-65:* Propoxyphene HCl caps 65-mg/ASA 389 mg/caffeine 32 mg. *Darvon-N w/ ASA:* Propoxyphene napsylate 100 mg/ASA 325 mg **SE:** OD can be lethal; ↓ BP, dizziness, sedation, GI upset, ↑ levels on LFTs

Propranolol (Inheral) **Uses:** *HTN, angina, MI, hyperthyroidism, essential tremor, hypertrophic subaortic stenosis, pheochromocytoma; prevents migraines & atrial arrhythmias* **Action:** β-Adrenergic receptor blocker, β_1, β_2; only β-blocker to block conversion of T_4 to T_3 **Dose:** *Adults. Angina:* 80–320 mg/d PO ÷ bid–qid or 80–160 mg/d SR. *Arrhythmia:* 10–80 mg PO tid–qid or 1 mg IV slowly, repeat q5min, 5 mg max. *HTN:* 40 mg PO bid or 60–80 mg/d SR, ↑ weekly to max 640 mg/d. *Hypertrophic subaortic stenosis:* 20–40 mg PO tid–qid. *MI:* 180–240 mg/d ÷ tid–qid. *Migraine prophylaxis:* 80 mg/d ÷ qid–tid, ↑ weekly 160–240 mg/d ÷ qid; wean if no response in 6 wk. *Pheochromocytoma:* 30–60 mg/d ÷ tid–qid. *Thyrotoxicosis:* 1–3 mg IV × 1; 10–40 mg PO q6h. *Tremor:* 40 mg PO bid, ↑ PRN 320 mg max. *Peds. Arrhythmia:* 0.5–1.0 mg/kg/d ÷ tid–qid, ↑ weekly q3–7d to 60 mg/d max; 0.01–0.1 mg/kg IV over 10 min, 1 mg max. *HTN:* 0.5–1.0 mg/kg ÷ bid–qid, ↑ PRN q3–7d to 2 mg/kg/d max; ↓ in renal impair **Caution:** [C (1st tri, D if 2nd or 3rd tri), +] **Contra:** Uncompensated CHF, cardiogenic shock, bradycardia, heart block, PE, severe resp Dz **Supplied:** Tabs 10, 20, 40, 60, 80 mg; SR caps 60, 80, 120, 160 mg; oral soln 4, 8, 80 mg/mL; inj 1 mg/mL **SE:** Bradycardia, ↓ BP, fatigue, GI upset, ED

Propylthiouracil [PTU] **Uses:** *Hyperthyroidism* **Action:** ↓ Production of T_3 & T_4 & conversion of T_4 to T_3 **Dose:** *Adults. Initial:* 100 mg PO q8h (may need up to 1200 mg/d); after pt euthyroid (6–8 wk), taper dose by ½ q4–6wk to maint, 50–150 mg/24 h; can usually D/C in 2–3 y; ↓ in elderly *Peds. Initial:* 5–7 mg/kg/24 h PO ÷ q8h. *Maint:* ⅓–⅔ of initial dose **Caution:** [D, –] **Contra:** Allergy **Supplied:** Tabs 50 mg **SE:** Fever, rash, leukopenia, dizziness, GI upset, taste perversion, SLE-like syndrome **Notes:** Monitor pt clinically, check TFT

Protamine (generic) **Uses:** *Reverse heparin effect* **Action:** Neutralize heparin by forming a stable complex **Dose:** Based on degree of heparin reversal; give IV slowly; 1 mg reverses approx. 100 Units of heparin given in the preceding 3–4 h, 50 mg max **Caution:** [C, ?] **Contra:** Allergy **Supplied:** Inj 10 mg/mL **SE:** Follow coags; anticoag effect if given w/o heparin; ↓ BP, bradycardia, dyspnea, hemorrhage

Pseudoephedrine (Sudafed, Novafed, Afrinol, others) [OTC]
Uses: *Decongestant* Action: Stimulates α-adrenergic receptors w/ vasoconstriction Dose: *Adults.* 30–60 mg PO q6–8h; SR caps 120 mg PO q12h. *Peds.* 4 mg/kg/24 h PO ÷ qid; ↓ in renal insuff Caution: [B, ?] Contra: Poorly controlled HTN or CAD Dz & in MAOIs Supplied: Tabs 30, 60 mg; caps 60 mg; SR tabs 120, 240 mg; SR caps 120 mg; liq 7.5 mg/0.8 mL, 15, 30 mg/5 mL SE: HTN, insomnia, tachycardia, arrhythmias, nervousness, tremor Notes: Found in many OTC cough/cold preparations; OTC restricted in many states

Psyllium (Metamucil, Serutan, Effer-Syllium) Uses: *Constipation & colonic diverticular Dz* Action: Bulk laxative Dose: 1 tsp (7 g) in glass of H_2O PO qd–tid Caution: [B, ?] Effer-Syllium (effervescent Psyllium) usually contains K^+; caution w/ renal failure; phenylketonuria (in products w/ aspartame) Contra: Suspected bowel obstruction Supplied: Granules 4, 25 g/tsp; powder 3.5 g/packet SE: D, abdominal cramps, bowel obstruction, constipation, bronchospasm

Pyrazinamide (generic) Uses: *Active TB in combo w/ other agents* Action: Bacteriostatic; unknown mechanism Dose: *Adults.* 15–30 mg/kg/24 h PO ÷ tid–qid; max 2 g/d. *Peds.* 15–30 mg/kg/d PO ÷ qd–bid; ↓ w/ renal/hepatic impair Caution: [C, +/–] Contra: Severe hepatic damage, acute gout Supplied: Tabs 500 mg SE: Hepatotox, malaise, GI upset, arthralgia, myalgia, gout, photosensitivity Notes: Use in combo w/ other anti-TB drugs; consult *MMWR* for the latest TB recommendations; dosage regimen differs for directly observed therapy

Pyridoxine [Vitamin B₆] Uses: *Rx & prevention of vitamin B_6 deficiency* Action: Vitamin B_6 supl Dose: *Adults. Deficiency:* 10–20 mg/d PO. *Drug-induced neuritis:* 100–200 mg/d; 25–100 mg/d prophylaxis. *Peds.* 5–25 mg/d × 3 wk Caution: [A (C if doses exceed RDA), +] Contra: Component allergy Supplied: Tabs 25, 50, 100 mg; inj 100 mg/mL SE: Allergic Rxns, HA, N

Quazepam (Doral) [C-IV] Uses: *Insomnia* Action: Benzodiazepine Dose: 7.5–15 mg PO hs PRN; ↓ in elderly & hepatic failure Caution: [X, ?/–] NA glaucoma Contra: PRG, sleep apnea Supplied: Tabs 7.5, 15 mg SE: Sedation, hangover, somnolence, resp depression Notes: Do not D/C abruptly

Quetiapine (Seroquel) WARNING: ↑ mortality in elderly with dementia-related psychosis Uses: *Acute exacerbations of schizophrenia* Action: Serotonin & dopamine antagonism Dose: 150–750 mg/d; initiate at 25–100 mg bid–tid; slowly ↑ dose; ↓ dose for hepatic & geriatric pts Caution: [C, –] Contra: Component allergy Supplied: Tabs 25, 100, 200 mg SE: Reports of confusion w/ nefazodone; HA, somnolence, weight gain, orthostatic ↓ BP, dizziness, cataracts, neuroleptic malignant syndrome, tardive dyskinesia, QT prolongation

Quinapril (Accupril) WARNING: ACE inhibitors used during the 2nd & 3rd tri of PRG can cause fetal injury & death Uses: *HTN, CHF, DN, post-MI* Action: ACE inhibitor Dose: 10–80 mg PO qd ×1; ↓ in renal impair Caution: [D, +] Contra: ACE inhibitor sensitivity or angioedema Supplied: Tabs 5, 10, 20, 40 mg SE: Dizziness, HA, ↓ BP, impaired renal Fxn, angioedema, taste perversion, cough

Quinidine (Quinidex, Quinaglute) Uses: *Prevention of tachydysrhythmias, malaria* Action: Class 1A antiarrhythmic Dose: *Adults. AF/flutter conversion:* After digitalization, 200 mg q2–3h × 8 doses;↑ qd to 3–4 g max or nl rhythm. *Peds.* 15–60 mg/kg/24 h PO in 4–5 ÷ doses; ↓ in renal impair Caution: [C, +] w/ ritonavir Contra: Digitalis tox & AV block; conduction disorders Supplied: Sulfate: Tabs 200, 300 mg; SR tabs 300 mg. Gluconate: SR tabs 324 mg; inj 80 mg/mL SE: Extreme ↓ BP may be seen w/ IV administration; syncope, QT prolongation, GI upset, arrhythmias, fatigue, cinchonism (tinnitus, hearing loss, delirium, visual changes), fever, hemolytic anemia, thrombocytopenia, rash Notes: Check levels (Table 2, page 200); sulfate salt 83% quinidine; gluconate salt 62% quinidine; use in combo w/ drug that slows AV conduction (eg, digoxin, diltiazem, β-blocker)

Quinupristin–Dalfopristin (Synercid) Uses: *Vancomycin-resistant Infxns due to E. faecium & other gram(+)'s* Action: ↓ early & late phases of ribosomal protein synthesis. Spectrum: Vancomycin-resistant Enterococcus faecium, methicillin-susceptible Staphylococcus aureus, Streptococcus pyogenes; not active against Enterococcus faecalis Dose: *Adults & Peds.* 7.5 mg/kg IV q8–12h (use central line if possible); incompatible w/ NS or heparin; flush IV w/ dextrose; ↓ in hepatic failure Caution: [B, M] Contra: Allergy Supplied: Inj 500 mg (150 mg quinupristin/350 mg dalfopristin) SE: Hyperbilirubinemia, inf site Rxns & pain, arthralgia, myalgia Notes: Multiple drug interactions (eg, cyclosporine)

Rabeprazole (Aciphex) Uses: *PUD, GERD, ZE* Action: Proton-pump inhibitor Dose: 20 mg/d; may ↑ to 60 mg/d; do not crush tabs Caution: [B, ?/–] Supplied: Tabs 60 mg SE: HA, fatigue, GI upset

Raloxifene (Evista) Uses: *Prevent osteoporosis* Action: Partial antagonist of estrogen, behaves like estrogen Dose: 60 mg/d Caution: [X, –] Contra: Thromboembolism, PRG Supplied: Tabs 60 mg SE: Chest pain, insomnia, rash, hot flashes, GI upset, hepatic dysfunction

Ramipril (Altace) WARNING: ACE inhibitors used during the 2nd & 3rd tri of PRG can cause fetal injury & death Uses: *HTN, CHF, DN, post-MI* Action: ACE inhibitor Dose: 2.5–20 mg/d PO ÷ qd–bid; ↓ in renal failure Caution: [D, +] Contra: ACE-inhibitor-induced angioedema Supplied: Caps 1.25, 2.5, 5, 10 mg SE: Cough, HA, dizziness, ↓ BP, renal impair, angioedema Notes: OK in combo w/ diuretics

Ranitidine Hydrochloride (Zantac) Uses: *Duodenal ulcer, active benign ulcers, hypersecretory conditions, & GERD* Action: H₂-receptor antagonist Dose: *Adults. Ulcer:* 150 mg PO bid, 300 mg PO hs, or 50 mg IV q6–8h; or 400 mg IV/d cont inf, then maint of 150 mg PO hs. *Hypersecretion:* 150 mg PO bid, up to 600 mg/d. *GERD:* 300 mg PO bid; maint 300 mg PO hs. *Dyspepsia:* 75 mg PO qd–bid. *Peds.* 0.75–1.5 mg/kg/dose IV q6–8h or 1.25–2.5 mg/kg/dose PO q12h; ↓ in renal failure Caution: [B, +] Contra: Component allergy Supplied: Tabs 75 [OTC], 150, 300 mg; Effervescent tabs 150 mg; syrup 15 mg/mL; inj 25 mg/mL SE: Dizziness, sedation, rash, GI upset Notes: PO & parenteral doses differ

Rasburicase (Elitek) Uses: *Reduce ↑ uric acid due to tumor lysis (peds)* **Action:** Catalyzes uric acid **Dose:** *Peds.* 0.15 or 0.20 mg/kg IV over 30 min, qd × 5 **Caution:** [C, ?/–] Falsely ↓ uric acid values **Contra:** Anaphylaxis, screen for G6PD deficiency to avoid hemolysis, methemoglobinemia **Supplied:** 1.5 mg inj **SE:** Fever, neutropenia, GI upset, HA, rash

Repaglinide (Prandin) Uses: *Type 2 DM* **Action:** ↑ pancreatic insulin release **Dose:** 0.5–4 mg ac, PO start 1–2 mg, ↑ to 16 mg/d max; take pc **Caution:** [C, ?/–] **Contra:** DKA, type 1 DM **Supplied:** Tabs 0.5, 1, 2 mg **SE:** HA, hyper-/hypoglycemia, GI upset

Reteplase (Retavase) Uses: *Post-AMI* **Action:** Thrombolytic agent **Dose:** 10 Units IV over 2 min, 2nd dose in 30 min, 10 Units IV over 2 min **Caution:** [C, ?/–] **Contra:** Internal bleeding, spinal surgery/trauma, Hx CNS vascular malformations, uncontrolled ↓ BP, sensitivity to thrombolytics **Supplied:** Inj 10.8 Units/2 mL **SE:** Bleeding, allergic reactions

Ribavirin (Virazole) Uses: *RSV Infxn in infants; hepatitis C (in combo w/ interferon alfa-2b)* **Action:** Unknown **Dose:** *RSV:* 6 g in 300 mL sterile H$_2$O, inhale over 12–18 h. *Hep C:* 600 mg PO bid in combo w/ interferon alfa-2b (see Rebetron, page 112) **Caution:** [X, ?] **Contra:** PRG, autoimmune hepatitis, CrCl <50 mL/min **Supplied:** Powder for aerosol 6 g; caps 200 mg **SE:** May accumulate on soft contact lenses; fatigue, HA, GI upset, anemia, myalgia, alopecia, bronchospasm **Notes:** Aerosolized by a SPAG; monitor Hbg/Hct; PRG test monthly

Rifabutin (Mycobutin) Uses: *Prevent M. avium complex Infxn in AIDS pts w/ CD4 count <100* **Action:** ↓ DNA-dependent RNA polymerase activity **Dose:** *Adults.* 150–300 mg/d PO. *Peds. 1 y:* 15–25 mg/kg/d PO *2–10 y:* 4.4–18.8 mg/kg/d PO. *14–16 y:* 2.8–5.4 mg/kg/d PO **Caution:** [B; ?/–] WBC <1000/mm³ or platelets <50,000/mm³; ritonavir **Contra:** Allergy **Supplied:** Caps 150 mg **SE:** Discolored urine, rash, neutropenia, leukopenia, myalgia, ↑ LFTs **Notes:** SEs/interactions similar to rifampin

Rifampin (Rifadin) Uses: *TB & Rx & prophylaxis of N. meningitidis, H. influenzae, or S. aureus carriers*; adjunct for severe S. aureus **Action:** ↓ DNA-dependent RNA polymerase **Dose:** *Adults. N. meningitidis & H. influenzae carrier:* 600 mg/d PO for 4 d. *TB:* 600 mg PO or IV qd or 2 ×/wk w/ combo regimen. *Peds.* 10–20 mg/kg/dose PO or IV qd–bid; ↓ in hepatic failure **Caution:** [C, +] Amprenavir, multiple drug interactions **Contra:** Allergy, presence of active N. meningitidis Infxn, concomitant use of saquinavir/ritonavir **Supplied:** Caps 150, 300 mg; inj 600 mg **SE:** Orange-red discoloration of bodily fluids, ↑ LFTs, flushing, HA **Notes:** Never use as single agent w/ active TB

Rifapentine (Priftin) Uses: *Pulmonary TB* **Action:** ↓ DNA-dependent RNA polymerase. *Spectrum: M. tuberculosis* **Dose:** *Intensive phase:* 600 mg PO 2×/wk for 2 mo; separate doses by 3 or more days. *Continuation phase:* 600 mg/wk for 4 mo; part of 3–4 drug regimen **Caution:** [C, red-orange breast milk] ↓ protease inhibitor efficacy, antiepileptics, β-blockers, CCBs **Contra:** Allergy to rifamycins **Supplied:** 150-mg tabs **SE:** Neutropenia, hyperuricemia, HTN, HA, dizziness, rash, GI upset, blood dyscrasias, ↑ LFTs, hematuria, discolored secretions **Notes:** Monitor LFTs

Rifaximin (Xifaxan) Uses: * Travelers' diarrhea (noninvasive strains of *E coli*) in patients > 12 y* **Action:** Not absorbed, derivative of rifamycin. *Spectrum: E coli* **Dose:** 1 tab PO qd × 3 d **Caution:** [C, ?/-] Allergy (rash, angioedema, urticaria); pseudomembranous colitis **Contra:** Allergy to rifamycins **Supplied:** Tabs 200 mg **SE:** Flatulence, HA, abdominal pain, GI distress, fever **Notes:** D/C if Sx worsen or persist > 24–48 h, or w/ fever or blood in stool

Rimantadine (Flumadine) Uses: * Prophylaxis & Rx of influenza A viral Infxns* **Action:** Antiviral **Dose:** **Adults & Peds >9 y.** 100 mg PO bid. **Peds 1–9 y.** 5 mg/kg/d PO, 150 mg/d max; qd w/ severe renal/hepatic impair & elderly; initiate w/in 48 h of Sx onset **Caution:** [C, –] w/ cimetidine; avoid in PRG or breast-feeding **Contra:** Component & amantadine allergy **Supplied:** Tabs 100 mg; syrup 50 mg/5 mL **SE:** Orthostatic ↓ BP, edema, dizziness, GI upset, ↓ Sz threshold

Rimexolone (Vexol Ophthalmic) Uses: *Postop inflammation & uveitis* **Action:** Steroid **Dose:** **Adults & Peds >2 y.** Uveitis: 1–2 gtt/h daytime & q2h at night, taper to 1 gtt q4h. *Postop:* 1–2 gtt qid ≤ 2 wk **Caution:** [C, ?/–] Ocular Infxns **Supplied:** Susp 1%; **SE:** Blurred vision, local irritation **Notes:** Taper dose

Risedronate (Actonel) Uses: *Paget Dz; treat/prevent glucocorticoid-induced/postmenopausal osteoporosis* **Action:** Bisphosphonate; ↓ osteoclast-mediated bone resorption **Dose:** *Paget Dz:* 30 mg/d PO for 2 mo. *Osteoporosis Rx/prevention:* 5 mg qd or 35 mg qwk; 30 min before 1st food/drink of the day; stay upright for at least 30 min after **Caution:** [C, ?/–] Ca supls & antacids ↓ absorption **Contra:** Allergy, ↓ Ca^{2+}, esophageal abnormalities, unable to stand/sit for 30 min, CrCl < 30 mL/min **Supplied:** Tabs 5, 30, 35 mg **SE:** HA, D, abdominal pain, arthralgia; flu-like Sxs, rash, esophagitis, bone pain **Notes:** Monitor LFT, Ca^{2+}, PO_3^{3+}, K^+

Risperidone (Risperdal) **WARNING:** ↑ mortality in elderly with dementia-related psychosis Uses: *Psychotic disorders (schizophrenia),* dementia of the elderly, bipolar disorder, mania, Tourette disorder, autism **Action:** Benzisoxazole antipsychotic **Dose:** **Adults.** 0.5–6 mg PO bid. **Peds/Adolescents.** 0.25 mg PO bid, ↑ q5–7d; ↓ start dose w/ elderly, renal/hepatic impair **Caution:** [C, –], ↑ ↓ BP w/ antihypertensives, clozapine **Contra:** Component allergy **Supplied:** Tabs 0.25, 0.5, 1, 2, 3, 4 mg; soln 1 mg/mL **SE:** Orthostatic ↓ BP, EPS w/ high dose, tachycardia, arrhythmias, sedation, dystonias, neuroleptic malignant syndrome, sexual dysfunction, constipation, xerostomia, blood dyscrasias, cholestatic jaundice, weight gain **Notes:** Several weeks to see effect

Ritonavir (Norvir) Uses: *HIV* **Actions:** Protease inhibitor; ↓ maturation of immature noninfectious virions to mature infectious virus **Dose:** **Adults.** Initial 300 mg PO bid, titrate over 1 wk to 600 mg PO bid (titration will ↓ GI SE) **Peds ≥2 y.** 250 mg/m² titrate to 400 mg bid (dose adjust w/ amprenavir, indinavir, nelfinavir, & saquinavir); (w/ food) **Caution:** [B, +] w/ ergotamine, amiodarone, bepridil, flecainide, propafenone, quinidine, pimozide, midazolam, triazolam **Contra:** W/ ergotamine, amiodarone, bepridil, flecainide, propafenone, quinidine, pimozide, midazolam, triazolam, St. John's wort **Supplied:** Caps 100 mg; soln 80 mg/mL **SE:** ↑ triglycerides, ↑ LFTs, N/V/D/C, abdominal pain, taste perversion, anemia, weakness, HA, fever, malaise, rash, paresthesias **Notes:** Refrigerate

Rivastigmine (Exelon) **Uses:** *Mild–moderate dementia in Alzheimer Dz* **Action:** Enhances cholinergic activity **Dose:** 1.5 mg bid; ↑ to 6 mg bid, w/ ↑ at 2-wk intervals (w/ food) **Caution:** [B, ?] β-Blockers, CCBs, smoking, neuromuscular blockade, digoxin **Contra:** Allergy to rivastigmine or carbamates **Supplied:** Caps 1.5, 3, 4.5, 6 mg; soln 2 mg/mL **SE:** Dose-related GI effects, N/V/D; dizziness, insomnia, fatigue, tremor, diaphoresis, HA **Notes:** Swallow capsules whole, do not break, chew, or crush; avoid EtOH

Rizatriptan (Maxalt, Maxalt MLT) (See Table 11, page 218)

Rocuronium (Zemuron) **Uses:** *Skeletal muscle relaxation during rapid-sequence intubation, surgery, or mechanical ventilation* **Action:** Nondepolarizing neuromuscular blocker **Dose:** *Rapid sequence intubation:* 0.6–1.2 mg/kg IV. *Continuous inf:* 4–16 mcg/kg/min IV; ↓ in hepatic impair **Caution:** [C, ?] Aminoglycosides, vancomycin, tetracycline, polymyxins enhance blockade **Contra:** Component or pancuronium allergy **Supplied:** 10 mg/mL 5,10 mL vials **SE:** BP changes, tachycardia

Rofecoxib (Vioxx) Withdrawn from market due to safety concerns

Ropinirole (Requip) **Uses:** *Rx of Parkinson Dz* **Action:** Dopamine agonist **Dose:** Initial 0.25 mg PO tid, weekly ↑ 0.25 mg/dose, to 3 mg max **Caution:** [C, ?/–] Severe CV, renal, or hepatic impair **Contra:** Component allergy **Supplied:** Tabs 0.25, 0.5, 1, 2, 5 mg **SE:** Syncope, postural ↓ BP, N/V, HA, somnolence, hallucinations, dyskinesias **Notes:** D/C w/ 7-d taper

Rosiglitazone (Avandia) **Uses:** *Type 2 DM* **Action:** ↑ insulin sensitivity **Dose:** 4–8 mg/d PO or in 2 ÷ doses (w/o regard to meals) **Caution:** [C, –] Not for DKA; w/ ESRD (renal elimination) **Contra:** Active liver Dz **Supplied:** Tabs 2, 4, 8 mg **SE:** Weight gain, hyperlipidemia, HA, edema, fluid retention, exacerbated CHF, hyper-/hypoglycemia, hepatic damage

Rosuvastatin (Crestor) **Uses:** *Rx primary hypercholesterolemia & mixed dyslipidemia* **Action:** HMG-CoA reductase inhibitor **Dose:** 5–40 mg PO qd; max 5 mg/d w/ cyclosporine, 10 mg/d w/ gemfibrozil or CrCl < 30 mL/min (avoid Al-/Mg-based antacids for 2 h after) **Caution:** [X,?/–] **Contra:** Active liver Dz or unexplained ↑ LFT **Supplied:** Tabs 5, 10, 20, 40 mg **SE:** Myalgia, constipation, asthenia, abdominal pain, nausea, myopathy, rarely rhabdomyolysis **Notes:** May ↑ warfarin effect; monitor LFTs at baseline, 12 wk, then q6mo; ↓ dose in Asian patients

Salmeterol (Serevent) **Uses:** *Asthma, exercise-induced asthma, COPD* **Action:** Sympathomimetic bronchodilator, β₂-agonist **Dose:** *Adults & Peds ≥12 y.*

1 diskus-dose inhaled bid **Caution:** [C, ?/–] **Contra:** Acute asthma; w/in 14 d of MAOI **Supplied:** Dry powder discus **SE:** HA, pharyngitis, tachycardia, arrhythmias, nervousness, GI upset, tremors **Notes:** Not for acute attacks; also prescribe short-acting β-agonist

Saquinavir (Fortovase) Uses: *HIV Infxn* **Action:** HIV protease inhibitor **Dose:** 1200 mg PO tid w/in 2 h pc (dose adjust w/ ritonavir, delavirdine, lopinavir, & nelfinavir) **Contra:** Allergy, sun exposure w/o sunscreen/clothing, triazolam, midazolam, ergots, rifampin **Supplied:** Caps 200 mg **SE:** Dyslipidemia, lipodystrophy, rash, hyperglycemia, GI upset, weakness, hepatic dysfunction **Notes:** Take 2h after meal, avoid direct sunlight

Sargramostim [GM-CSF] (Prokine, Leukine) Uses: *Myeloid recovery following BMT or chemo* **Action:** Recombinant GF, Activates mature granulocytes & macrophages **Dose:** *Adults & Peds.* 250 mcg/m²/d IV for 21 d (BMT) **Caution:** [C, ?/–] Lithium, corticosteroids **Contra:** >10% blasts, allergy to yeast, concurrent chemo/RT **Supplied:** Inj 250, 500 mcg **SE:** Bone pain, fever, ↓ BP, tachycardia, flushing, GI upset, myalgia **Notes:** Rotate inj sites; use APAP PRN for pain

Scopolamine, Scopolamine Transdermal (Scopace, Transderm-Scop) Uses: *Prevent N/V associated w/ motion sickness, anesthesia, opiates; mydriatic,* cycloplegic, Rx iridiocyclitis **Action:** Anticholinergic, antiemetic **Dose:** 1 patch behind ear q3d; apply > 4 h before exposure: 0.4–0.8 PO, repeat PRN q4–6h; ↓ in elderly **Caution:** [C, +] APAP, levodopa, ketoconazole, digitalis, KCl **Contra:** NA glaucoma, GI or GU obstruction, thyrotoxicosis, paralytic ileus **Supplied:** Patch 1.5 mg, tabs 0.4 mg, ophth 0.25% **SE:** Xerostomia, drowsiness, blurred vision, tachycardia, constipation **Notes:** Do not blink excessively after eye gt, wait 5 min before other eye gtt; activity w/ patch requires several hours

Secobarbital (Seconal) (C-II) Uses: *Insomnia,* preanesthetic agent **Action:** Rapid-acting barbiturate **Dose:** *Adults.* 100–200 mg, 100–300 mg preop. *Peds.* 2–6 mg/kg/dose, 100 mg/max, ↓ in elderly **Caution:** [D, +] CYP2C9, 3A3/4, 3A5–7 inducer (page 220); ↑ tox w/ other CNS depressants **Contra:** Porphyria, PRG **Supplied:** Caps 100 mg **SE:** Tolerance in 1–2 wk; resp depression, CNS depression, porphyria, photosensitivity

Selegiline (Eldepryl) Uses: Parkinson Dz **Action:** MAOI **Dose:** 5 mg PO bid; ↓ in elderly **Caution:** [C, ?] Meperidine, SSRI, TCAs **Contra:** Concurrent meperidine **Supplied:** Tabs/caps 5 mg **SE:** Nausea, dizziness, orthostatic ↓ BP, arrhythmias, tachycardia, edema, confusion, xerostomia **Notes:** ↓ carbidopa/levodopa if used in combo

Selenium Sulfide (Exsel Shampoo, Selsun Blue Shampoo, Selsun Shampoo) Uses: *Scalp seborrheic dermatitis,* scalp itching & flaking due to *dandruff*; tinea versicolor **Action:** Antiseborrheic **Dose:** *Dandruff, seborrhea:* Massage 5–10 mL into wet scalp, leave on 2–3 min, rinse, repeat; use

2×/wk, then once q1–4wk PRN. *Tinea versicolor:* Apply 2.5% qd for 7 d on area & lather w/ small amounts of water; leave on skin 10 min, then rinse **Caution:** [C, ?] **Contra:** Open wounds **Supplied:** Shampoo [OTC] 1, 2.5% **SE:** Dry or oily scalp, lethargy, hair discoloration, local irritation **Notes:** Do not use more than 2×/wk

Sertaconazole (Ertaczo) **Uses:** *Topical Rx interdigital tinea pedis* **Action:** Imidazole antifungal. *Spectrum: Trichophyton rubrum, T. mentagrophytes, Epidermophyton floccosum* **Dose: Adults & Peds > 12.** Apply between toes & immediate surrounding healthy skin bid × 4 wk **Caution:** [C, ?] **Contra:** Component allergy **Supplied:** 2% cream **SE:** Contact dermatitis, dry/burning skin, tenderness **Notes:** Use in immunocompetent pts

Sertraline (Zoloft) **WARNING:** Closely monitor pts for worsening depression or emergence of suicidality, particularly in ped pts **Uses:** *Depression, panic disorders, obsessive–compulsive disorder (OCD), posttraumatic stress disorders (PTSD),* social anxiety disorder, eating disorders, premenstrual disorders **Action:** ↓ neuronal uptake of serotonin **Dose: Adults.** *Depression:* 50–200 mg/d PO. *PTSD:* 25 mg PO qd ×1 wk, then 50 mg PO qd, 200 mg/d max. **Peds.** *6–12 y:* 25 mg PO qd. *13–17 y:* 50 mg PO qd **Caution:** [C, ?/–] w/ haloperidol (serotonin syndrome), sumatriptan, linezolid, hepatic impair **Contra:** MAOI use w/in 14 d; concomitant pimozide **Supplied:** Tabs 25, 50, 100 mg **SE:** Can activate manic/hypomanic state; weight loss; insomnia, somnolence, fatigue, tremor, xerostomia, N/D, ejaculatory dysfunction, ↓ libido, hepatotox

Sevelamer (Renagel) **Uses:** ↓ serum phosphorus in ESRD **Action:** Binds intestinal PO_4^{3+} **Dose:** 2–4 capsules PO tid w/ meals; adjust based on PO_4^{3+} **Caution:** [C, ?] **Contra:** Bowel obstruction **Supplied:** Capsules 403 mg **SE:** BP changes, N/V/D, dyspepsia, thrombosis **Notes:** Do not open or chew capsules; may ↓ fat-soluble vitamin absorption; 800 mg sevelamer = 667 mg Ca acetate

Sibutramine (Meridia) [C-IV] **Uses:** *Obesity* **Action:** Blocks uptake of norepinephrine, serotonin, dopamine **Dose:** 10 mg/d PO, may ↓ to 5 mg after 4 wk **Caution:** [C, –] SSRIs, lithium, dextromethorphan, opioids **Contra:** MAOI w/in 14 d, uncontrolled HTN, arrhythmias **Supplied:** Caps 5, 10, 15 mg **SE:** HA, insomnia, xerostomia, constipation, rhinitis, tachycardia, HTN **Notes:** Use w/ low-calorie diet, monitor BP & HR

Sildenafil (Viagra, Revatio) **Uses:** *Viagra:* *Erectile dysfunction,* *Revatio:* *Pulmonary artery HTN* **Action:** ↓ Phosphodiesterase type 5 (responsible for cGMP breakdown); ↑ cGMP activity, causing smooth muscle relaxation & ↑ flow to the corpus cavernosum and pulmonary vasculature; possible antiproliferative effect on pulmonary artery smooth muscle; **Dose:** 25–100 mg PO 1 h before sexual activity, max ×1 qd; if >65 y; avoid fatty foods w/ dose; Revatio 20 mg PO tid **Caution:** [B, ?] CYP3A4 inhibitors **Contra:** W/ nitrates; retinitis pigmentosa; hepatic/severe renal impair **Supplied:** Tabs (Viagra) 25, 50, 100 mg, tabs (Revatio) 20 mg **SE:** HA; flushing; dizziness; blue haze visual disturbance (usually reversible) **Notes:** Cardiac events in absence of nitrates debatable

Silver Nitrate (Dey-Drop, others) Uses: *Removal of granulation tissue & warts; prophylaxis in burns* Action: Caustic antiseptic & astringent Dose: *Adults & Peds.* Apply to moist surface 2–3×/wk for several wks or until effect Caution: [C, ?] Contra: Do not use on broken skin Supplied: Topical impregnated applicator sticks, oint 10%, soln 10, 25, 50%; ophth 1% amp SE: May stain tissue black, usually resolves; local irritation, methemoglobinemia Notes: D/C if redness or irritation develop; no longer used in US for newborn prevention of GC conjunctivitis

Silver Sulfadiazine (Silvadene) Uses: *Prevention & Rx of Infxn in 2nd- & 3rd-degree burns* Action: Bactericidal Dose: *Adults & Peds.* Aseptically cover the area w/ ¹⁄₁₆-in. coating bid Caution: [B unless near term, ?/–] Contra: Infants < 2 mo, PRG near term Supplied: Cream 1% SE: Itching, rash, skin discoloration, blood dyscrasias, hepatitis, allergy Notes: Systemic absorption w/ extensive application

Simethicone (Mylicon) [OTC] Uses: Flatulence Action: Defoaming action Dose: *Adults & Peds.* 40–125 mg PO pc & hs PRN Caution: [C, ?] Contra: Intestinal perforation or obstruction Supplied: [OTC] Tabs 80, 125 mg; caps 125 mg; gt 40 mg/0.6 mL SE: N/D Notes: Available in combo products OTC

Simvastatin (Zocor) Uses: ↓ Cholesterol Action: HMG-CoA reductase inhibitor Dose: 5–80 mg PO; w/ meals; ↓ in renal insuff Caution: [X, –] Avoid concurrent use of gemfibrozil Contra: PRG, liver Dz Supplied: Tabs 5, 10, 20, 40 mg SE: HA, GI upset, myalgia, myopathy (muscle pain, tenderness or weakness with creatine kinase 10× ULN), hepatitis Notes: Follow LFTs

Sirolimus [Rapamycin] (Rapamune) WARNING: Can cause immunosuppression & Infxns Uses: Prophylaxis of organ rejection Action: ↓ T-lymphocyte activation Dose: *Adults >40 kg.* 6 mg PO on day 1, then 2 mg/d PO. *Adults <40 kg & Peds ≥13 y.* 3 mg/m² load, then 1 mg/m²/d (in H₂O/orange juice; no grapefruit juice while on sirolimus); take 4 h after cyclosporine; ↓ in hepatic impair Caution: [C, ?/–] Grapefruit juice, ketoconazole Contra: Component allergy Supplied: Soln 1 mg/mL, tab 1 mg SE: HTN, edema, CP, fever, HA, insomnia, acne, rash, ↑ cholesterol, GI upset, ↑ or ↓ K⁺, Infxns, blood dyscrasias, arthralgia, tachycardia, renal impair, hepatic artery thrombosis, graft loss & death in de novo liver transplant Notes: Levels not needed except in liver failure (trough 9–17 ng/mL)

Smallpox Vaccine (Dryvax) Uses: Immunization against smallpox (variola virus) Action: Active immunization (live attenuated vaccinia virus) Dose: *Adults (routine nonemergency) or all ages (emergency):* 2–3 punctures w/ bifurcated needle dipped in vaccine into deltoid, posterior triceps muscle; check site for Rxn in 6–8 d; if major Rxn, site scabs, & heals, leaving scar; if mild/equivocal Rxn, repeat w/ 15 punctures Caution: [X, N/A] Contra: *Nonemergency use:* Febrile illness, immunosuppression, Hx eczema & their household contacts. *Emergency:* No absolute contraindications Supplied: Vial for reconstitution: 100 million pock-forming Units/mL **SE:** Malaise, fever, regional lymphadenopathy, encephalopathy, rashes, spread of inoculation to other sites administered; Stevens–Johnson syndrome, eczema vaccinatum w/ severe disability

Sodium Bicarbonate [NaHCO₃] Uses: *Alkalinization of urine,* RTA, *metabolic acidosis, ↑ K⁺, TCA OD* **Action:** Alkalinizing agent **Dose:** *Adults. Cardiac arrest:* Initiate ventilation, 1 mEq/kg/dose IV; repeat 0.5 mEq/kg in 10 min once or based on acid–base status. *Metabolic acidosis:* 2–5 mEq/kg IV over 8 h & PRN based on acid–base status. *Alkalinize urine:* 4 g (48 mEq) PO, then 1–2 g q4h; adjust based on urine pH; 2 amp/1 L D₅W at 100–250 mL/h IV, monitor urine pH & serum bicarbonate. *Chronic renal failure:* 1–3 mEq/kg PO. *Distal RTA:* 1 mEq/kg/d PO. *Peds >1 y: Cardiac arrest:* See Adult dosage. *Peds <1 y: ECC:* Initiate ventilation, 1:1 dilution 1 mEq/mL dosed 1 mEq/kg IV; can repeat w/ 0.5 mEq/kg in 10 min ×1 or based on acid–base status. *Chronic renal failure:* See Adult dosage. *Distal RTA:* 2–3 mEq/kg/d PO. *Proximal RTA:* 5–10 mEq/kg/d; titrate based on serum bicarbonate. *Urine alkalinization:* 84–840 mg/kg/d (1–10 mEq/kg/d) in ÷ doses; adjust based on urine pH **Caution:** [C, ?] **Contra:** Alkalosis, ↑ Na⁺, severe pulmonary edema, ↓ Ca²⁺ **Supplied:** Powder, tabs; 300 mg = 3.6 mEq; 325 mg = 3.8 mEq; 520 mg = 6.3 mEq; 600 mg = 7.3 mEq; 650 mg = 7.6 mEq; inj 1 mEq/mL vial or amp **SE:** Belching, edema, flatulence, ↑ Na⁺, metabolic alkalosis **Notes:** 1 g neutralizes 12 mEq of acid; 50 mEq bicarb = 50 mEq Na; can make 3 amps in 1 L D₅W to = D₅NS w/ 150 mEq bicarb

Sodium Citrate (Bicitra) Uses: Alkalinize urine; dissolve uric acid & cysteine stones **Action:** Urinary alkalinizer **Dose:** *Adults.* 2–6 tsp (10–30 mL) diluted in 1–3 oz H₂O pc & hs. *Peds.* 1–3 tsp (5–15 mL) diluted in 1–3 oz H₂O pc & hs; best after meals **Caution:** [C, +] **Contra:** Aluminum-based antacids; severe renal impair or Na-restricted diets **Supplied:** 15- or 30-mL unit dose: 16 (473 mL) or 4 (118 mL) fl oz **SE:** Tetany, metabolic alkalosis, ↑ K⁺, GI upset; avoid use of multiple 50-mL amps; can cause ↑ Na⁺/hyperosmolality **Notes:** 1 mL = 1 mEq Na & 1 mEq bicarb

Sodium Oxybate (Xyrem) [C-III] Uses: *Narcolepsy-associated cataplexy* **Action:** Inhibitory neutrotransmitter **Dose:** *Adults & Peds ≥ 16 y:* 2.25 g PO qhs, second dose 2.5–4 h later; may ↑ 9 g/d max **Caution:** [B, ?/–] **Contra:** Succinic semialdehyde dehydrogenase deficiency; potentiates EtOH **Supplied:** 500 mg/mL 180-mL PO soln **SE:** Confusion, depression, diminished level of consciousness, incontinence, significant vomiting, resp depression, psychiatric Sxs **Notes:** May lead to dependence; synonym for γ-hydroxybutyrate (GHB), abused as a "date rape drug"; controlled distribution (prescriber & pt registration); must be administered when pt in bed

Sodium Phosphate (Visicol) Uses: Bowel prep prior to colonoscopy **Action:** Hyperosmotic laxative **Dose:** 3 tabs PO w/ at least 8 oz clear liq every 15 min (20 tabs total night before procedure; 3–5 h before colonoscopy, repeat) **Caution:** [C, ?] Renal impair, electrolyte disturbances **Contra:** Megacolon, bowel obstruction, CHF, ascites, unstable angina, gastric retention, bowel perforation, colitis, hypomotility. **Supplied:** Tablets 2 g **SE:** QT prolongation, D, ↑ Na⁺, flatulence, cramps

Sodium Polystyrene Sulfonate (Kayexalate)
Uses: *↑ K⁺* **Action:** Na⁺/K⁺ ion-exchange resin **Dose:** *Adults.* 15–60 g PO or 30–60 g PR q6h based on serum K⁺. **Peds.** 1 g/kg/dose PO or PR q6h based on serum K⁺ (given w/ agent, eg, sorbitol, to promote movement through the bowel) **Caution:** [C, M] **Contra:** ↑ Na⁺ **Supplied:** Powder; susp 15 g/60 mL sorbitol **SE:** Can cause ↑ Na⁺, ↓ K⁺, Na retention, GI upset, fecal impaction **Notes:** Enema acts more quickly than PO; PO most effective

Solifenacin (VESIcare)
Uses: OAB **Action:** Antimuscarinic **Dose:** 5 mg PO qd, 10 mg max **Caution:** [C, ?/-] Bladder outflow or GI obstruction, ulcerative colitis, MyG, renal/hepatic impair, QT prolongation risk **Contra:** NA glaucoma, urinary/gastric retention **Supplied:** Tabs 5, 10 mg **SE:** Constipation, xerostomia **Notes:** Interacts w/ azole antifungals; do not ↑ dose w/ severe renal/moderate hepatic impair

Sorbitol (generic)
Uses: *Constipation* **Action:** Laxative **Dose:** 30–60 mL PO of a 20–70% soln PRN **Caution:** [B, +] **Contra:** Anuria **Supplied:** Liq 70% **SE:** Edema, electrolyte losses, lactic acidosis, GI upset, xerostomia **Notes:** May be vehicle for many liq formulations (eg, zinc, Kayexalate)

Sotalol (Betapace)
WARNING: Monitor pts for 1st 3 d of Rx to ↓ risks of arrhythmia **Uses:** *Ventricular arrhythmias, AF* **Action:** β-Adrenergic-blocking agent **Dose:** *Adults.* 80 mg PO bid; may be ↑ to 240–320 mg/d. **Peds.** *Neonates:* 9 mg/m² tid. *1–19 mo:* 20 mg/m² tid. *20–23 mo:* 29.1 mg/m² tid. *≥ 2 y:* 30 mg/m² tid; ↓ in renal failure **Caution:** [B (1st tri) (D if 2nd or 3rd tri), +] **Contra:** Asthma, bradycardia, prolonged QT interval, 2nd- or 3rd-degree heart block w/o pacemaker, cardiogenic shock, uncontrolled CHF, CrCl <40 mL/min **Supplied:** Tabs 80, 120, 160, 240 mg **SE:** Bradycardia, CP, palpitations, fatigue, dizziness, weakness, dyspnea **Notes:** Betapace should not be substituted for Betapace AF because of significant differences in labeling

Sotalol (Betapace AF)
WARNING: To minimize risk of induced arrhythmia, pts initiated/reinitiated on Betapace AF should be placed for a minimum of 3 d (on their maint dose) in a facility that can provide cardiac resuscitation, continuous ECG monitoring, & calculations of CrCl; Betapace should not be substituted for Betapace AF because of labeling differences **Uses:** *Maintain sinus rhythm for symptomatic A fib/flutter* **Action:** β-Adrenergic-blocking agent **Dose:** *Adults.* Initial CrCl >60 mL/min: 80 mg PO q12h. CrCl 40–60 mL/min: 80 mg PO q2h; ↑ to 120 mg during hospitalization; monitor QT interval 2–4 h after each dose, w/ dose reduction or D/C if QT interval >500 ms. **Peds.** *Neonates:* 9 mg/m² tid. *1–19 mo:* 20 mg/m² tid. *20–23 mo:* 29.1 mg/m² tid. *≥ 2 y:* 30 mg/m² tid; all dosage ranges may be doubled as max daily dose; allow ≥ 36 h between dosage titrations **Caution:** [B (1st tri; D if 2nd or 3rd tri), +] if converting from previous antiar-

rhythmic therapy **Contra:** Asthma, bradycardia, prolonged QT interval, 2nd- or 3rd-degree heart block w/o pacemaker, cardiogenic shock, uncontrolled CHF, CrCl <40 mL/min **Supplied:** Tabs 80, 120, 160 mg **SE:** Bradycardia, CP, palpitations, fatigue, dizziness, weakness, dyspnea **Notes:** Follow renal Fxn & QT interval

Sparfloxacin (Zagam) Uses: *Community-acquired pneumonia, acute exacerbations of chronic bronchitis reported **Action:** Quinolone; ↓ DNA gyrase **Dose:** 400 mg PO day 1, then 200 mg q24h × 10 d; ↓ in renal impair **Caution:** [C, ?/−] W/ theophylline, caffeine, sucralfate, warfarin, & antacids **Contra:** w/QT prolongation & drugs that prolong QT interval **Supplied:** Tabs 200 mg **SE:** Phototox (even daylight through windows); restlessness, N/V/D, rash, ruptured tendons, ↑ LFTs, sleep disorders, confusion, convulsions **Notes:** Protect from sunlight up to 5 d after last dose

Spironolactone (Aldactone) Uses: *Hyperaldosteronism, ascites from CHF or cirrhosis* **Action:** Aldosterone antagonist; K⁺-sparing diuretic **Dose:** *Adults.* 25–100 mg PO qid; CHF (NYHA class III–IV) 25–50 mg/d. *Peds.* 1–3.3 mg/kg/24 h PO ÷ bid–qid. *Neonates.* 0.5–1 mg/kg/dose q8h; w/ food **Caution:** [D, +] **Contra:** ↑ K⁺, renal failure, anuria **Supplied:** Tabs 25, 50, 100 mg **SE:** ↑ K⁺ & gynecomastia, arrhythmia, sexual dysfunction, confusion, dizziness

Stavudine (Zerit) WARNING: Lactic acidosis & severe hepatomegaly w/ steatosis & pancreatitis Uses: *Advanced HIV* **Action:** Reverse transcriptase inhibitor **Dose:** *Adults.* >60 kg: 40 mg bid. <60 kg: 30 mg bid. *Peds. Birth–13 d:* 0.5 mg/kg q12h. *>14 d & <30 kg:* 1 mg/kg q12h. *≥30 kg:* Adult dose; ↓ in renal failure **Caution:** [C, +] **Contra:** Allergy **Supplied:** Caps 15, 20, 30, 40 mg; soln 1 mg/mL **SE:** Peripheral neuropathy, HA, chills, fever, malaise, rash, GI upset, anemias, lactic acidosis, ↑ LFTs, pancreatitis **Notes:** Take w/ plenty of H₂O

Steroids, Systemic (See also Table 4, page 206) The following relates only to the commonly used systemic glucocorticoids Uses: *Endocrine disorders* (adrenal insuff), *rheumatoid disorders, collagen–vascular Dzs, dermatologic Dzs, allergic states, cerebral edema,* nephritis, nephrotic syndrome, immunosuppression for transplantation, ↑ Ca²⁺, malignancies (breast, lymphomas), preop (in any pt who has been on steroids in the previous year, known hypoadrenalism, preop for adrenalectomy; inj into joints/tissue **Action:** Glucocorticoid **Dose:** Varies w/ use & institutional protocols. *Adrenal insuff, acute: Adults.* Hydrocortisone: 100 mg IV; then 300 mg/d ÷ q6h; convert to 50 mg PO q8h ×6 doses, taper to 30–50 mg/d ÷ bid. *Peds. Hydrocortisone:* 1–2 mg/kg IV, then 150–250 mg/d ÷ tid. *Adrenal insuff, chronic (physiologic replacement):* May need mineralocorticoid supl such as Florinef. *Adults.* Hydrocortisone 20 mg PO qAM, 10 mg PO qPM; cortisone 0.5–0.75 mg/kg/d ÷ bid; cortisone 0.25–0.35 mg/kg/d IM; dexamethasone 0.03–0.15 mg/kg/d or 0.6–0.75 mg/m²/d ÷ q6–12h PO, IM, IV. *Peds. Hydrocortisone:* 0.5–0.75 mg/kg/d PO tid; hydrocortisone succinate 0.25–0.35 mg/kg/d IM. *Asthma, acute: Adults.* Methylprednisolone 60 mg PO/IV q6h or dexamethasone 12 mg IV q6h. *Peds.* Prednisolone 1–2 mg/kg/d or prednisone 1–2 mg/kg/d ÷

qd–bid for up to 5 d; methylprednisolone 2–4 mg/kg/d IV ÷ tid; dexamethasone 0.1–0.3 mg/kg/d divided q6h. *Congenital adrenal hyperplasia:* **Peds.** Initial hydrocortisone 30–36 mg/m²/d PO ÷ ⅓ dose qAM, ⅔ dose qPM; maint 20–25 mg/m²/d ÷ bid. *Extubation/airway edema:* **Adults.** Dexamethasone 0.5–1 mg/kg/d IM/IV ÷ q6h (start 24 h prior to extubation; continue × 4 more doses). **Peds.** Dexamethasone 0.1–0.3 mg/kg/d ÷ q6h × 3–5 d (start 48–72h before extubation) *Immunosuppressive/antiinflammatory:* **Adults & Older Peds.** Hydrocortisone: 15–240 mg PO, IM, IV q12h; *methylprednisolone:* 4–48 mg/d PO, taper to lowest effective dose; *methylprednisolone Na succinate:* 10–80 mg/d IM. **Adults.** *Prednisone or prednisolone:* 5–60 mg/d PO ÷ qd–qid. **Infants & Younger Children.** Hydrocortisone 2.5–10 mg/kg/d PO ÷ q6–8h; 1–5 mg/kg/d IM/IV ÷ bid. *Nephrotic syndrome:* **Peds.** Prednisolone or prednisone 2 mg/kg/d PO tid–qid until urine is protein-free for 5 d, use up to 28 d; for persistent proteinuria, 4 mg/kg/dose PO qod max 120 mg/d for an additional 28 d; maint 2 mg/kg/dose qod for 28 d; taper over 4–6 wk (max 80 mg/d). *Septic shock* (controversial): **Adults.** Hydrocortisone 500 mg–1 g IM/IV q2–6h. **Peds.** Hydrocortisone 50 mg/kg IM/IV, repeat q4–24 h PRN. *Status asthmaticus:* **Adults & Peds.** Hydrocortisone 1–2 mg/kg/dose IV q6h; then ↓ by 0.5–1 mg/kg q6h. *Rheumatic Dz:* **Adults.** *Intraarticular:* Hydrocortisone acetate 25–37.5 mg large joint, 10–25 mg small joint; methylprednisolone acetate 20–80 mg large joint, 4–10 mg small joint. *Intrabursal:* Hydrocortisone acetate 25–37.5 mg. *Intraganglial:* Hydrocortisone acetate 25–37.5 mg. *Tendon sheath:* Hydrocortisone acetate 5–12.5 mg. *Periop steroid coverage:* Hydrocortisone 100 mg IV night before surgery, 1 h preop, intraop, & 4, 8, & 12 h postop; postop d #1 100 mg IV q6h; postop d #2 100 mg IV q8h; postop d #3 100 mg IV q12h; postop d #4 50 mg IV q12h; postop d #5 25 mg IV q12h; resume prior PO dosing if chronic use or D/C if only periop coverage required. *Cerebral edema:* Dexamethasone 10 mg IV; then 4 mg IV q4–6h **Caution:** [C, ?/–] **Contra:** Active varicella Infxn, serious Infxn except TB, fungal Infxns **Supplied:** See Table 4, page 206. **SE:** All can cause ↑ appetite, hyperglycemia, ↓ K⁺, osteoporosis, nervousness, insomnia, "steroid psychosis," adrenal suppression **Notes:** Hydrocortisone succinate for systemic, acetate for intraarticular; never abruptly D/C steroids, taper dose

Streptokinase (Streptase, Kabikinase) **Uses:** *Coronary artery thrombosis, acute massive PE, DVT, & some occluded vascular grafts* **Action:** Activates plasminogen to plasmin that degrades fibrin **Dose:** **Adults.** *PE:* Load 250,000 Units peripheral IV over 30 min, then 100,000 Units/h for 24–72 h. *Coronary artery thrombosis:* 1.5 million units IV over 60 min. *DVT or arterial embolism:* Load as w/ PE, then 100,000 Units/h for 72 h. **Peds.** 3500–4000 Units/kg over 30 min, followed by 1000–1500 Units/kg/h. *Occluded catheter* (controversial): 10,000–25,000 Units in NS to final volume of catheter (leave in place for 1h, aspirate & flush catheter w/NS) **Caution:** [C, +] **Contra:** Streptococcal Infxn or streptokinase in last 6 mo, active bleeding, CVA, TIA, spinal surgery, or trauma in last month, vascular anomalies, severe hepatic or renal Dz, endocarditis,

pericarditis, severe uncontrolled HTN **Supplied:** Powder for inj 250,000, 600,000, 750,000, 1,500,000 Units **SE:** Bleeding, ↓ BP, fever, bruising, rash, GI upset, hemorrhage, anaphylaxis **Notes:** If maint inf inadequate to maintain thrombin clotting time 2–5× control, see insert for adjustments; antibodies remain 3–6 mo following dose

Streptomycin **Uses:** *TB,* streptococcal or enterococcal endocarditis **Action:** Aminoglycoside; interferes w/ protein synthesis **Dose:** *Adults. Endocarditis:* 1 g q12h 1–2 wk, then 500 mg q12h 1–4 wk; *TB:* 15 mg/kg/d (up to 1 g), directly observed therapy (DOT) 2×wk 20–30 mg/kg/dose (max 1.5gm), DOT 3×wk 25–30 mg/kg/dose (max 1g). *Peds.* 15 mg/kg/d; DOT 2×wk 20–40 mg/kg/dose (max 1 g); DOT 3×wk 25–30 mg/kg/dose (max 1 g); ↓ in renal failure, either IM or IV over 30–60 min **Caution:** [D, +] **Contra:** PRG **Supplied:** Inj 400 mg/mL (1-g vial) **SE:** ↑ incidence of vestibular & auditory tox, neurotox, nephrotox **Notes:** Monitor levels max 20–30 mcg/mL, trough < 5 mcg/mL; toxic peak > 50, trough > 10

Streptozocin (Zanosar) **Uses:** *Pancreatic islet cell tumors* & carcinoid tumors **Action:** DNA–DNA (interstrand) cross-linking; DNA, RNA, & protein synthesis inhibitor **Dose:** Per protocol; ↓ in renal failure **Caution:** [D, ?/–] **Contra:** Caution in renal failure, PRG **Supplied:** Inj 1 g **SE:** N/V, duodenal ulcers; myelosuppression rare (20%) & mild; nephrotox (proteinuria & azotemia often heralded by hypophosphatemia) dose-limiting; hypo-/hyperglycemia; inj site Rxns **Notes:** Monitor renal Fxn

Succimer (Chemet) **Uses:** *Lead poisoning (levels >45 mcg/mL)* **Action:** Heavy-metal chelating agent **Dose:** *Adults & Peds.* 10 mg/kg/dose q8h × 5 d, then 10 mg/kg/dose q12h for 14 d; ↓ in renal impair **Caution:** [C, ?] **Contra:** Allergy **Supplied:** Caps 100 mg **SE:** Rash, fever, GI upset, hemorrhoids, metallic taste, drowsiness, ↑ LFTs **Notes:** Monitor lead levels, maintain hydration, may open capsules

Succinylcholine (Anectine, Quelicin, Sucostrin) **Uses:** *Adjunct to general anesthesia to facilitate ET intubation & to induce skeletal muscle relaxation during surgery or mechanical ventilation* **Action:** Depolarizing neuromuscular blocking agent **Dose:** *Adults.* 1–1.5 mg/kg IV over 10–30 s, followed by 0.04–0.07 mg/kg PRN or 10–100 mcg/kg/min inf. *Peds.* 1–2 mg/kg IV, followed by 0.3–0.6 mg/kg/dose q5min or use of CI not OK; ↓ in severe liver Dz **Caution:** [C, M] **Contra:** If risk for malignant hyperthermia; myopathy; recent major burn, multiple trauma, extensive skeletal muscle denervation **Supplied:** Inj 20, 50, 100 mg/mL; powder for inj 500 mg, 1 g/vial **SE:** May precipitate malignant hyperthermia, resp depression, or prolonged apnea; multiple drugs potentiate; observe for CV effects (arrhythmias, ↓ BP, brady/tachycardia); ↑ intraocular pressure, postop stiffness, salivation, myoglobinuria **Notes:** May be given IVP or inf or IM in the deltoid

Sucralfate (Carafate) **Uses:** *Duodenal ulcers,* gastric ulcers, stomatitis, GERD, preventing stress ulcers, esophagitis **Action:** Forms ulcer-adherent complex that protects against acid, pepsin, & bile acid **Dose:** *Adults.* 1 g PO qid, 1 h prior to meals & hs. **Peds.** 40–80 mg/kg/d ÷ q6h; continue 4–8 wk unless healing demonstrated by x-ray or endoscopy; separate from other drugs by 2 h; on empty stomach ac **Caution:** [B, +] **Contra:** Component allergy **Supplied:** Tabs 1 g; susp 1 g/10 mL **SE:** Constipation frequent; D, dizziness, xerostomia **Notes:** Aluminum may accumulate in renal failure

Sulfacetamide (Bleph-10, Cetamide, Sodium Sulamyd) Uses:
Conjunctival Infxns **Action:** Sulfonamide antibiotic **Dose:** 10% oint apply qid & hs; soln for keratitis apply q2–3h based on severity **Caution:** [C, M] **Contra:** Sulfonamide sensitivity; age <2 mo **Supplied:** Oint 10%; soln 10, 15, 30% **SE:** Irritation, burning; blurred vision, brow ache, Stevens–Johnson syndrome, photosensitivity

Sulfacetamide & Prednisolone (Blephamide, others) Uses:
Steroid-responsive inflammatory ocular conditions w/ Infxn or a risk of Infxn **Action:** Antibiotic & antiinflammatory **Dose:** *Adults & Peds >2 y.* Apply oint to lower conjunctival sac qd–qid; soln 1–3 gtt 2–3 h while awake **Caution:** [C, ?/–] Sulfonamide sensitivity; age <2 mon **Supplied:** Oint sulfacetamide 10%/prednisolone 0.5%, sulfacetamide 10%/prednisolone 0.2%, sulfacetamide 10%/prednisolone 0.25%; susp sulfacetamide 10%/prednisolone 0.25%, sulfacetamide 10%/prednisolone 0.5%, sulfacetamide 10%/prednisolone 0.2% **SE:** Irritation, burning, blurred vision, brow ache, Stevens–Johnson syndrome, photosensitivity **Notes:** Ophth susp can be used as an otic agent

Sulfasalazine (Azulfidine, Azulfidine EN) Uses:
Ulcerative colitis, RA, juvenile RA, active Crohn Dz, ankylosing spondylitis, psoriasis **Action:** Sulfonamide; actions unclear **Dose:** *Adults.* Initial, 1 g PO tid–qid; ↑ to a max of 8 g/d in 3–4 ÷ doses; maint 500 mg PO qid. *Peds.* Initial, 40–60 mg/kg/24 h PO ÷ q4–6h; maint, 20–30 mg/kg/24 h PO ÷ q6h. *RA >6 y:* 30–50 mg/kg/d in 2 doses, start w/ ¼–⅓ maint dose, ↑ weekly until dose reached at 1 mo, 2 g/d max; ↓ in renal failure **Caution:** [B (D if near term), M] **Contra:** Sulfonamide or salicylate sensitivity, porphyria, GI or GU obstruction; avoid in hepatic impair **Supplied:** Tabs 500 mg; EC tabs 500 mg; PO susp 250 mg/5 mL **SE:** Can cause severe GI upset; discolors urine; dizziness, HA, photosensitivity, oligospermia, anemias, Stevens–Johnson syndrome **Notes:** May cause yellow-orange skin discoloration or stain contact lenses; avoid long sunlight exposure

Sulfinpyrazone (Anturane) Uses:
Acute & chronic gout **Action:** ↓ renal tubular absorption of uric acid **Dose:** 100–200 mg PO bid for 1 wk, ↑ PRN to maint of 200–400 mg bid; max 800 mg/d; take w/ food or antacids, & plenty of fluids; avoid salicylates **Caution:** [C (D if near term), ?/–] **Contra:** Renal impair, avoid salicylates; peptic ulcer; blood dyscrasias, near term PRG, allergy **Supplied:** Tabs 100 mg; caps 200 mg **SE:** N/V, stomach pain, urolithiasis, leukopenia **Notes:** Take w/ plenty of H_2O

Sulindac (Clinoril) WARNING:
May ↑ risk of cardiovascular events & GI bleeding **Uses:** *Arthritis & pain* **Action:** NSAID; ↓ prostaglandins **Dose:** 150–200 mg bid w/ food **Caution:** [B (D if 3rd tri or near term), ?] **Contra:** NSAID or ASA

sensitivity, ulcer, GI bleeding **Supplied:** Tabs 150, 200 mg **SE:** Dizziness, rash, GI upset, pruritus, edema, ↓ renal blood flow, renal failure (May have fewer renal effects than other NSAIDs), peptic ulcer, GI bleeding

Sumatriptan (Imitrex) **Uses:** Rx acute migraine attacks **Action:** Vascular serotonin receptor agonist **Dose:** *Adults.* *SQ:* 6 mg SQ as a single dose PRN; repeat PRN in 1 h to a max of 12 mg/24 h. *PO:* 25 mg, repeat in 2 h, PRN, 100 mg/d max PO dose; max 300 mg/d. *Nasal spray:* 1 spray into 1 nostril, repeat in 2 h to 40 mg/24 h max. *Peds.* *Nasal spray:* 6–9 y: 5–20 mg/d. 12–17 y: 5–20 mg, up to 40 mg/d **Caution:** [C, M] **Contra:** Angina, ischemic heart Dz, uncontrolled HTN, ergot use, MAOI use w/in 14 d **Supplied:** Inj 6 mg/mL; orally disintegrating tabs 25, 50, 100 mg; nasal spray 5, 20 mg **SE:** Pain & bruising at site; dizziness, hot flashes, paresthesias, CP, weakness, numbness, coronary vasospasm, HTN

Tacrine (Cognex) **Uses:** *Mild–moderate Alzheimer dementia* **Action:** Cholinesterase inhibitor **Dose:** 10–40 mg PO qid to 160 mg/d; separate doses from food **Caution:** [C, ?] **Contra:** Previous tacrine-induced jaundice **Supplied:** Caps 10, 20, 30, 40 mg **SE:** ↑ LFT, HA, dizziness, GI upset, flushing, confusion, ataxia, myalgia, bradycardia **Notes:** Serum conc >20 ng/mL have more SE; monitor LFTs

Tacrolimus (FK 506) (Prograf, Protopic) **Uses:** *Prophylaxis against organ rejection,* eczema **Action:** Macrolide immunosuppressant **Dose:** *Adults.* *IV:* 0.05–0.1 mg/kg/d cont inf. *PO:* 0.15–0.3 mg/kg/d ÷ 2 doses. *Peds.* *IV:* 0.03–0.05 mg/kg/d as cont inf. *PO:* 0.15–0.2 mg/kg/d PO ÷ q 12 h. *Adults & Peds.* *Eczema:* Apply bid, continue 1 wk after clearing; ↓ in hepatic/renal impair **Caution:** [C, –] Do not use w/ cyclosporine; avoid topical if < 2 yrs of age **Contra:** Component allergy **Supplied:** Caps 1, 5 mg; inj 5 mg/mL; oint 0.03, 0.1% **SE:** Neurotox & nephrotox, HTN, edema, HA, insomnia, fever, pruritus, ↓ K⁺/↑ K⁺, hyperglycemia, GI upset, anemia, leukocytosis, tremors, paresthesias, pleural effusion, Szs, lymphoma **Notes:** Monitor levels; reports of ↑ cancer risk; topical use for short term/second line

Tadalafil (Cialis) **Uses:** *Erectile dysfunction* **Action:** Phosphodiesterase 5 inhibitor **Dose:** *Adults.* 10 mg PO before sexual activity w/o regard to meals (20 mg max); ↓ 5 mg (10 mg max) in renal & hepatic insuff **Caution:** [B, –] **Contra:** Nitrates, α-blockers (except tamsulosin), severe hepatic insuff **Supplied:** 5-, 10-, 20-mg tabs **SE:** HA, flushing, dyspepsia, rhinitis, back pain, myalgia **Notes:** Longest acting of class (36 h)

Talc (Sterile Talc Powder) **Uses:** *↓ recurrence of malignant pleural effusions (pleurodesis)* **Action:** Sclerosing agent **Dose:** Mix slurry: 50 mL NS w/ 5-g vial, mix, distribute 25 mL into two 60-mL syringes, volume to 50 mL/syringe w/ NS. Infuse each into chest tube, flush w/ 25 mL NS. Keep tube clamped; have pt change positions q15min for 2 h, unclamp tube **Caution:** [X, –] **Contra:** Planned further surgery on site **Supplied:** 5 g powder **SE:** Pain, Infxn **Notes:** May add 10–20 mL 1% lidocaine/syringe; must have chest tube placed, monitor closely while tube clamped (tension pneumothorax), not antineoplastic

Tamoxifen (Nolvadex) Uses: *Breast CA [postmenopausal, estrogen receptor(+)], reduction of breast CA in high-risk women, metastatic male breast CA,* mastalgia, pancreatic CA, gynecomastia, ovulation induction **Action:** Nonsteroidal antiestrogen; mixed agonist–antagonist effect **Dose:** 20–40 mg/d (typically 10 mg bid or 20 mg/d) **Caution:** [D, –]**Contra:** Caution in leukopenia, thrombocytopenia, hyperlipidemia **Supplied:** Tabs 10, 20 mg **SE:** Uterine malignancy & thrombotic events noted in breast CA prevention trials; menopausal Sxs (hot flashes, N/V) in premenopausal pts; vaginal bleeding & menstrual irregularities; skin rash, pruritus vulvae, dizziness, HA, peripheral edema; acute flare of bone metastasis pain & ↑ Ca^{2+}; retinopathy reported (high dose) **Notes:** ↑ risk of PRG in premenopausal women by inducing ovulation

Tamsulosin (Flomax) Uses: * BPH* **Action:** Antagonist of prostatic α-receptors **Dose:** 0.4 mg/d PO; do not crush, chew, or open caps **Caution:** [B, ?] **Contra:** Female gender **Supplied:** Caps 0.4, 0.8 mg **SE:** HA, dizziness, syncope, somnolence, ↓ libido, GI upset, retrograde ejaculation, rhinitis, rash, angioedema **Notes:** Not for use as antihypertensive

Tazarotene (Tazorac) Uses: *Facial acne vulgaris; stable plaque psoriasis up to 20% body surface area* **Action:** Keratolytic **Dose:** *Adults & Peds >12 y. Acne:* Cleanse face, dry, & apply thin film qd hs on acne lesions. *Psoriasis:* Apply hs **Caution:** [X, ?/–] **Contra:** Retinoid sensitivity **Supplied:** Gel 0.05, 0.1% **SE:** Burning, erythema, irritation, rash, photosensitivity, desquamation, bleeding, skin discoloration **Notes:** D/C w/ excessive pruritus, burning, skin redness or peeling occur until Sxs resolve

Tegaserod (Zelnorm) **WARNING:** Rare reports of ischemic colitis Uses: *Short-term Rx of constipation-predominant IBS in women*, chronic idiopathic constipation in pts < 65y **Action:** 5HT4 serotonin agonist **Dose:** 6 mg PO bid pc for 4–6 wk; may continue for 2nd course **Caution:** [B, ?/–] **Contra:** Severe renal, moderate–severe hepatic impair, Hx of bowel obstruction, gallbladder Dz, sphincter of Oddi dysfunction, abdominal adhesions **Supplied:** Tabs 2, 6 mg **SE:** Do not administer if D present, as GI motility ↑; D/C if abdominal pain worsens **Notes:** Maintain hydration

Telithromycin (Ketek) **WARNING:** May be associated with pseudomembranous colitis Uses: *Acute bacterial exacerbations of chronic bronchitis, acute bacterial sinusitis; mild–moderate community-acquired pneumonia* **Action:** Unique macrolide, blocks protein synthesis; bacteriocidal. **Spectrum:** *Staphylococcus aureus, Streptococcus pneumoniae, H. influenzae, M. catarrhalis, Chlamydophilia pneumoniae, M. pneumoniae* **Dose:** *Chronic bronchitis/sinusitis:* 800 mg (2 tabs) PO qd ×5; *Pneumonia:* 800 mg (2 tabs) PO qd × 7–10 d **Caution:** [C, M] pseudomembranous colitis, QTc interval prolongation, MyG exacerbations, visual disturbances, hepatic dysfunction; dosing in renal impair unknown **Contra:** Macrolide allergy, use w/ cisapride or pimozide **Supplied:** Tabs 400 mg **SE:** N/V/D, dizziness **Notes:** CYP450 inhibitor; multiple drug interactions

Telmisartan (Micardis) Uses: *HTN, CHF,* DN Action: Angiotensin II receptor antagonist Dose: 40–80 mg/d Caution: [C (1st tri; D 2nd & 3rd tri), ?/–] Contra: Angiotensin II receptor antagonist sensitivity Supplied: Tabs 40, 80 mg SE: Edema, GI upset, HA, angioedema, renal impair, orthostatic ↓ BP

Temazepam (Restoril) [C-IV] Uses: *Insomnia,* anxiety, depression, panic attacks Action: Benzodiazepine Dose: 15–30 mg PO hs PRN; ↓ in elderly Caution: [X, ?/–] Potentiates CNS depressive effects of opioids, barbs, EtOH, antihistamines, MAOIs, TCAs Contra: NA glaucoma Supplied: Caps 7.5, 15, 30 mg SE: Confusion, dizziness, drowsiness, hangover Notes: Abrupt D/C after >10 d use may cause withdrawal

Tenecteplase (TNKase) Uses: *Restore perfusion & ↓ mortality w/ AMI* Action: Thrombolytic; TPA Dose: 30–50 mg; see table:

Tenecteplase Dosing

Weight (kg)	TNKase (mg)	TNKase^a Volume (mL)
<60	30	6
60–69	35	7
70–79	40	8
80–89	45	9
≥90	50	10

^{a}From one vial of reconstituted TNKase.

Caution: [C, ?], ↑ bleeding w/ NSAIDs, ticlodipine, clopidogrel, GPIIb/IIIa antagonists Contra: Bleeding, CVA, major surgery (intracranial, intraspinal) or trauma w/in 2 mo Supplied: Inj 50 mg, reconstitute w/ 10 mL sterile H_2O SE: Bleeding, allergy Notes: Do not shake when reconstituting; do *not* use D_5W either in the IV line or to reconstitute

Tenofovir (Viread) Uses: *HIV Infxn* Action: Nucleotide RT inhibitor Dose: 300 mg PO qd w/ a meal Caution: [B, ?/–] Didanosine (separate admin times), lopinavir, ritonavir w/ known risk factors for liver Dz Contra: CrCl <60 mL/min; Supplied: Tabs 300 mg SE: GI upset, metabolic syndrome, hepatotox; separate didanosine doses by 2 h Notes: Take w/ fatty meal; combination product with emtricitabine known as Truvada

Tenofovir/Emtricitabine (Truvada) WARNING: Lactic acidosis & severe hepatomegaly with steatosis, including fatal cases, have been reported with the use of nucleoside analogs alone or in combo w/ other antiretrovirals. Not OK w/ chronic hepatitis; effects in patients co-infected with hepatitis B & HIV unknown **Uses:** *HIV Infxn* **Action:** Dual nucleotide RT inhibitor **Dose:** 300 mg PO qd w/ or w/o a meal **Caution:** W/ known risk factors for liver Dz [B, ?/–] **Contra:** CrCl <30 mL/min; **Supplied:** Tabs: 200 mg emtricitabine/300 mg tenofovir **SE:** GI upset, metabolic syndrome, hepatotox **Notes:** Take w/ fatty meal

Terazosin (Hytrin) **Uses:** *BPH & HTN* **Action:** α_1-Blocker (blood vessel & bladder neck/prostate) **Dose:** Initial, 1 mg PO hs; ↑ 20 mg/d max **Caution:** [C, ?] ↑ ↓ BP w/ BB, CCB, ACEI **Contra:** α-Antagonist sensitivity **Supplied:** Tabs 1, 2, 5, 10 mg; caps 1, 2, 5, 10 mg **SE:** ↓ BP & syncope following 1st dose; dizziness, weakness, nasal congestion, peripheral edema common; palpitations, GI upset **Notes:** Caution w/ 1st dose syncope; if for HTN, combine w/ thiazide diuretic

Terbinafine (Lamisil) **Uses:** *Onychomycosis, athlete's feet, jock itch, ringworm,* cutaneous candidiasis, pityriasis versicolor **Action:** ↓ squalene epoxidase resulting in fungal death **Dose:** *PO:* 250 mg/d PO for 6–12 wk. *Topical:* Apply to area; ↓ in renal/hepatic impair **Caution:** [B, –] May ↑ effects of drug metab by CYP2D6 **Contra:** Liver Dz or kidney failure **Supplied:** Tabs 250 mg; cream 1% **SE:** HA, dizziness, rash, pruritus, alopecia, GI upset, taste perversion, neutropenia, retinal damage, Stevens–Johnson syndrome **Notes:** Effect may take months due to need for new nail growth; do not use occlusive dressings

Terbutaline (Brethine, Bricanyl) **Uses:** *Reversible bronchospasm (asthma, COPD); inhibition of labor (tocolytic)* **Action:** Sympathomimetic **Dose:** *Adults. Bronchodilator:* 2.5–5 mg PO qid or 0.25 mg SQ; may repeat in 15 min (max 0.5 mg in 4 h). *Met-dose inhaler:* 2 inhal q4–6h. *Premature labor:* Acutely 2.5–10 mg/min/IV, gradually ↑ as tolerated q10–20min; maint 2.5–5 mg PO q4–6h until term *Peds. PO:* 0.05–0.15 mg/kg/dose PO tid; max 5 mg/24h; ↓ in renal failure **Caution:** [B, +] ↑ tox w/ MAOIs, TCAs; diabetes, HTN, hyperthyroidism **Contra:** Tachycardia, component allergy **Supplied:** Tabs 2.5, 5 mg; inj 1 mg/mL; met-dose inhaler **SE:** HTN, hyperthyroidism; high dose may precipitate β_1-adrenergic effects; nervousness, trembling, tachycardia, HTN, dizziness

Terconazole (Terazol 7) **Uses:** *Vaginal fungal Infxns* **Action:** Topical antifungal **Dose:** 1 applicatorful or 1 supp intravag hs for 3–7 d **Caution:** [C, ?] **Contra:** Component allergy **Supplied:** Vaginal cream 0.4%, vaginal supp 80 mg **SE:** Vulvar/vaginal burning **Notes:** Insert high into vagina

Teriparatide (Forteo) **Uses:** *Severe/refractory osteoporosis* **Action:** PTH (recombinant) **Dose:** 20 mcg SQ qd in thigh or abdomen **Caution:** [C, ?/–] **Contra:** w/ Paget Dz, prior radiation, bone metastases, ↑ Ca^{2+}; caution in urolithiasis **Supplied:** 3-mL prefilled device (discard after 28 d) **SE:** Symptomatic orthostatic ↓ BP on administration, N/D, ↑ Ca, leg cramps **Notes:** Not OK for use > 2 y; osteosarcoma in animals

Testosterone (AndroGel, Androderm, Striant, Testim, Testoderm) [CIII] **Uses:** *Male hypogonadism* **Action:** Testosterone replacement; ↑ lean body mass, libido **Dose:** All daily *AndroGel:* 5 g gel. *Androderm:* two 2.5-

mg or one 5-mg patch qd. *Striant:* 30-mg buccal tabs bid. *Testim:* one 5-g gel tube. *Testoderm:* one 4- or 6-mg scrotal patch **Caution:** [N/A, N/A] **Supplied:** *Andro-Gel, Testim:* 5-gm gel (50-mg test); *Androderm:* 2.5-, 5-mg patches; *Striant:* 30-mg buccal tabs; *Testoderm:* 4- or 6-mg scrotal patch **SE:** Site Rxns, acne, edema, weight gain, gynecomastia, HTN, ↑ sleep apnea, prostate enlargement **Notes:** Injectable testosterone enanthate (Delatestryl; Testro-L.A.) & cypionate (Depo-Testosterone) require inj every 14–28 d with highly variable serum levels; PO agents (methyltestosterone & oxandrolone) associated w/ hepatitis/hepatic tumors; transdermal/mucosal forms preferred

Tetanus Immune Globulin

Uses: *Passive tetanus immunization * (suspected contaminated wound w/ unknown immunization status, see also Table 9, page 216) **Action:** Passive immunization **Dose:** *Adults & Peds.* 250–500 Units IM (higher dose w/ delayed Rx) **Caution:** [C, ?] **Contra:** Thimerosal sensitivity **Supplied:** Inj 250-unit vial or syringe **SE:** Pain, tenderness, erythema at inj site; fever, angioedema, muscle stiffness, anaphylaxis **Notes:** May begin active immunization series at different inj site if required

Tetanus Toxoid

Uses: *Tetanus prophylaxis* See also Table 9, page 216 **Action:** Active immunization **Dose:** Based on previous immunization status **Caution:** [C, ?] **Contra:** Chloramphenicol use, neurologic Sxs w/ previous use, active Infxn (for routine primary immunization) **Supplied:** Inj tetanus toxoid, fluid, 4–5 Lf Units/0.5 mL; tetanus toxoid, adsorbed, 5, 10 Lf Units/0.5 mL **SE:** Local erythema, induration, sterile abscess; chills, fever, neurologic disturbances

Tetracycline (Achromycin V, Sumycin)

Uses: *Broad-spectrum antibiotic* **Action:** Bacteriostatic; ↓ protein synthesis. *Spectrum:* Gram(+): *Staphylococcus, Streptococcus.* Gram(–): *H. pylori.* Atypicals: *Chlamydia, Rickettsia,* & *Mycoplasma* **Dose:** *Adults.* 250–500 mg PO bid–qid. *Peds >8 y.* 25–50 mg/kg/24 h PO q6–12h; ↓ in renal/hepatic impair **Caution:** [D, +] **Contra:** PRG, antacids, dairy products; children ≤8 y **Supplied:** Caps 100, 250, 500 mg; tabs 250, 500 mg; PO susp 250 mg/5 mL **SE:** Photosensitivity, GI upset, renal failure, pseudotumor cerebri, hepatic impair **Notes:** Can stain tooth enamel & depress bone formation in children

Thalidomide (Thalomid)

Uses: *Erythema nodosum leprosum (ENL),* graft-versus-host Dz, aphthous ulceration in HIV(+) pts **Action:** ↓ Neutrophil chemotaxis, ↓ monocyte phagocytosis **Dose:** *GVHD:* 100–1600 mg PO qd. *Stomatitis:* 200 mg bid for 5 d, then 200 mg qd up to 8 wk. *ENL:* 100–300 mg PO qhs **Cautions:** [X, –] May ↑ HIV viral load; Hx Szs **Contra:** PRG; sexually active males not using latex condoms, or females not using 2 forms of contraception **SE:** Dizziness, drowsiness, rash, fever, orthostasis, Stevens–Johnson syndrome, peripheral neuropathy, Szs **Supplied:** 50-mg cap **Notes:** MD must register w/ STEPS risk management program; informed consent necessary; immediately D/C if rash develops

Theophylline (Theo24, TheoChron)

Uses: *Asthma, bronchospasm* **Action:** Relaxes smooth muscle of the bronchi & pulmonary blood vessels **Dose:** *Adults.* 900 mg PO ÷ q6h; SR products may be ÷ q8–12h (maint). *Peds.* 16–22

mg/kg/24 h PO ÷ q6h; SR products may be ÷ q8–12h (maint); ↓ in hepatic failure **Caution:** [C, +] Multiple interactions (eg, caffeine, smoking, carbamazepine, barbiturates, β-blockers, ciprofloxacin, E-mycin, INH, loop diuretics) **Contra:** Arrhythmia, hyperthyroidism, uncontrolled Szs **Supplied:** Elixir 80, 150 mg/15 mL; liq 80, 160 mg/15 mL; caps 100, 200, 250 mg; tabs 100, 125, 200, 225, 250, 300 mg; SR caps 50, 75, 100, 125, 200, 250, 260, 300 mg; SR tabs 100, 200, 250, 300, 400, 450, 500 mg **SE:** N/V, tachycardia, & Szs; nervousness, arrhythmias **Notes:** See levels, Table 2 (page 200)

Thiamine [Vitamin B₁] **Uses:** *Thiamine deficiency (beriberi), alcoholic neuritis, Wernicke encephalopathy* **Action:** Dietary supl **Dose:** *Adults. Deficiency:* 100 mg IM for 2 wk, then 5–10 mg/d PO for 1 mo. *Wernicke encephalopathy:* 100 mg IV single dose, then 100 mg/d IM for 2 wk. *Peds.* 10–25 mg/d IM for 2 wk, then 5–10 mg/24 h PO for 1 mo **Caution:** [A (C if doses exceed RDA), +] **Contra:** Component allergy **Supplied:** Tabs 5, 10, 25, 50, 100, 500 mg; inj 100, 200 mg/mL **SE:** Angioedema, paresthesias, rash, anaphylaxis w/ rapid IV **Notes:** IV use associated w/ anaphylactic Rxn;give IV slowly

Thiethylperazine (Torecan) **Uses:** *N/V* **Action:** Antidopaminergic antiemetic **Dose:** 10 mg/d PO, PR, or IM qd–tid; ↓ in hepatic failure **Caution:** [X, ?] **Contra:** Phenothiazine & sulfite sensitivity, PRG **Supplied:** Tabs 10 mg; supp 10 mg; inj 5 mg/mL **SE:** EPS, xerostomia, drowsiness, orthostatic ↓ BP, tachycardia, confusion

6-Thioguanine [6-TG] (Tabloid) **Uses:** *AML, ALL, CML* **Action:** Purine-based antimetabolite (substitutes for natural purines interfering w/ nucleotide synthesis) **Dose:** 2–3 mg/kg/d; ↓ in severe renal/hepatic impair **Caution:** [D, –] **Contra:** Resistance to mercaptopurine **Supplied:** Tabs 40 mg **SE:** Myelosuppression (leucopenia/thrombocytopenia), N/V/D, anorexia, stomatitis, rash, hyperuricemia, rare hepatotox

Thioridazine (Mellaril) WARNING: Dose-related QT prolongation **Uses:** *Schizophrenia,* psychosis **Action:** Phenothiazine antipsychotic **Dose:** *Adults.* Initial, 50–100 mg PO tid; maint 200–800 mg/24 h PO in 2–4 ÷ doses. *Peds >2 y.* 0.5–3 mg/kg/24 h PO in 2–3 ÷ doses **Caution:** [C, ?] Phenothiazines, QT_c-prolonging agents, aluminum **Contra:** Phenothiazine sensitivity **Supplied:** Tabs 10, 15, 25, 50, 100, 150, 200 mg; PO conc 30, 100 mg/mL; PO susp 25, 100 mg/5 mL **SE:** Low incidence of EPS; ventricular arrhythmias; ↓ BP, dizziness, drowsiness, neuroleptic malignant syndrome, Szs, skin discoloration, photosensitivity, constipation, sexual dysfunction, blood dyscrasias, pigmentary retinopathy, hepatic impair **Notes:** Avoid EtOH, dilute PO conc in 2–4 oz liq

Thiothixene (Navane) **Uses:** *Psychotic disorders* **Action:** Antipsychotic **Dose:** *Adults & Peds >12 y. Mild–moderate psychosis:* 2 mg PO tid, up to 20–30 mg/d. *Severe psychosis:* 5 mg PO bid; ↑ to a max of 60 mg/24 h PRN. *IM use:* 16–20 mg/24 h ÷ bid–qid; max 30 mg/d. *Peds <12 y.* 0.25 mg/kg/24 h PO ÷ q6–12h **Caution:** [C, ?] **Contra:** Phenothiazine sensitivity **Supplied:** Caps 1, 2, 5, 10, 20 mg; PO conc 5 mg/mL; inj 2, 5 mg/mL **SE:** Drowsiness, EPS most common; ↓ BP, dizziness, drowsiness, neuroleptic malignant syndrome, Szs, skin discoloration, photosensitivity, constipation, sexual dysfunction, blood dyscrasias, pigmentary retinopathy, hepatic impair **Notes:** Dilute PO conc immediately before administration

Tiagabine (Gabitril) Uses: *Adjunct in Rx of partial Szs,* bipolar disorder **Action:** Inhibition of GABA **Dose:** *Adults & Peds ≥ 12 y.* Initial 4 mg PO, ↑ by 4 mg during 2nd wk; ↑ PRN by 4–8 mg/d based on response, 56 mg/d max **Caution:** [C, M] **Contra:** Component allergy **Supplied:** Tabs 4, 12, 16, 20 mg **SE:** Dizziness, HA, somnolence, memory impair, tremors **Notes:** Use gradual withdrawal; used in combo w/ other anticonvulsants

Ticarcillin (Ticar) Uses: *Infxns due to gram(–) bacteria (Klebsiella, Proteus, E. coli, Enterobacter, P. aeruginosa, & Serratia) involving the skin, bone, resp & urinary tract, abdomen, sepsis* **Action:** 4th-gen PCN, bactericidal; ↓ cell wall synthesis. *Spectrum:* Some gram(+) (strep, fair enterococcus, not MRSA), gram(–); enhanced w/aminoglycoside use, good anaerobes (*Bactericides*) **Dose:** *Adults.* 3 g IV q4–6h. *Peds.* 200–300 mg/kg/d IV ÷ q4–6h; ↓ in renal failure **Caution:** [B, +] PCN sensitivity **Supplied:** Inj **SE:** Interstitial nephritis, anaphylaxis, bleeding, rash, hemolytic anemia **Notes:** Used in combo w/ aminoglycosides

Ticarcillin/Potassium Clavulanate (Timentin) Uses: *Infxns of the skin, bone, resp & urinary tract, abdomen, sepsis* **Action:** 4th-gen PCN; bactericidal; ↓ cell wall synthesis; clavulanic acid blocks β-lactamase. *Spectrum:* Good gram(+), not MRSA; good gram(–) & anaerobes **Dose:** *Adults.* 3.1 g IV q4–6h. *Peds.* 200–300 mg/kg/d IV ÷ q4–6h; ↓ in renal failure **Caution:** [B, +/–] PCN sensitivity **Supplied:** Inj **SE:** Hemolytic anemia **Notes:** Often used in combo w/ aminoglycosides; penetrates CNS with meningeal irritation; may cause false + proteinuria

Ticlopidine (Ticlid) **WARNING:** Neutropenia/agranulocytosis, TTP, aplastic anemia reported Uses: *↓ risk of thrombotic stroke,* protect grafts status post CABG, diabetic microangiopathy, ischemic heart Dz, DVT prophylaxis, graft prophylaxis after renal transplant **Action:** Plt aggregation inhibitor **Dose:** 250 mg PO bid w/ food **Caution:** [B, ?/–], ↑ tox of ASA, anticoagulation, NSAIDs, theophylline **Contra:** Bleeding, hepatic impair, neutropenia, thrombocytopenia **Supplied:** Tabs 250 mg **SE:** Bleeding, GI upset, rash, ↑ on LFTs **Notes:** Follow CBC 1st 3 mo

Tigecycline (Tygacil) Uses: *Rx complicated skin & soft tissue Infxns, & complicated intraabdominal Infxns* **Action:** New class: related to tetracycline; *Spectrum:* Broad gram(+), gram(–), anaerobic, some mycobacterial; *E. coli, Enterococcus faecalis* (vanco-susceptible isolates), *Staphylococcus aureus* (meth-susceptible/resistant), *Streptococcus (agalactiae, anginosus* grp, *pyogenes), Citrobacter freundii, Enterobacter cloacae, B. fragilis* group, *C. perfringens, Peptostreptococcus* **Dose:** *Adults.* 100 mg, then 50 mg q12h IV over 30–60 min every 12 h **Caution:** [D, ?] hepatic impair, monotherapy w/ intestinal perf, not OK in peds **Contra:** Component sensitivity **Supplied:** Inj **SE:** N/V, inj site Rxn

Timolol (Blocadren) **WARNING:** Exacerbation of ischemic heart Dz w/
abrupt D/C **Uses:** *HTN & MI* **Action:** β-Adrenergic receptor blocker, β$_1$, β$_2$
Dose: *HTN:* 10–20 mg bid, up to 60 mg/d. *MI:* 10 mg bid **Caution:** [C (1st tri; D if
2nd or 3rd tri), +] **Contra:** CHF, cardiogenic shock, bradycardia, heart block,
COPD, asthma **Supplied:** Tabs 5, 10, 20 mg **SE:** Sexual dysfunction, arrhythmia,
dizziness, fatigue, CHF

Timolol, Ophthalmic (Timoptic) **Uses:** *Glaucoma* **Action:** β-
Blocker **Dose:** 0.25% 1 gt bid; ↓ to qd when controlled; use 0.5% if needed; 1 gt/d
gel **Caution:** [C (1st tri; D 2nd or 3rd), ?/+] **Supplied:** Soln 0.25/0.5%; Timoptic
XE (0.25, 0.5%) gel-forming soln **SE:** Local irritation

Tinidazole (Tindamax) **WARNING:** Off-label use discouraged (animal
carcinogenicity w/ other drugs in class) **Uses:** *Adults/children >3 y. * Trichomoniasis & giardiasis; intestinal amebiasis or amebic liver abscess * **Action:** Antiprotozo-
zoal nitroimidazole **Spectrum:** *Trichomonas vaginalis, Giardia duodenalis,
Entamoeba histolytica* **Dose:** *Adults. Trichomoniasis:* 2 g PO; treat partner; *Giardiasis:* 2 g PO; *Amebiasis:* 2 g PO qd ×3; *Amebic liver abscess:* 2 g PO qd ×3–5;
Peds. *Trichomoniasis:* 50 mg/kg PO, 2 g/day max; *Giardiasis:* 50 mg/kg PO, 2 g
max; *Amebiasis:* 50 mg/kg PO qd ×3, 2 g/day max; *Amebic liver abscess:* 50
mg/kg PO qd ×3–5, 2 g/day max (w/food) **Caution:** [C, D in 1st trimester; –] May
be cross-resistant with metronidazole; Sz/peripheral neuropathy may require D/C;
w/CNS/hepatic impair **Contra:** Metronidazole allergy, 1st trimester PRG, w/
EtOH use **Supplied:** Tabs 250, 500 **SE:** CNS disturbances; blood dyscrasias, taste
disturbances, N/V, darkens urine **Notes:** D/C EtOH during & 3 d after Rx; potentiates warfarin & lithium; clearance ↓ w/other drugs; crush & disperse in cherry
syrup for peds; removed by HD

Tinzaparin (Innohep) **Uses:** *Rx of DVT w/ or w/o PE* **Action:** LMW
heparin **Dose:** 175 Units/kg SQ qd at least 6 d until warfarin dose stabilized **Caution:** [B, ?] Pork allergy, active bleeding, mild–moderate renal dysfunction **Contra:** Allergy to sulfites, heparin, benzyl alcohol, HIT **Supplied:** 20,000 Units/mL
SE: Bleeding, bruising, thrombocytopenia, inj site pain, ↑ LFTs **Notes:** Monitor
via Anti-Xa levels; no effect on: bleeding time, plt Fxn, PT, aPTT

Tioconazole (Vagistat) **Uses:** *Vaginal fungal Infxns* **Action:** Topical
antifungal **Dose:** 1 applicatorful intravag hs (single dose) **Caution:** [C, ?] **Contra:**
Component allergy **Supplied:** Vaginal oint 6.5% **SE:** Local burning, itching, soreness, polyuria **Notes:** Insert high into vagina

Tiotropium (Spiriva) **Uses:** Bronchospasm w/ COPD, bronchitis, emphysema **Action:** Synthetic anticholinergic like atropine **Dose:** 1 cap/d inhaled using
HandiHaler, *do not* use w/ spacer **Caution:** [C, ?/–] BPH, NA glaucoma, MyG,
renal impair **Contra:** Acute bronchospasm **Supplied:** Caps 18 mcg **SE:** URI, xerostomia **Notes:** Monitor FEV$_1$ or peak flow

Tirofiban (Aggrastat) **Uses:** *Acute coronary syndrome* **Action:** Glycoprotein IIB/IIIa inhibitor **Dose:** Initial 0.4 mcg/kg/min for 30 min, followed by 0.1

mcg/kg/min; use in combo w/ heparin; ↓ in renal insuff **Caution:** [B, ?/–] **Contra:** Bleeding, intracranial neoplasm, vascular malformation, stroke/surgery/trauma w/in last 30 d, severe HTN **Supplied:** Inj 50, 250 mcg/mL **SE:** Bleeding, bradycardia, coronary dissection, pelvic pain, rash

Tobramycin (Nebcin) Uses: *Serious gram(–) Infxns* Action: Aminoglycoside; ↓ protein synthesis. *Spectrum:* Gram(–) bacteria (including *Pseudomonas*) **Dose:** *Adults.* 1–2.5 mg/kg/dose IV q8h. *Peds.* 2.5 mg/kg/dose IV q8h; ↓ w/ renal insuff **Caution:** [C, M] **Contra:** Aminoglycoside sensitivity **Supplied:** Inj 10, 40 mg/mL **SE:** Nephrotox & ototox **Notes:** Follow CrCl & levels for dosage adjustments (Table 2, page 200)

Tobramycin Ophthalmic (AKTob, Tobrex) Uses: *Ocular bacterial Infxns* Action: Aminoglycoside **Dose:** 1–2 gtt q4h; oint bid–tid; if severe, use oint q3–4h, or 2 gtt q30–60min, then less frequently **Caution:** [C, M] **Contra:** Aminoglycoside sensitivity **Supplied:** Oint & soln tobramycin 0.3% **SE:** Ocular irritation

Tobramycin & Dexamethasone Ophthalmic (TobraDex) Uses: *Ocular bacterial Infxns associated w/ significant inflammation* Action: Antibiotic w/ antiinflammatory **Dose:** 0.3% oint apply q3–8h or soln 0.3% apply 1–2 gtt q1–4h **Caution:** [C, M] **Contra:** Aminoglycoside sensitivity **Supplied:** Oint & soln tobramycin 0.3% & dexamethasone 0.1% **SE:** Local irritation/edema **Notes:** Use under ophthalmologist's direction

Tolazamide (Tolinase) Uses: *Type 2 DM* Action: Sulfonylurea; ↑ pancreatic insulin release; ↑ peripheral insulin sensitivity; ↓ hepatic glucose output **Dose:** 100–500 mg/d (no benefit >1 g/d) **Caution:** [C, +/–] Elderly, hepatic or renal impair **Supplied:** Tabs 100, 250, 500 mg; soln 1 mg/mL **NSE:** HA, dizziness, GI upset, rash, hyperglycemia, photosensitivity, blood dyscrasias

Tolazoline (Priscoline) Uses: *Peripheral vasospastic disorders* Action: Competitively blocks α-adrenergic receptors **Dose:** *Adults.* 10–50 mg IM/IV/SQ qid. *Neonates.* 1–2 mg/kg IV over 10–15 min, then 1–2 mg/kg/h (adjust w/ ↓ renal Fxn) **Caution:** [C, ?] **Contra:** CAD **Supplied:** Inj 25 mg/mL **SE:** ↓ BP, peripheral vasodilation, tachycardia, arrhythmias, GI upset & bleeding, blood dyscrasias, renal failure

Tolbutamide (Orinase) Uses: *Type 2 DM* Action: Sulfonylurea; ↑ pancreatic insulin release; ↑ peripheral insulin sensitivity; ↓ hepatic glucose output **Dose:** 500–1000 mg bid; ↓ in hepatic failure **Caution:** [C, +] **Contra:** Sulfonylurea sensitivity **Supplied:** Tabs 500 mg **SE:** HA, dizziness, GI upset, rash, photosensitivity, blood dyscrasias, hypoglycemia

Tolcapone (Tasmar) Uses: *Adjunct to carbidopa/levodopa in Parkinson Dz* Action: Catechol-O-methyltransferase inhibitor slows metabolism of levodopa **Dose:** 100 mg PO w/ first daily levodopa/carbidopa dose, then dose 6 & 12 h later; ↓ in renal impair **Caution:** [C, ?] **Contra:** Hepatic impair; nonselective MAOI **Supplied:** Tablets 100 mg, 200 mg **SE:** Constipation, xerostomia, vivid dreams, hallucinations, anorexia, N/D, orthostasis, liver failure **Notes:** Do not abruptly D/C or ↓ dose; monitor LFTs

Tolmetin (Tolectin)   WARNING: May ↑ risk of cardiovascular events & GI bleeding **Uses:** *Arthritis & pain* **Action:** NSAID; ↓ prostaglandins **Dose:** 200–600 mg PO tid; 2000 mg/d max **Caution:** [C (D in 3rd tri or near term), +] **Contra:** NSAID or ASA sensitivity **Supplied:** Tabs 200, 600 mg; caps 400 mg **SE:** Dizziness, rash, GI upset, edema, GI bleeding, renal failure

Tolnaftate (Tinactin) [OTC]   **Uses:** *Tinea pedis, cruris, corporis, manus, versicolor* **Action:** Topical antifungal **Dose:** Apply to area bid for 2–4 wk **Caution:** [C, ?] **Contra:** Nail & scalp Infxns **Supplied:** OTC 1% liq; gel; powder; cream; soln **SE:** Local irritation **Notes:** Avoid ocular contact, Infxn should improve in 7–10 d

Tolterodine (Detrol, Detrol LA)   **Uses:** *OAB (frequency, urgency, incontinence)* **Action:** Anticholinergic **Dose:** Detrol 1–2 mg PO bid; Detrol LA 2–4 mg/d **Caution:** [C, ?/–] w/ CYP2D6 & 3A3/4 inhibitor **Contra:** Urinary retention, gastric retention, or uncontrolled NA glaucoma **Supplied:** Tabs 1, 2 mg; Detrol LA tabs 2, 4 mg **SE:** Xerostomia, blurred vision

Topiramate (Topamax)   **Uses:** *Adjunctive Rx for complex partial Szs & tonic–clonic Szs,* bipolar disorder, neuropathic pain, migraine prophylaxis **Action:** Anticonvulsant **Dose:** *Adults. Seizures:* Total dose 400 mg/d; see insert for 8-wk titration schedule. *Migraine prophylaxis:* titrate 100 m/d total *Peds 2–16 y:* Initial, 1–3 mg/kg/d PO qhs; titrate per insert to 5–9 mg/kg/d; ↓ in renal failure **Caution:** [C, ?/–] **Contra:** Component allergy **Supplied:** Tabs 25, 100, 200 mg; caps sprinkles 15, 25, 50 mg **SE:** Metabolic acidosis, kidney stones; fatigue, dizziness, psychomotor slowing, memory impair, GI upset, tremor, nystagmus; weight loss, acute secondary glaucoma requiring drug D/C **Notes:** Metabolic acidosis responsive to dose ↓ or D/C; D/C requires taper

Topotecan (Hycamtin)   WARNING: Chemo precautions, BM suppression possible **Uses:** *Ovarian CA (cisplatin-refractory), small-cell lung CA,* sarcoma, ped non-small-cell lung CA **Action:** Topoisomerase I inhibitor; ↓ DNA synthesis **Dose:** 1.5 mg/m^2/d as a 1-h IV inf ×5 days, repeat q3wk; ↓ in renal failure **Caution:** [D, –] **Contra:** PRG, breast-feeding **Supplied:** 4-mg vials **SE:** Myelosuppression, N/V/D, drug fever, skin rash

Torsemide (Demadex)   **Uses:** *Edema, HTN, CHF, & hepatic cirrhosis* **Action:** Loop diuretic; ↓ reabsorption of Na$^+$ & Cl$^-$ in ascending loop of Henle & distal tubule **Dose:** 5–20 mg/d PO or IV **Caution:** [B, ?] **Contra:** Sulfonylurea sensitivity **Supplied:** Tabs 5, 10, 20, 100 mg; inj 10 mg/mL **SE:** Orthostatic ↓ BP, HA, dizziness, photosensitivity, electrolyte imbalance, blurred vision, renal impair **Notes:** 20 mg torsemide = 40 mg furosemide

Tramadol (Ultram)   **Uses:** *Moderate–severe pain* **Action:** Centrally acting analgesic **Dose:** *Adults.* 50–100 mg PO q4–6h PRN, 400 mg/d max. *Peds.* 0.5–1 mg/kg PO q 4–6h PRN **Caution:** [C, ?/–] **Contra:** Opioid dependency; MAOIs; sensitivity to codeine **Supplied:** Tabs 50 mg **SE:** Dizziness, HA, somnolence, GI upset, resp depression, anaphylaxis **Notes:** ↓ Sz threshold; tolerance or dependence may develop

Tramadol/Acetaminophen (Ultracet) Uses: *Short-term Rx acute pain (<5 d)* **Action:** Centrally acting analgesic; nonnarcotic analgesic **Dose:** 2 tabs PO q4–6h PRN; 8 tabs/d max. *Elderly/renal impair:* Lowest possible dose; 2 tabs q12h max if CrCl <30 **Caution:** [C, –] Szs, hepatic/renal impair, or Hx addictive tendencies **Contra:** Acute intox **Supplied:** Tab 37.5 mg tramadol/325 mg APAP **SE:** SSRIs, TCAs, opioids, MAOIs ↑ risk of Szs; dizziness, somnolence, tremor, HA, N/V/D, constipation, xerostomia, liver tox, rash, pruritus, ↑ sweating, physical dependence **Notes:** Avoid EtOH

Trandolapril (Mavik) WARNING: Use in PRG in 2nd/3rd tri can result in fetal death **Uses:** *HTN,* CHF, LVD, post-AMI **Action:** ACE inhibitor **Dose:** **HTN:** 2–4 mg/d. **CHF/LVD:** 4 mg/d; ↓ in severe renal/hepatic impair **Caution:** [D, +] ACE inhibitor sensitivity, angioedema w/ ACE inhibitors **Supplied:** Tabs 1, 2, 4 mg **SE:** ↓ BP, bradycardia, dizziness, ↑ K+, GI upset, renal impair, cough, angioedema **Notes:** Afro-Americans, min. dose is 2 mg vs 1 mg in Caucasians

Trastuzumab (Herceptin) Uses: *Metastatic breast CAs that overexpress the HER2/neu protein* breast cancer, adjuvant, w/ doxorubicin, cyclophosphamide, and paclitaxel if pt HER(+) breast cancer **Action:** MoAb; binds human epidermal GF receptor 2 protein (HER2); mediates cellular cytotox **Dose:** Per protocol **Caution:** [B, ?] CV dysfunction, allergy/inf Rxns **Contra:** None known **Supplied:** Inj form **SE:** Anemia, cardiomyopathy, nephrotic syndrome, pneumonitis **Notes:** Inf related Rxns minimized w/ acetaminophen, diphenhydramine, & meperidine

Trazodone (Desyrel) Uses: *Depression,* hypnotic, augment other antidepressants **Action:** Antidepressant; ↓ reuptake of serotonin & norepinephrine **Dose:** *Adults & Adolescents.* 50–150 mg PO qd–qid; max 600 mg/d. *Sleep:* 50 mg PO, qhs, PRN **Caution:** [C, ?/–] **Contra:** Component allergy **Supplied:** Tabs 50, 100, 150, 300 mg **SE:** Dizziness, HA, sedation, nausea, xerostomia, syncope, confusion, tremor, hepatitis, EPS **Notes:** Takes 1–2 wk for symptom improvement; may interact with CYP3A4 inhibitors to ↑ trazodone concentrations, carbamazepine to ↓ trazodone concentrations

Treprostinil Sodium (Remodulin) Uses: *NYHA class II–IV pulmonary arterial HTN* **Action:** Vasodilation, inhibits plt aggregation **Dose:** 0.625–1.25 ng/kg/min cont inf **Caution:** [B, ?/–] **Contra:** Component allergy **Supplied:** 1, 2.5, 5, 10 mg/mL inj **SE:** Additive effects w/ anticoagulants, antihypertensives; inf site Rxns **Notes:** Initiate in monitored setting; do not D/C or ↓ dose abruptly

Tretinoin, Topical [Retinoic Acid] (Retin-A, Avita, Renova) **Uses:** *Acne vulgaris, sun-damaged skin, wrinkles* (photo aging), some skin CAs **Action:** Exfoliant retinoic acid derivative **Dose:** *Adults & Peds >12 y.* Apply qd hs (w/ irritation, ↓ frequency). *Photoaging:* Start w/ 0.025%, ↑ to 0.1% over several months (apply only q3d if on neck area; dark skin may require bid application) **Caution:** [C, ?] **Contra:** Retinoid sensitivity **Supplied:** Cream 0.025, 0.05, 0.1%; gel 0.01, 0.025, 0.1%; microformulation gel 0.1%; liq 0.05% **SE:** Avoid sunlight;

edema; skin dryness, erythema, scaling, changes in pigmentation, stinging, photosensitivity

Triamcinolone (Azmacort) Uses: *Chronic asthma* Actions: Topical steroid Dose: Two inhalations tid–qid or 4 inhal bid Caution: [C, ?] SE: Cough, oral candidiasis Contra: Component allergy Supplied: Inhaler 100 mcg/met spray Notes: Instruct pts to rinse mouth after use; not for acute asthma

Triamcinolone & Nystatin (Mycolog-II) Uses: *Cutaneous candidiasis* Action: Antifungal & antiinflammatory Dose: Apply lightly to area bid; max 25 mg/d Caution: [C, ?] Contra: Varicella; systemic fungal Infxns Supplied: Cream & oint 15, 30, 60, 120 mg SE: Local irritation, hypertrichosis, changes in pigmentation Notes: For short-term use (<7 d)

Triamterene (Dyrenium) Uses: *Edema associated w/ CHF, cirrhosis* Action: K⁺-sparing diuretic Dose: Adults. 100–300 mg/24 h PO ÷ qd–bid. Peds. 2–4 mg/kg/d in 1–2 ÷ doses; ↓ in renal/hepatic impair Caution: [B (manufacturer; D expert opinion), ?/–] Contra: ↑ K⁺, renal impair, DM; caution w/ other K⁺-sparing diuretics Supplied: Caps 50, 100 mg SE: ↓ K⁺, blood dyscrasias, liver damage, other Rxns

Triazolam (Halcion) [C-IV] Uses: *Short-term management of insomnia* Action: Benzodiazepine Dose: 0.125–0.25 mg/d PO hs PRN; ↓ in elderly Caution: [X, ?/–] Contra: NA glaucoma; cirrhosis; concurrent amprenavir, ritonavir, or nelfinavir Supplied: Tabs 0.125, 0.25 mg SE: Tachycardia, CP, drowsiness, fatigue, memory impair, GI upset Notes: Additive CNS depression w/ EtOH & other CNS depressants

Triethanolamine (Cerumenex) [OTC] Uses: *Cerumen (ear wax) removal* Action: Ceruminolytic agent Dose: Fill ear canal & insert cotton plug; irrigate w/ H₂O after 15 min; repeat PRN Caution: [C, ?] Contra: Perforated tympanic membrane, otitis media Supplied: Soln 6, 12 mL SE: Local dermatitis, pain, erythema, pruritus

Triethylenetriphosphamide (Thio-Tepa, Tespa, TSPA) Uses: *Hodgkin Dz & NHLs; leukemia; breast, ovarian, & bladder CAs* (IV & intravesical therapy), preparative regimens for allogeneic & ABMT w/ high doses Action: Polyfunctional alkylating agent Dose: 0.5 mg/kg q1–4wk, 6 mg/m² IM or IV ×4 d q2–4wk, 15–35 mg/m² by cont IV infr over 48 h; 60 mg into the bladder & retained 2 h q1–4wk; 900–125 mg/m² in ABMT regimens (highest dose w/o ABMT is 180 mg/m²); 1–10 mg/m² (typically 15 mg) IT 1 or 2 ×/wk; 0.8 mg/kg in 1–2 L of soln may be instilled intraperitoneally; ↓ in renal failure Caution: [D, –] Contra: Component allergy Supplied: Inj 15 mg SE: Myelosuppression, N/V, dizziness, HA, allergy, paresthesias, alopecia

Trifluoperazine (Stelazine) Uses: *Psychotic disorders* Action: Phenothiazine; blocks postsynaptic CNS dopaminergic receptors in the brain Dose: Adults. 2–10 mg PO bid. Peds 6–12 y. 1 mg PO qd–bid initial, gradually ↑ to 15 mg/d; ↓ in elderly/debilitated pts Caution: [C, ?/–] Contra: Hx blood dyscrasias;

phenothiazine sensitivity **Supplied:** Tabs 1, 2, 5, 10 mg; PO conc 10 mg/mL; inj 2 mg/mL **SE:** Orthostatic ↓ BP, EPS, dizziness, neuroleptic malignant syndrome, skin discoloration, lowered Sz threshold, photosensitivity, blood dyscrasias **Notes:** PO conc must be diluted to 60 mL or more prior to administration; requires several weeks for onset of effects

Trifluridine (Viroptic) **Uses:** *Herpes simplex keratitis & conjunctivitis* **Action:** Antiviral **Dose:** 1 gt q2h (max 9 gtt/d); ↓ to 1 gt q4h after healing begins; Rx up to 14 d **Caution:** [C, M] **Contra:** Component allergy **Supplied:** Soln 1% **SE:** Local burning, stinging

Trihexyphenidyl (Artane) **Uses:** *Parkinson Dz* **Action:** Blocks excess acetylcholine at cerebral synapses **Dose:** 2–5 mg PO qd–qid **Caution:** [C, +] **Contra:** NA glaucoma, GI obstruction, MyG, bladder obstructions **Supplied:** Tabs 2, 5 mg; SR caps 5 mg; elixir 2 mg/5 mL **SE:** Dry skin, constipation, xerostomia, photosensitivity, tachycardia, arrhythmias

Trimethobenzamide (Tigan) **Uses:** *N/V* **Action:** ↓ medullary chemoreceptor trigger zone **Dose:** *Adults.* 250 mg PO or 200 mg PR or IM tid–qid PRN. *Peds.* 20 mg/kg/24 h PO or 15 mg/kg/24 h PR or IM in 3–4 ÷ doses **Caution:** [C, ?] **Contra:** Benzocaine sensitivity **Supplied:** Caps 100, 250 mg; supp 100, 200 mg; inj 100 mg/mL **SE:** Drowsiness, ↓ BP, dizziness; hepatic impair, blood dyscrasias, Szs, parkinsonian-like syndrome **Notes:** In the presence of viral Infxns, may mask emesis or mimic CNS effects of Reye syndrome

Trimethoprim (Trimpex, Proloprim) **Uses:** *UTI due to susceptible gram(+) & gram(–) organisms;* suppression of UTI **Action:** ↓ dihydrofolate reductase. *Spectrum:* Many gram(+) & (–) except *Bacteroides, Branhamella, Brucella, Chlamydia, Clostridium, Mycobacterium, Mycoplasma, Nocardia, Neisseria, Pseudomonas,* & *Treponema* **Dose:** *Adults.* 100 mg/d PO bid or 200 mg/d PO. *Peds.* 4 mg/kg/d in 2 ÷ doses; ↓ in renal failure **Caution:** [C, +] **Contra:** Megaloblastic anemia due to folate deficiency **Supplied:** Tabs 100, 200 mg; PO soln 50 mg/5 mL **SE:** Rash, pruritus, megaloblastic anemia, hepatic impair, blood dyscrasias **Notes:** Take w/ plenty of H_2O

Trimethoprim (TMP)–Sulfamethoxazole (SMX) [Co-Trimoxazole] (Bactrim, Septra) **Uses:** *UTI Rx & prophylaxis, otitis media, sinusitis, bronchitis* **Action:** SMX-inhibiting synthesis of dihydrofolic acid; TMP-inhibiting dihydrofolate reductase to impair protein synthesis. *Spectrum:* Includes *Shigella, P. jiroveci* (formerly *carinii*), & *Nocardia* Infxns, *Mycoplasma, Enterobacter* sp, *Staphylococcus, Streptococcus,* & more **Dose:** *Adults.* 1 DS tab PO bid or 5–20 mg/kg/24 h (based on TMP) IV in 3–4 ÷ doses. *P. jiroveci:* 15–20 mg/kg/d IV or PO (TMP) in 4 ÷ doses. *Nocardia:* 10–15 mg/kg/d IV or PO (TMP) in 4 ÷ doses. *UTI prophylaxis:* 1 PO qd. *Peds.* 8–10 mg/kg/24 h (TMP) PO ÷ into 2 doses or 3–4 doses IV; do not use in newborns; ↓ in renal failure; maintain hydration **Caution:** [B (D if near term), +] **Contra:** Sulfonamide sensitivity, porphyria, megaloblastic anemia w/ folate deficiency, significant hepatic impair **Supplied:**

Regular tabs 80 mg TMP/400 mg SMX; DS tabs 160 mg TMP/800 mg SMX; PO susp 40 mg TMP/200 mg SMX/5 mL; inj 80 mg TMP/ 400 mg SMX/5 mL **SE:** Allergic skin Rxns, photosensitivity, GI upset, Stevens–Johnson syndrome, blood dyscrasias, hepatitis **Notes:** Synergistic combo, interacts w/ warfarin

Trimetrexate (Neutrexin) WARNING: Must be used w/ leucovorin to avoid tox **Uses:** *Moderate–severe PCP* **Action:** ↓ dihydrofolate reductase **Dose:** 45 mg/m^2 IV q24h for 21 d; administer w/ leucovorin 20 mg/m^2 IV q6h for 24 d; ↓ in hepatic impair **Caution:** [D, ?/–] **Contra:** MTX sensitivity **Supplied:** Inj **SE:** Sz, fever, rash, GI upset, anemias, ↑ LFTs, peripheral neuropathy, renal impair **Notes:** Use cytotoxic cautions; inf over 60 min

Triptorelin (Trelstar Depot, Trelstar LA) Uses: *Palliation of advanced CAP* **Action:** LHRH analog; ↓ GNRH w/ continuous dosing; transient ↑ in LH, FSH, testosterone, & estradiol 7–10 d after first dose; w/ chronic/continuous use (usually 2–4 wk), sustained ↓ LH & FSH w/ ↓ testicular & ovarian steroidogenesis similar to surgical castration **Dose:** 3.75 mg IM monthly or 11.25 mg IM q3mo **Caution:** [X, N/A] **Contra:** Not indicated in females **Supplied:** Inj depot 3.75 mg; LA 11.25 mg **SE:** Dizziness, emotional lability, fatigue, HA, insomnia, HTN, D, vomiting, ED, retention, UTI, pruritus, anemia, inj site pain, musculoskeletal pain, osteoporosis, allergic Rxns

Trospium Chloride (Sanctura) Uses: *OAB* **Action:** Antimuscarinic, antispasmodic **Dose:** 20 mg PO bid, ↓ in renal impair or >75 y (on empty stomach or 1 h ac) **Caution:** [C, ?/-] BOO, GI obstruction, ulcerative colitis, MyG, renal/hepatic impair **Contra:** NA glaucoma, urinary/gastric retention **Supplied:** Tabs 20 mg **SE:** Constipation, xerostomia

Trovafloxacin (Trovan) WARNING: Trovan has been associated w/ serious liver injury leading to need for liver transplantation &/or death. **Uses:** *Life-threatening Infxns* including pneumonia, complicated intraabdominal, gynecologic/pelvic, or skin Infxns **Action:** Fluoroquinolone antibiotic; ↓ DNA gyrase. *Spectrum:* Broad-spectrum gram(+) & gram(–), including anaerobes; TB typically resistant **Dose:** 200 mg/d; ↓ in hepatic impair **Caution:** [C, –] in children **Contra:** Hepatic impair **Supplied:** Inj 5 mg/mL in 40 & 60 mL; tabs 100, 200 mg **SE:** Liver failure, dizziness, HA, nausea, rash **Notes:** Use restricted to hospitals; hepatotox led to restricted availability

Urokinase (Abbokinase) Uses: *PE, DVT, restore patency to IV catheters* **Action:** Converts plasminogen to plasmin; causes clot lysis **Dose:** *Adults & Peds. Systemic effect:* 4400 Units/kg IV over 10 min, then by 4400–6000 Units/kg/h for 12 h. *Restore catheter patency:* Inject 5000 Units into catheter & aspirate **Caution:** [B, +] **Contra:** Do not use w/in 10 d of surgery, delivery, or organ biopsy; bleeding, CVA, vascular malformation **Supplied:** Powder for inj 5000 Units/mL, 250,000-unit vial **SE:** Bleeding, ↓ BP, dyspnea, bronchospasm, anaphylaxis, cholesterol embolism

Valacyclovir (Valtrex) Uses: *Herpes zoster; genital herpes* **Action:** Prodrug of acyclovir; ↓ viral DNA replication. *Spectrum:* Herpes simplex I & II **Dose:** 1 g PO tid. *Genital herpes:* 500 mg bid × 7 d. *Herpes prophylaxis:* 500–1000 mg/d; ↓ in renal failure **Caution:** [B, +] **Supplied:** Caplets 500 mg **SE:** HA, GI upset, dizziness, pruritus, photophobia

Valdecoxib (Bextra) Uses: *RA, osteoarthritis, primary dysmenorrhea* **Action:** COX-2 inhibition **Dose:** *Arthritis:* 10 mg PO qd. *Dysmenorrhea:* 20 mg PO bid, PRN **Caution:** [C, ?] Asthma, urticaria, allergic-type reactions after ASA or NSAIDs, sulfonamide allergy **Supplied:** Tabs 10, 20 mg **SE:** ↑ LFT, GI ulceration or bleeding; dizziness, edema, HTN, peptic ulcer, renal failure; serious allergic reactions have occurred, including Stevens–Johnson syndrome

Valganciclovir (Valcyte) Uses: *CMV* **Action:** Ganciclovir prodrug; ↓ viral DNA synthesis **Dose:** Induction, 900 mg PO bid w/ food × 21 d, then 900 mg PO qd; ↓ in renal dysfunction **Caution:** [C, ?/–] Use w/ imipenem/cilastatin, nephrotoxic drugs **Contra:** Allergy to acyclovir, ganciclovir, valganciclovir; ANC < 500/mm³; plt < 25 K; Hgb < 8 g/dL **Supplied:** Tabs 450 mg **SE:** BM suppression **Notes:** Monitor CBC & Cr

Valproic Acid (Depakene, Depakote) Uses: *Rx epilepsy, mania; prophylaxis of migraines,* Alzheimer behavior disorder **Action:** Anticonvulsant; ↑ availability of GABA **Dose:** *Adults & Peds. Szs:* 30–60 mg/kg/24 h PO ÷ tid (after initiation of 10–15 mg/kg/24 h). *Mania:* 750 mg in 3 ÷ doses, ↑ 60 mg/kg/d max. *Migraines:* 250 mg bid, ↑ 1000 mg/d max; ↓ in hepatic impair **Caution:** [D, +] **Contra:** Severe hepatic impair **Supplied:** Caps 250 mg; syrup 250 mg/5 mL **SE:** Somnolence, dizziness, GI upset, diplopia, ataxia, rash, thrombocytopenia, hepatitis, pancreatitis, prolonged bleeding times, alopecia, weight gain, hyperammonemic encephalopathy reported in pts w/ urea cycle disorders **Notes:** Monitor LFTs & serum levels (Table 2, page 200); phenobarbital & phenytoin may alter levels

Valsartan (Diovan) WARNING: Use during 2nd/3rd tri of PRG can cause fetal harm Uses: *HTN, CHF, DN* **Action:** Angiotensin II receptor antagonist **Dose:** 80–160 mg/d **Caution:** [C (1st tri; D 2nd & 3rd tri), ?/–] W/ K⁺-sparing diuretics or K⁺ supls **Contra:** Severe hepatic impair, biliary cirrhosis/obstruction, primary hyperaldosteronism, bilateral renal artery stenosis **Supplied:** Caps 80, 160 mg **SE:** ↓ BP, dizziness

Vancomycin (Vancocin, Vancoled) Uses: *Serious MRSA Infxns; enterococcal Infxns; PO Rx of C. difficile pseudomembranous colitis* **Action:** ↓ Cell wall synthesis. *Spectrum:* Gram(+) bacteria & some anaerobes (includes MRSA, *Staphylococcus* sp, *Enterococcus* sp, *Streptococcus* sp, *C. difficile*) **Dose:** *Adults.* 1 g IV q12h; for colitis 125–500 mg PO q6h. *Peds.* 40–60 mg/kg/24 h IV in ÷ doses q6–12 h. *Neonates.* 10–15 mg/kg/dose q12h; (↓ in renal insuff) **Caution:** [C, M] **Contra:** Component allergy; avoid in Hx hearing loss **Supplied:** Caps 125, 250 mg; powder for PO soln; powder for inj 500 mg, 1000 mg, 10 g/vial **SE:** Ototoxic & nephrotoxic; GI upset (PO), neutropenia **Notes:** See drug levels (Table 2, page 200); not absorbed PO, local effect in gut only; give IV dose slowly (over 1–3 h) to prevent "red-man syndrome" (red flushing of head, neck, upper torso); IV product may be given PO for colitis

Vardenafil (Levitra)   WARNING: May prolong QT$_c$ interval **Uses:** *ED* **Action:** Phosphodiesterase 5 inhibitor **Dose:** 10 mg PO 60 min before sexual activity; 2.5 mg if administered w/ CYP3A4 inhibitors; max ×1 ≤20 mg **Caution:** [B, –] W/ CV, hepatic, or renal Dz **Contra:** Nitrates **Supplied:** 2.5-mg, 5-mg, 10-mg, 20-mg tabs **SE:** ↓ BP, HA, dyspepsia, priapism **Notes:** Concomitant α-blockers may cause ↓ BP

Varicella Virus Vaccine (Varivax)   Uses: *Prevent varicella (chickenpox)* **Action:** Active immunization; live attenuated virus **Dose:** *Adults & Peds.* 0.5 mL SQ, repeat 4–8 wk **Caution:** [C, M] **Contra:** Immunocompromise; neomycin-anaphylactoid Rxn, blood dyscrasias; immunosuppressive drugs; avoid PRG 3 mo after **Supplied:** Powder for inj **SE:** Mild varicella Infxn; fever, local Rxns, irritability, GI upset **Notes:** OK for all children & adults who have not had chickenpox

Vasopressin [Antidiuretic Hormone, ADH] (Pitressin)   Uses: *DI; Rx postop abdominal distension*; adjunct Rx of GI bleeding & esophageal varices; pulseless VT & VF, adjunct systemic vasopressor (IV drip) **Action:** Posterior pituitary hormone, potent GI vasoconstrictor, potent peripheral vasoconstrictor **Dose:** *Adults & Peds. DI:* 2.5–10 Units SQ or IM tid-qid. *GI hemorrhage:* 0.2–0.4 Units/min; ↓ in cirrhosis; caution in vascular Dz. *VT/VF:* 40 Units IVP × 1. *Vasopressor:* 0.01–0.1 Units/kg/min **Caution:** [B, +] **Contra:** Allergy **Supplied:** Inj 20 Units/mL **SE:** HTN, arrhythmias, fever, vertigo, GI upset, tremor **Notes:** Addition of vasopressor to concurrent norepinephrine or epi infs

Vecuronium (Norcuron)   Uses: *Skeletal muscle relaxation during surgery or mechanical ventilation* **Action:** Nondepolarizing neuromuscular blocker **Dose:** *Adults & Peds.* 0.08–0.1 mg/kg IV bolus; maint 0.010–0.015 mg/kg after 25–40 min; additional doses q12–15min PRN; ↓ in severe renal/hepatic impair **Caution:** [C, ?] Drug interactions cause ↑ effect (eg, aminoglycosides, tetracycline, succinylcholine) **Supplied:** Powder for inj 10 mg **SE:** Bradycardia, ↓ BP, itching, rash, tachycardia, CV collapse **Notes:** Fewer cardiac effects than pancuronium

Venlafaxine (Effexor)   WARNING: Closely monitor for worsening depression or emergence of suicidality, particularly in ped pts **Uses:** *Depression, generalized anxiety,* social anxiety disorder;* obsessive–compulsive disorder, chronic fatigue syndrome, ADHD, autism **Action:** Potentiation of CNS neurotransmitter activity **Dose:** 75–375 mg/d ÷ into 2–3 equal doses; ↓ in renal/hepatic impair **Caution:** [C, ?/–] **Contra:** MAOIs **Supplied:** Tabs 25, 37.5, 50, 75, 100 mg; ER caps 37.5, 75, 150 mg **SE:** HTN, ↑ mean HR, HA, somnolence, GI upset, sexual dysfunction; actuates mania or Szs **Notes:** Avoid EtOH

Verapamil (Calan, Isoptin) Uses: *Angina, HTN, PSVT, AF, atrial flutter,* migraine prophylaxis, hypertrophic cardiomyopathy, bipolar Dz Action: CCB Dose: *Adults. Arrhythmias:* 2nd line for PSVT w/ narrow QRS complex & adequate BP 2.5–5 mg IV over 1–2 min; repeat 5–10 mg in 15–30 min PRN (30 mg max). *Angina:* 80–120 mg PO tid, ↑ 480 mg/24 h max. *HTN:* 80–180 mg PO tid or SR tabs 120–240 mg PO qd to 240 mg bid. *Peds. <1 y:* 0.1–0.2 mg/kg IV over 2 min (may repeat in 30 min). *1–16y:* 0.1–0.3 mg/kg IV over 2 min (may repeat in 30 min); 5 mg max. *PO: 1–5 y:* 4–8 mg/kg/d in 3 ÷ doses. *>5 y:* 80 mg q6–8h; ↓ in renal/hepatic impair Caution: [C, +] Amiodarone/β-blockers/flecainide can cause bradycardia; statins, midazolam, tacrolimus, theophylline levels may be ↑ Contra: Conduction disorders, cardiogenic shock; caution w/ elderly pts Supplied: Tabs 40, 80, 120 mg; SR tabs 120, 180, 240 mg; SR caps 120, 180, 240, 360 mg; inj 5 mg/2 mL SE: Gingival hyperplasia, constipation, ↓ BP, bronchospasm, heart rate or conduction disturbances

Vinblastine (Velban, Velbe) WARNING: Chemotherapeutic agent; handle w/ caution Uses: *Hodgkin Dz & NHLs, mycosis fungoides, CAs (testis, renal cell, breast, non-small-cell lung, AIDS-related Kaposi sarcoma,* choriocarcinoma), histiocytosis Action: ↓ microtubule assembly Dose: 0.1–0.5 mg/kg/wk (4–20 mg/m^2); ↓ in hepatic failure Caution: [D, ?] Contra: Intrathecal use Supplied: Inj 1 mg/mL SE: Myelosuppression (especially leukopenia), N/V (rare), constipation, neurotox (like vincristine but less frequent), alopecia, rash; myalgia, tumor pain

Vincristine (Oncovin, Vincasar PFS) WARNING: Chemotherapeutic agent; handle w/ caution***Fatal if administered intrathecally*** Uses: *ALL, breast & small-cell lung CA, sarcoma (eg, Ewing tumor, rhabdomyosarcoma), Wilms tumor, Hodgkin Dz & NHLs, neuroblastoma, multiple myeloma* Action: Promotes disassembly of mitotic spindle, causing metaphase arrest Dose: 0.4–1.4 mg/m^2 (single doses 2 mg/max); ↓ in hepatic failure Caution: [D, ?] Contra: Intrathecal use Supplied: Inj 1 mg/mL SE: Neurotox commonly dose limiting, jaw pain (trigeminal neuralgia), fever, fatigue, anorexia, constipation & paralytic ileus, bladder atony; no significant myelosuppression w/ standard doses; tissue necrosis w/ extravasation

Vinorelbine (Navelbine) WARNING: Chemotherapeutic agent; handle w/ caution Uses: *Breast & non-small-cell lung CA* (alone or w/ cisplatin) Action: ↓ polymerization of microtubules, impairing mitotic spindle formation; semisynthetic vinca alkaloid Dose: 30 mg/m^2/wk; ↓ in hepatic failure Caution: [D, ?] Contra: Intrathecal use Supplied: Inj 10 mg SE: Myelosuppression (leukopenia), mild GI effects, infrequent neurotox (6–29%); constipation & paresthesias (rare); tissue damage from extravasation

Vitamin B$_1$ See Thiamine (page 178)
Vitamin B$_6$ See Pyridoxine (page 159)
Vitamin B$_{12}$ See Cyanocobalamin (page 64)

Vitamin K See Phytonadione (page 152)

Voriconazole (VFEND) Uses: *Invasive aspergillosis, serious fungal Infxns* **Action:** ↓ ergosterol synthesis. *Spectrum:* Several types of fungus: *Aspergillus, Scedosporium* sp, *Fusarium* sp **Dose:** *Adults & Peds ≥ 12 y.* IV: 6 mg/kg q12h × 2, then 4 mg/kg bid; may ↓ to 3 mg/kg/dose. *PO:* <40 kg: 100 mg q12h, up to 150 mg; >40 kg: 200 mg q 12 h, up to 300 mg; ↓ in mild–moderate hepatic impair; IV only one dose w/ renal impair (PO empty stomach) **Caution:** [D, ?/–] **Contra:** Severe hepatic impair **Supplied:** Tabs 50, 200 mg; 200-mg inj **SE:** Visual changes, fever, rash, GI upset, ↑ LFTs **Notes:** Screen for multiple drug interactions (eg, ↑ dose w/ phenytoin)

Warfarin (Coumadin) Uses: *Prophylaxis & Rx of PE & DVT, AF w/ embolization,* other postop indications **Action:** ↓ Vitamin K-dependent production of clotting factors in this order: VII-IX-X-II **Dose:** *Adults.* Titrate to keep INR 2.0–3.0 for most; mechanical valves INR is 2.5–3.5. *ACCP guidelines:* 5 mg initial (unless rapid therapeutic INR needed), may use 7.5–10 mg; if pt elderly or has other bleeding risk factors ↓. *Alternative:* 10–15 mg PO, IM, or IV qd for 1–3 d; maint 2–10 mg/d PO, IV, or IM; follow daily INR initial to adjust dosage (see Table 10, page 217). *Peds.* 0.05–0.34 mg/kg/24 h PO, IM, or IV; follow PT/INR to adjust dosage; monitor vitamin K intake; ↓ in hepatic impair/elderly **Caution:** [X, +] **Contra:** Severe hepatic/renal Dz, bleeding, peptic ulcer, PRG **Supplied:** Tabs 1, 2, 2.5, 3, 4, 5, 6, 7.5, 10 mg; inj **SE:** Bleeding due to overanticoagulation (PT >3× control or INR >5.0–6.0) or injury & INR w/in therapeutic range; bleeding, alopecia, skin necrosis, purple toe syndrome **Notes:** INR preferred test; to rapidly correct overanticoagulation, use vitamin K, FFP or both; highly teratogenic; do *not* use in PRG. Caution pt on taking w/ other meds, especially ASA. *Common warfarin interactions:* Potentiated by APAP, EtOH (w/ liver Dz), amiodarone, cimetidine, ciprofloxacin, cotrimoxazole, erythromycin, fluconazole, flu vaccine, isoniazid, itraconazole, metronidazole, omeprazole, phenytoin, propranolol, quinidine, tetracycline. Inhibited by barbiturates, carbamazepine, chlordiazepoxide, cholestyramine, dicloxacillin, nafcillin, rifampin, sucralfate, high-vitamin K foods

Zafirlukast (Accolate) Uses: *Adjunctive Rx of asthma* **Action:** Selective & competitive inhibitor of leukotrienes **Dose:** *Adults & Peds ≥ 12 y.* 20 mg bid. *Peds 5–11 y.* 10 mg PO bid (empty stomach) **Caution:** [B, –] Interacts w/ warfarin, ↑ INR **Contra:** Component allergy **Supplied:** Tabs 20 mg **SE:** Hepatic dysfunction, usually reversible on D/C; HA, dizziness, GI upset; Churg–Strauss syndrome **Notes:** Not for acute asthma

Zalcitabine (Hivid) **WARNING:** Use w/ caution in pts w/ neuropathy, pancreatitis, lactic acidosis, hepatitis Uses: *HIV* **Action:** Antiretroviral agent **Dose:** *Adults.* 0.75 mg PO tid. *Peds.* 0.015–0.04 mg/kg PO q 6 h; ↓ in renal failure **Caution:** [C, +] **Contra:** Component allergy **Supplied:** Tabs 0.375, 0.75 mg **SE:** Peripheral neuropathy, pancreatitis, fever, malaise, anemia, hypo/hyperglycemia, hepatic impair **Notes:** May be used in combo w/ zidovudine

Zaleplon (Sonata) [C-IV] Uses: *Insomnia* Action: A nonbenzodiazepine sedative/hypnotic, a pyrazolopyrimidine Dose: 5–20 mg hs PRN; ↓ in renal/hepatic insuff, elderly Caution: [C, ?/–] w/ mental/psychological conditions Contra: Component allergy Supplied: Caps 5, 10 mg SE: HA, edema, amnesia, somnolence, photosensitivity Notes: Take immediately before desired onset

Zanamivir (Relenza) Uses: *Influenza A & B* Action: ↓ viral neuraminidase Dose: Adults & Peds >7 y. 2 inhal (10 mg) bid for 5 d; initiate w/in 48 h of Sxs Caution: [C, M] Contra: Pulmonary Dz Supplied: Powder for inhal 5 mg SE: Bronchospasm, HA, GI upset Notes: Uses a Diskhaler for administration

Ziconotide (Prialt) WARNING: Psychiatric, cognitive, neurologic impair may develop over several weeks; monitor frequently; may necessitate D/C Uses: *IT Rx of severe, refractory, chronic pain* Action: N-type CCB in spinal cord Dose: 2.6 mcg/d IT at 0.1 mcg/h; may ↑ 0.8 mcg/h to total 19.2 mcg/d by day 21 Caution: [C, ?/-] Reversible psychiatric/neurologic impair Contra: Psychosis Supplied: Inj 25, 100 mg/mL SE: Dizziness, N/V, confusion, abnormal vision; may require dosage adjustment Notes: May D/C abruptly; uses specific pumps; do not ↑ more frequently than 2–3 ×/wk

Zidovudine (Retrovir) WARNING: Neutropenia, anemia, lactic acidosis, & hepatomegaly w/ steatosis Uses: *HIV Infxn, prevention of maternal transmission of HIV* Action: ↓ RT Dose: Adults. 200 mg PO tid or 300 mg PO bid or 1–2 mg/kg/dose IV q4h. PRG: 100 mg PO 5×/d until labor starts; during labor 2 mg/kg over 1 h followed by 1 mg/kg/h until clamping of the cord. Peds. 160 mg/m²/dose q8h; ↓ in renal failure Caution: [C, ?/–] Contra: Allergy Supplied: Caps 100 mg; tabs 300 mg; syrup 50 mg/5 mL; inj 10 mg/mL SE: Hematologic tox, HA, fever, rash, GI upset, malaise

Zidovudine & Lamivudine (Combivir) WARNING: Neutropenia, anemia, lactic acidosis, & hepatomegaly w/ steatosis Uses: *HIV Infxn* Action: Combo of RT inhibitors Dose: Adults & Peds >12 y. 1 tab PO bid; ↓ in renal failure Caution: [C, ?/–] Contra: Component allergy Supplied: Caps zidovudine 300 mg/lamivudine 150 mg SE: Hematologic tox, HA, fever, rash, GI upset, malaise, pancreatitis Notes: Combo product ↓ daily pill burden

Zileuton (Zyflo) Uses: *Chronic Rx of asthma* Action: Inhibitor of 5-lipoxygenase Dose: Adults & Peds ≥ 12 y. 600 mg PO qid Caution: [C, ?/–] Contra: Hepatic impair Supplied: Tabs 600 mg SE: Hepatic damage, HA, GI upset, leukopenia Notes: Monitor LFTs every month × 3, then q2–3 mo; take on regular basis; not for acute asthma

Ziprasidone (Geodon) WARNING: ↑ mortality in elderly with dementia-related psychosis Uses: *Schizophrenia, acute agitation* Action: Atypical antipsychotic Dose: 20 mg PO bid, may ↑ in 2-d intervals up to 80 mg bid; agitation 10–20 mg IM PRN up to 40 mg/d; separate 10 mg doses by 2 h & 20 mg doses by 4h (w/ food) Caution: [C, –] w/ ↓ Mg²⁺, ↓ K⁺ Contra: QT prolongation, recent

MI, uncompensated heart failure, meds that prolong QT interval **Supplied:** Caps 20, 40, 60, 80 mg; Inj 20 mg/mL **SE:** Bradycardia; rash, somnolence, resp disorder, EPS, weight gain, orthostatic ↓ BP **Notes:** Monitor electrolytes

Zoledronic Acid (Zometa) Uses: *↑ Ca^{2+} of malignancy (HCM),* ↓ skeletal-related events in CAP, multiple myeloma, & metastatic bone lesions **Action:** Bisphosphonate; ↓ osteoclastic bone resorption **Dose:** *HCM:* 4 mg IV over at least 15 min; may re-treat in 7 d if adequate renal Fxn. *Bone lesions/myeloma:* 4 mg IV over at least 15 min, repeat q3–4wk PRN; prolonged w/ Cr ↑ **Caution:** [C, ?/–] Loop diuretics, aminoglycosides; ASA-sensitive asthmatics; avoid invasive dental procedures in cancer patients; renal dysfunction **Contra:** Bisphosphonate allergy **Supplied:** Vial 4 mg **SE:** Adverse effects ↑ w/ renal dysfunction; fever, flu-like syndrome, GI upset, insomnia, anemia; electrolyte abnormalities, osteonecrosis of jaw **Notes:** Requires vigorous prehydration; do not exceed recommended doses/inf duration to ↓ dose-related renal dysfunction; follow Cr; avoid oral surgery; dental examination recommended prior to therapy; ↓ dose w/ renal dysfunction

Zolmitriptan (Zomig, Zomig XMT, Zomig Nasal) Uses: *Acute Rx migraine* **Action:** Selective serotonin agonist; causes vasoconstriction **Dose:** Initial 2.5 mg PO, may repeat after 2 h, 10 mg max in 24 h; nasal 5 mg; HA returns, repeated after 2 h 10 mg max 24 h **Caution:** [C, ?/–] **Contra:** Ischemic heart Dz, Prinzmetal angina, uncontrolled HTN, accessory conduction pathway disorders, ergots, MAOIs **Supplied:** Tabs 2.5, 5 mg; Rapid tabs (ZMT) 2.5 mg; nasal 5.0, 2.5, 1.0, 0.5 mg, **SE:** Dizziness, hot flashes, paresthesias, chest tightness, myalgia, diaphoresis

Zolpidem (Ambien, Ambien CR) [C-IV] Uses: *Short-term Rx of insomnia* **Action:** Hypnotic agent **Dose:** 5–10 mg or 12.5 mg CR PO hs PRN; ↓ in elderly (use 6.25 mg CR), hepatic insuff **Caution:** [B, –] **Contra:** Breast-feeding **Supplied:** Tabs 5, 10 mg; CR 6.25, 12.5 mg **SE:** HA, dizziness, drowsiness, nausea, myalgia **Notes:** May be habit-forming; CR delivers a rapid then a longer lasting dose

Zonisamide (Zonegran) Uses: *Adjunct Rx complex partial Szs* **Action:** Anticonvulsant **Dose:** Initial 100 mg/d PO; may ↑ to 400 mg/d **Caution:** [C, –] ↑ tox w/ CYP3A4 inhibitor; ↓ levels w/ concurrent carbamazepine, phenytoin, phenobarbital, valproic acid **Contra:** Allergy to sulfonamides; oligohidrosis & hypothermia in peds **Supplied:** Caps 100 mg **SE:** Dizziness, drowsiness, confusion, ataxia, memory impair, paresthesias, psychosis, nystagmus, diplopia, tremor; anemia, leukopenia; GI upset, nephrolithiasis, Stevens–Johnson syndrome; monitor for ↓ sweating & ↑ body temperature **Notes:** Swallow capsules whole

NATURAL and HERBAL AGENTS

The following is a guide to some common herbal products. These may be sold separately or in combination with other products. According to the FDA: "manufacturers of dietary supplements can make claims about how their products affect the structure or function of the body, but they may not claim to prevent, treat, cure, mitigate, or diagnose a disease without prior FDA approval"*

Black Cohosh Uses: Sx of menopause (eg, hot flashes), PMS, hypercholesterolemia, peripheral arterial Dz; has antiinflammatory & sedative effects **Efficacy:** May have short-term benefit on menopausal Sx **Dose:** 40–160 mg PO qd. **Caution:** May further ↓ lipids &/or BP w/ prescription meds **Contra:** PRG (miscarriage, prematurity reports) **SE:** OD can cause N/V, dizziness, nervous system & visual changes, bradycardia, & (possibly) Szs, liver damage/failure

Chamomile Uses: Antispasmodic, sedative, antiinflammatory, astringent, antibacterial. **Dose:** 10–15 g PO qd (3 g dried flower heads tid–qid between meals; can steep in 250 mL hot H_2O) **Caution:** W/ allergy to chrysanthemums, ragweed, asters (family Compositae) **SE:** Contact dermatitis; allergy; anaphylaxis **Interactions:** W/ anticoagulants, additive w/ sedatives (benzodiazepines); delayed gastric absorption of meds if taken together (↓ GI motility)

Cranberry (Vaccinium macrocarpon) Uses: Prevention & Rx UTI. **Efficacy:** Possibly effective **Dose:** 150 mg/d PO **Caution:** May ↑ kidney stones in susceptible individuals **SE:** None known **Interactions:** None significant

Dong Quai (Angelica polymorpha, sinensis) Uses: Uterine stimulant; menstrual cramps, irregular menses, & menopausal Sx; antiinflammatory, vasodilator, CNS stimulant, immunosuppressant, analgesic, antipyretic, antiasthmatic **Efficacy:** Possibly effective for menopausal Sx **Dose:** 9–12 g PO tab bid. **Caution:** Avoid in PRG & lactation. **SE:** D, photosensitivity, skin cancer. **Interactions:** Anticoagulants (↑ INR in pts on warfarin).

Echinacea (Echinacea purpurea) Uses: Immune system stimulant; prevention/Rx of colds, flu; supportive care chronic infections of the resp/lower urinary tract **Efficacy:** Not well established; may ↓ severity & duration of URI **Dose:** 6–9 mL expressed juice or 2–5 g dried root PO **Caution:** Do not use w/ progressive systemic or immune Dzs (eg, TB, collagen–vascular disorders, MS); may interfere with immunosuppressive therapy, not OK w/ PRG; do not use > 8

*Based on data in Haist SA and Robbins JB: *Internal Medicine on Call*, 4th ed, 2005 McGraw-Hill. See also www.fda.gov.

consecutive wk); possible immunosuppression) **SE:** N; rash **Interactions:** Anabolic steroids, amiodarone, MTX, corticosteroids, cyclosporine.

Ephedra/MaHuang
Uses: Stimulant, aid in weight loss, bronchial dilation. **Dose:** ***Not OK due to reported deaths.*** (> 100 mg/d can be life-threatening). US sales banned by FDA in 2004 **Caution:** Adverse cardiac events, strokes, death **SE:** Nervousness, HA, insomnia, palpitations, V, hyperglycemia **Interactions:** Digoxin, antihypertensives, antidepressants, diabetic medications

Evening Primrose Oil
Uses: PMS, diabetic neuropathy, ADHD **Efficacy:** Possibly for PMS, not for menopausal Sx **Dose:** 2–4 g/d PO **SE:** Indigestion, N, soft stools, HA **Interactions:** ↑ Phenobarbital metabolism, ↓ Sz threshold

Feverfew (*Tanacetum parthenium*)
Uses: Prevent/Rx migraine; fever; menstrual disorders; arthritis; toothache; insect bites **Efficacy:** Weak for migraine prevention **Dose:** 125 mg of dried leaf (w/ at least 0.2% of parthenolide) PO **Caution:** Do not use in PRG **SE:** Oral ulcers, gastric disturbance, swollen lips, abdominal pain; long-term SE unknown. **Interactions:** ASA, warfarin

Garlic (*Allium sativum*)
Uses: Antioxidant; hyperlipidemia, HTN; antiinfective (antibacterial, antifungal); tick repellant (oral) **Efficacy:** ↓ Cholesterol by 4–6%; soln ↓ BP; possible ↑ GI/CAP risk **Dose:** 400–1200 mg powder (2–5 mg allicin) PO **Caution:** Do not use in PRG (abortifacient); D/C 7 d pre-op (bleeding risk) **SE:** ↑ Insulin levels, ↑ lipid/cholesterol levels, anemia, oral burning sensation, N/V/D **Interactions:** Warfarin & ASA (↓ plt aggregation), additive w/ DM agents (↑ hypoglycemia). CYP 450 3A4 inducer (may ↑ cyclosporine, HIV antivirals, oral contraceptives)

Ginger (*Zingiber officinale*)
Uses: Prevent motion sickness; N/V due to anesthesia **Efficacy:** Benefit in ↓ N/V w/motion or PRG; weak for postop or chemo **Dose:** 1–4 g rhizome or 0.5–2 g powder PO qd **Caution:** Consult physician in pt w/ gallstones; excessive dose (↑ depression, & may interfere w/ cardiac Fxn or anticoagulants) **SE:** Heartburn **Interactions:** Excessive consumption may interfere with cardiac, DM, or anticoagulant meds (↓ plt aggregation)

Ginkgo Biloba
Uses: Memory deficits, dementia, anxiety, improvement Sx peripheral vascular Dz, vertigo, tinnitus, asthma/bronchospasm, antioxidant, premenstrual Sx (especially breast tenderness), impotence, SSRI-induced sexual dysfunction **Dose:** 60–80 mg standardized dry extract PO bid–tid **Efficacy:** Small cognition benefit w/ dementia; no other demonstrated benefit in healthy adults **Caution:** ↑ Bleeding risk (antagonism of plt-activating factor), concerning w/ antiplatelet agents (D/C 3 d preop); reports of ↑ Sz risk **SE:** GI upset, HA, dizziness, heart palpitations, rash **Interactions:** ASA, salicylates, warfarin

Ginseng
Uses: "Energy booster," stress reduction, enhance brain activity & physical endurance (adaptogenic), antioxidant, aid in glucose control **Efficacy:** Not established **Dose:** 1–2 g of root or 100–300 mg of extract (7% ginsenosides) PO TID **Caution:** W/ cardiac Dz, DM, hypotension, HTN, mania, schizophrenia, w/ corticosteroids; avoid in PRG; D/C 7 d preop (bleeding risk) **SE:** Controversial "ginseng abuse syndrome" w/ high dose (nervousness, excitation, HA, insomnia);

palpitations, vaginal bleeding, breast nodules, hypoglycemia **Interactions:** Warfarin, antidepressants & caffeine (↑ stimulant effect), DM meds (↑ hypoglycemia)

Glucosamine Sulfate (Chitosamine) and Chondroitin Sulfate

Uses: Osteoarthritis (glucosamine: rate-limiting step in glycosaminoglycan synthesis), ↑ cartilage rebuilding; chondroitin: biological polymer, flexible matrix between protein filaments in cartilage; draws fluids/nutrients into joint, "shock absorption") **Efficacy:** Controversial **Dose:** Glucosamine 500 PO tid, chondroitin 400 mg PO tid **Caution:** None known **SE:** ↑ Insulin resistance in DM; concentrated in cartilage, theoretically unlikely to cause toxic/teratogenic effects **Interactions:** *Glucosamine:* None. *Chondroitin:* Monitor anticoagulant therapy

Kava Kava (Kava Kava Root Extract, *Piper methysticum*)

Uses: Anxiety, stress, restlessness, insomnia **Efficacy:** Possible mild anxiolytic **Dose:** Standardized extract (70% kavalactones) 100 mg PO bid–tid **Caution:** Hepatotox risk, banned in Europe/Canada. Not OK in PRG, lactation. D/C 24 h preop (may ↑ sedative effect of anesthetics) **SE:** Mild GI disturbances; rare allergic skin/rash reactions, may ↑ cholesterol; ↑ LFT /jaundice; vision changes, red eyes, puffy face, muscle weakness **Interactions:** Avoid w/ sedatives, alcohol, stimulants, barbiturates (may potentiate CNS effect)

Melatonin

Uses: Insomnia, jet lag, antioxidant, immunostimulant **Efficacy:** Sedation most effective w/ elderly patients w/ ↑ endogenous melatonin levels; some evidence for jet lag **Dose:** 1–3 mg 20 min before HS (w/ CR 2 h before hs) **Caution:** Use synthetic rather than animal pineal gland, "heavy head," HA, depression, daytime sedation, dizziness **Interactions:** β-Blockers, steroids, NSAIDs, benzodiazepines

Milk Thistle (*Silybum marianum*)

Uses: Prevent/Rx liver damage (eg, from alcohol, toxins, cirrhosis, chronic hepatitis); preventive w/ chronic toxin exposure (painters, chemical workers, etc) **Efficacy:** Use before exposure more effective than use after damage has occurred **Dose:** 70–200 mg PO tid **SE:** GI intolerance **Interactions:** None

Saw Palmetto (*Serenoa repens*)

Uses: Rx BPH (weak 5-α-reductase inhibitor) **Efficacy:** Small–significant benefit for prostatic Sx **Dose:** 320 mg qd **Caution:** Hormonal effects, avoid in PRG, w/ women of childbearing years **SE:** Mild GI upset, mild HA, D w/ large amounts **Interactions:** ↑ Iron absorption; ↑ estrogen replacement effects

St. John's Wort (*Hypericum perforatum*)

Uses: Mild–moderate depression, anxiety, gastritis, insomnia, vitiligo; antiinflammatory; immune stimulant/anti-HIV/antiviral **Efficacy:** Variable; benefit in mild–moderate depression in several trials, but not always seen in clinical practice **Dose:** 2–4 g of herb or 0.2–1 mg of total hypericin (standardized extract) qd. Common preps: 300 mg PO tid (0.3% hypericin) **Caution:** Excessive doses may potentiate MAOI, cause allergic reaction, not OK in PRG **SE:** Photosensitivity, xerostomia, dizziness, constipation, confusion, fluctuating mood w/ chronic use **Interactions:** Do not use w/ prescription antidepressants, (especially MAOI); ↑ cyclosporine efficacy (may cause rejection), digoxin (may exacerbate CHF), protease inhibitors, theophylline, oral contraceptives; cytochrome P-450 3A4 enzyme inducer; potency can vary between products/batches

Valerian (*Valeriana officinalis*)   **Uses:** Anxiolytic, sedative, restlessness, dysmenorrheal **Efficacy:** Probably effective sedative (reduces sleep latency) **Dose:** 2–3 g extract PO qd–bid (Combined w/ OTC sleep product Alluna) **Caution:** None known **SE:** Sedation, hangover effect, HA, cardiac disturbances, GI upset **Interactions:** Caution w/ other sedating agents (eg, alcohol, or prescription sedatives): may cause drowsiness w/ impaired Fxn

Yohimbine (*Pausinystalia yohimbe*)   **Uses:** Improve sexual vigor, Rx ED **Efficacy:** Variable **Dose:** 5 mg PO tid (use w/ physician supervision) **Caution:** Do not use w/ renal/hepatic Dz; may exacerbate schizophrenia/mania (if pt predisposed). α_2-Adrenergic antagonist ($\downarrow$ BP, abdominal distress, weakness w/ high doses), OD can be fatal; salivation, dilated pupils, arrhythmias **SE:** Anxiety, tremors, dizziness, high BP, $\uparrow$ heart rate **Interactions:** Do not use w/ antidepressants (eg, MAOIs or similar agents)

Unsafe Herbs with Known Toxicity

Agent	Toxicities
Aconite	Salivation, N/V, blurred vision, cardiac arrhythmias
Aristolochic acid	Nephrotox
Calamus	Possible carcinogenicity
Chaparral	Hepatotox, possible carcinogenicity, nephrotox
"Chinese herbal mixtures"	May contain MaHuang or other dangerous herbs
Coltsfoot	Hepatotox, possibly carcinogenic
Comfrey	Hepatotox, carcinogenic
Ephedra/MaHuang	Adverse cardiac events, stroke, Sz
Juniper	High allergy potential, D, Sz, nephrotox
Kava kava	Hepatotox
Licorice	Chronic daily amounts (> 30 g/mo) can result in $\downarrow$ K^+, Na/fluid retention w/HTN, myoglobinuria, hyporeflexia
Life root	Hepatotox, liver cancer
MaHuang/Ephedra	Adverse cardiac events, stroke, Sz
Pokeweed	GI cramping, N/D/V, labored breathing, $\downarrow$ BP, Sz
Sassafras	V, stupor, hallucinations, dermatitis, abortion, hypothermia, liver cancer
Usnic acid	Hepatotox
Yohimbine	Hypotension, abdominal distress, CNS stimulation (mania/& psychosis in predisposed individuals)

Tables

TABLE 1
Quick Guide to Dosing of Acetaminophen Based on the Tylenol Product Line

	Suspension[a] Drops and Original Drops 80 mg/0.8 mL Dropperful	Chewable[a] Tablets 80-mg tabs	Suspension[a] Liquid and Original Elixir 160 mg/5 mL	Junior[a] Strength 160-mg Caplets/ Chewables	Regular[b] Strength 325-mg Caplets/ Tablets	Extra Strength[b] 500-mg Caplets/ Gelcaps
Birth–3 mo/ 6–11 lb/ 2.5–5.4 kg	$\frac{1}{2}$ dppr[c] (0.4 mL)					
4–11 mo/ 12–17 lb/ 5.5–7.9 kg	1 dppr[c] (0.8 mL)		$\frac{1}{2}$ tsp			
12–23 mo/ 18–23 lb/ 8.0–10.9 kg	1$\frac{1}{2}$ dppr[c] (1.2 mL)		$\frac{3}{4}$ tsp			
2–3 y/24–35 lb/ 11.0–15.9 kg	2 dppr[c] (1.6 mL)	2 tab	1 tsp			
4–5 y/36–47 lb/ 16.0–21.9 kg		3 tab	1$\frac{1}{2}$ tsp			

6–8 y/48–59 lb/ 22.0–26.9 kg	4 tab	2 tsp	2 cap/tab
9–10 y/60–71 lb/ 27.0–31.9 kg	5 tab	2½ tsp	2½ cap/ tab
11 y/72–95 lb/ 32.0–43.9 kg	6 tab	4 tsp	3 cap/tab
Adults & children ≥ 12 y ≥ 96 lb ≥ 44.0 kg			4 cap/tab
			1 or 2 caps/ tabs
			2 caps/ gel

[a]Doses should be administered 4 or 5 times daily. Do not exceed 5 doses in 24 h.

[b]No more than 8 dosage units in any 24-h period. Not to be taken for pain for more than 10 days or for fever for more than 3 days unless directed by a physician.

[c]Dropperful.

199

TABLE 2
Common Drug Levels[a]

Drug	When to Sample	Therapeutic Levels	Usual Half-Life	Potentially Toxic Levels
Antibiotics				
Gentamicin, Tobramycin	*Peak:* 30 min after 30-min infusion (peak level not necessary if extended-interval dosing: 6 mg/kg/dose) *Trough:* <0.5 h before next dose	*Peak:* 5–8 mcg/mL *Trough:* <2 mcg/mL <1.0 mcg/mL for extended intervals (6 mg/kg/dose) (peak levels not needed with extended-interval dosing)	2 h	Peak: >12 mcg/mL
Amikacin Vancomycin	Same as above *Peak:* 1 h after 1-h infusion *Trough:* <0.5 h before next dose	*Peak:* 20–30 mcg/mL *Peak:* 30–40 mcg/mL	2 h 6–8 h	Peak: >35 mcg/mL Peak: >50 mcg/mL Trough: >15 mcg/mL

Anticonvulsants

Carbamazepine	Trough: just before next oral dose	8–12 mcg/mL (monotherapy) 4–8 mcg/mL (polytherapy)	15–20 h	Trough: >12 mcg/mL
Ethosuximide	Trough: just before next oral dose	40–100 mcg/mL	30–60 h	Trough: >100 mcg/mL
Phenobarbital	Trough: just before next dose	15–40 mcg/mL	40–120 h	Trough: >40 mcg/mL
Phenytoin	May use free phenytoin to monitor[b] Trough: just before next dose	10–20 mcg/mL	Concentration-dependent	>20 mcg/mL
Primidone	Trough: just before next dose (primidone is metabolized to phenobarb; order levels separately)	5–12 mcg/mL	10–12 h	>12 mcg/mL
Valproic acid	Trough: just before next dose	50–100 mcg/mL	5–20 h	>100 mcg/mL

TABLE 2
(Continued)

Drug	When to Sample	Therapeutic Levels	Usual Half-Life	Potentially Toxic Levels
Bronchodilators				
Caffeine	*Trough:* just before next dose	Adults 5–15 mcg/mL Neonates 6–11 mcg/mL	Adults 3–4 h Neonates 30–140 h	20 mcg/mL
Theophylline (IV)	IV: 12–24 h after infusion started	5–15 mcg/mL	Nonsmoking adults 8 h Children and smoking adults 4 h	>20 mcg/mL
Theophylline (PO)	*Peak levels:* not recommended *Trough level:* just before next dose	5–15 mcg/mL		
Cardiovascular Agents				
Amiodarone	*Trough:* just before next dose	1–2.5 mcg/mL	30–100 days	>2.5 mcg/mL

202

Digoxin	Trough: just before next dose (levels drawn earlier than 6 h after a dose will be artificially elevated)	0.8–2.0 ng/mL	36 h	>2 ng/mL
Disopyramide	Trough: just before next dose	2–5 mcg/mL	4–10 h	>5 mcg/mL
Flecainide	Trough: just before next dose	0.2–1 mcg/mL	11–14 h	>1 mcg/mL
Lidocaine	Steady-state levels are usually achieved after 6–12 h	1.2–5 mcg/mL	1.5 h	>6 mcg/mL
Procainamide	Trough: just before next oral dose	4–10 mcg/mL NAPA + procaine: 5–30 mcg/mL	Procaine: 3–5 h NAPA: 6–10 h	>10 mcg/mL NAPA + procaine: >30 mcg/mL
Quinidine	Trough: just before next oral dose	2–5 mcg/mL	6 h	0.5 mcg/mL
Other Agents				
Amitriptyline plus nortriptyline	Trough: just before next dose	120–250 ng/mL		
Nortriptyline	Trough: just before next dose	50–140 ng/mL		
Lithium	Trough: just before next dose	0.5–1.5 mEq/mL	18–20 h	>1.5 mEq/mL

TABLE 2
(Continued)

Drug	When to Sample	Therapeutic Levels	Usual Half-Life	Potentially Toxic Levels
Imipramine plus desipramine	*Trough:* just before next dose	150–300 ng/mL		
Desipramine	*Trough:* just before next dose	50–300 ng/mL		
Methotrexate	By protocol	<0.5 mcmol/L after 48 h		
Cyclosporine	*Trough:* just before next dose	Highly variable *Renal:* 150–300 ng/mL (RIA) *Hepatic:* 150–300 ng/mL	Highly variable	
Doxepin	*Trough:* just before next dose	100–300 ng/mL		
Trazodone	*Trough:* just before next dose	900–2100 ng/mL		

^aResults of therapeutic drug monitoring *must* be interpreted in light of the complete clinical situation. For information on dosing or interpretation of drug levels contact the pharmacist or an order for a pharmacokinetic consult may be written in the patient's chart. Modified and reproduced with permission from the *Pharmacy and Therapeutics Committee Formulary*, 41st ed., Thomas Jefferson University Hospital, Philadelphia, PA.

^bMore reliable in cases of uremia and hypoalbuminemia.

204

TABLE 3
Local Anesthetic Comparison Chart for Commonly Used Injectable Agents

Agent	Proprietary Names	Onset	Duration	Maximum Dose mg/kg	Maximum Dose Volume in 70-kg Adult[a]
Bupivacaine	Marcaine	7–30 min	5–7 h	3	70 mL of 0.25% solution
Lidocaine	Xylocaine, Anestacon	5–30 min	2 h	4	28 mL of 1% solution
Lidocaine with epinephrine (1:200,000)		5–30 min	2–3 h	7	50 mL of 1% solution
Mepivacaine	Carbocaine	5–30 min	2–3 h	7	50 mL of 1% solution
Procaine	Novocaine	Rapid	30 min–1 h	10–15	70–105 mL of 1% solution

[a]To calculate the maximum dose if not a 70-kg adult, use the fact that a 1% solution has 10 mg of drug per milliliter.

205

TABLE 4
Comparison of Systemic Steroids

Drug	Relative Equivalent Dose (mg)	Mineralo-corticoid Activity	Duration (h)	Route
Betamethasone	0.75	0	36–72	PO, IM
Cortisone (Cortone)	25	2	8–12	PO, IM
Dexamethasone (Decadron)	0.75	0	36–72	PO, IV
Hydrocortisone (Solu-Cortef, Hydrocortone)	20	2	8–12	PO, IM, IV
Methylprednisolone acetate (Depo-Medrol)	4	0	36–72	PO, IM, IV
Methylprednisolone succinate (Solu-Medrol)	4	0	8–12	PO, IM, IV
Prednisone (Deltasone)	5	1	12–36	PO
Prednisolone (Delta-Cortef)	5	1	12–36	PO, IM, IV

TABLE 5
Topical Steroid Preparations

Agent	Common Trade Names	Potency	Apply
Alclometasone dipropionate	Aclovate, cream, oint 0.05%	Low	bid/tid
Amcinonide	Cyclocort, cream, lotion, oint 0.1%	High	bid/tid
Betamethasone			
Betamethasone valerate	Valisone, lotion 0.01%	Low	qd/bid
Betamethasone valerate	Valisone cream 0.01, 0.1%, oint, lotion 0.1%	Intermediate	qd/bid
Betamethasone dipropionate	Diprosone cream 0.05%	High	qd/bid
Betamethasone dipropionate	Diprosone aerosol 0.1%	Ultrahigh	qd/bid
Betamethasone dipropionate, augmented	Diprolene oint, gel 0.05%	Ultrahigh	bid (2 wk max)
Clobetasol propionate	Temovate, gel, oint, scalp, soln 0.05%	Ultrahigh	qd-qid
Clocortolone pivalate	Cloderm cream 0.1%	Intermediate	bid-qid
Desonide	DesOwen, cream, oint, lotion 0.05%	Low	
Desoximetasone			
Desoximetasone 0.05%	Topicort LP cream, gel 0.05%	Intermediate	
Desoximetasone 0.25%	Topicort cream, oint	High	bid-qid
Dexamethasone base	Aeroseb-Dex aerosol 0.01%	Low	
	Decadron cream 0.1%		
Diflorasone diacetate	Psorcon cream, oint 0.05%	Ultrahigh	bid/qid
Fluocinolone			
Fluocinolone acetonide 0.01%	Synalar cream, soln 0.01%	Low	bid/tid
Fluocinolone acetonide 0.025%	Synalar oint, cream 0.025%	Intermediate	bid/tid

(continued)

207

TABLE 5
(Continued)

Agent	Common Trade Names	Potency	Apply
Fluocinolone acetonide 0.2%	Synalar-HP cream 0.2%	High	bid/tid
Fluocinonide 0.05%	Lidex, anhydrous cream, gel, soln 0.05%	High	bid/tid oint
	Lidex-E aqueous cream 0.05%		
Flurandrenolide	Cordran cream, oint 0.025%	Intermediate	bid/tid
	cream, lotion, oint 0.05%	Intermediate	bid/tid
	tape, 4 mcg/cm²	Intermediate	qd
Fluticasone propionate	Cutivate cream 0.05%, oint 0.005%	Intermediate	bid
Halobetasol	Ultravate cream, oint 0.05%	Very high	bid
Halcinonide	Halog cream 0.025%, emollient base 0.1% cream, oint, sol 0.1%	High	qd/tid
Hydrocortisone			
Hydrocortisone	Cortizone, Caldecort, Hycort, Hytone, etc.	Low	tid/qid
	aerosol 1%, cream 0.5, 1, 2.5%, gel 0.5%, oint 0.5, 1, 2.5%, lotion 0.5, 1, 2.5%, paste 0.5%, soln 1%		
Hydrocortisone acetate	Corticaine cream, oint 0.5, 1%	Low	tid/qid
Hydrocortisone butyrate	Locoid oint, soln 0.1%	Intermediate	bid/tid
Hydrocortisone valerate	Westcort cream, oint 0.2%	Intermediate	bid/tid

Mometasone furoate	Elocon 0.1% cream, oint, lotion	Intermediate	qd
Prednicarbate	Dermatop 0.1% cream	Intermediate	bid
Triamcinolone			
Triamcinolone acetonide 0.025%	Aristocort, Kenalog cream, oint, lotion 0.025%	Low	tid/qid
Triamcinolone acetonide 0.1%	Aristocort, Kenalog cream, oint, lotion 0.1% Aerosol 0.2-mg/2-sec spray	Intermediate	tid/qid
Triamcinolone acetonide 0.5%	Aristocort, Kenalog cream, oint 0.5%	High	tid/qid

TABLE 6
Comparison of Insulins

Type of Insulin	Onset (h)	Peak (h)	Duration (h)
Ultra Rapid			
Apidra (glulisine)	Immediate	0.5–1.5	3–5
Humalog (lispro)	Immediate	0.5–1.5	3–5
NovoLog (insulin aspart)	Immediate	0.5–1.5	3–5
Rapid			
Regular Iletin II	0.25–0.5	2–4	5–7
Humulin R	0.5	2–4	6–8
Novolin R	0.5	2.5–5	5–8
Velosulin	0.5	2–5	6–8
Intermediate			
NPH Iletin II	1–2	6–12	18–24
Lente Iletin II	1–2	6–12	18–24
Humulin N	1–2	6–12	14–24
Novolin L	2.5–5	7–15	18–24
Novolin 70/30	0.5	7–12	24
Prolonged			
Ultralente	4–6	14–24	28–36
Humulin U	4–6	8–20	24–28
Lantus (insulin glargine)	4–6	No peak	24
Combination Insulins			
Humalog Mix (lispro protamine/ lispro)	0.25–0.5	1–4	24

TABLE 7
Commonly Used Oral Contraceptives[a]

Monophasics

Drug (Manufacturer)	Estrogen (mcg)	Progestin (mg)
Alesse 21, 28 (Wyeth)	Ethinyl estradiol (20)	Levonorgestrel (0.1)
Apri 28 (Barr)	Ethinyl estradiol (30)	Desogestrel (0.15)
Aviane 28 (Barr)	Ethinyl estradiol (20)	Levonorgestrel (0.1)
Brevicon 28 (Watson)	Ethinyl estradiol (35)	Norethindrone (0.5)
Cryselle 28 (Barr)	Ethinyl estradiol (30)	Norgestrel (0.3)
Demulen 1/35 21, 28 (Pfizer)	Ethinyl estradiol (35)	Ethynodiol diacetate (1)
Demulen 1/50 21, 28 (Pfizer)	Ethinyl estradiol (50)	Ethynodiol diacetate (1)
Desogen 28 (Organon)	Ethinyl estradiol (30)	Desogestrel (0.15)
Estrostep 28 (Warner-Chilcott)[b]	Ethinyl estradiol (20, 30, 35)	Norethindrone acetate (1)
Junel Fe 1/20, 21, 28 (Barr)	Ethinyl estradiol (20)	Norethindrone acetate (1)
Junel Fe 1.5/30 21, 28 (Barr)	Ethinyl estradiol (30)	Norethindrone acetate (1.5)
Kariva 28 (Barr)	Ethinyl estradiol (20, 0, 10)	Desogestrel (0.15)
Lessina 28 (Barr)	Ethinyl estradiol (20)	Levonorgestrel (0.1)
Levlen 28 (Berlex)	Ethinyl estradiol (30)	Levonorgestrel (0.15)
Levlite 28 (Berlex)	Ethinyl estradiol (20)	Levonorgestrel (0.1)
Levora 28 (Watson)	Ethinyl estradiol (30)	Levonorgestrel (0.15)
Loestrin Fe 1.5/30 21, 28 (Warner-Chilcott)	Ethinyl estradiol (30)	Norethindrone acetate (1.5)
Loestrin Fe 1/20 21, 28 (Warner-Chilcott)	Ethinyl estradiol (20)	Norethindrone acetate (1)
Lo/Ovral 21, 28 (Wyeth)	Ethinyl estradiol (30)	Norgestrel (0.3)
Low-Ogestrel 28 (Watson)	Ethinyl estradiol (30)	Norgestrel (0.3)
Microgestin Fe 1/20 21, 28 (Watson)	Ethinyl estradiol (20)	Norethindrone acetate (1)
Microgestin Fe 1.5/30 21, 28 (Watson)	Ethinyl estradiol (30)	Norethindrone acetate (1.5)

TABLE 7
(Continued)

Drug (Manufacturer)	Estrogen (mcg)	Progestin (mg)
Mircette 28 (Organon)	Ethinyl estradiol (20, 0, 10)	Desogestrel (0.15)
Modicon 28 (Ortho-McNeil)	Ethinyl estradiol (35)	Norethindrone (0.5)
MonoNessa 28 (Watson)	Ethinyl estradiol (35)	Norgestimate (0.25)
Necon 1/50 28 (Watson)	Mestranol (50)	Norethindrone (1)
Necon 0.5/35 28 (Watson)	Ethinyl estradiol (35)	Norethindrone (0.5)
Necon 1/35 28 (Watson)	Ethinyl estradiol (35)	Norethindrone (1)
Nordette 21, 28 (King)	Ethinyl estradiol (30)	Levonorgestrel (0.15)
Nortrel 0.5/35 28 (Barr)	Ethinyl estradiol (35)	Norethindrone (0.5)
Nortrel 1/35 21, 28 (Barr)	Ethinyl estradiol (35)	Norethindrone (1)
Norinyl 1/35 28 (Watson)	Ethinyl estradiol (35)	Norethindrone (1)
Norinyl 1/50 28 (Watson)	Mestranol (50)	Norethindrone (1)
Ogestrel 28 (Watson)	Ethinyl estradiol (50)	Norgestrel (0.5)
Ortho-Cept 28 (Ortho-McNeil)	Ethinyl estradiol (30)	Desogestrel (0.15)
Ortho-Cyclen 28 (Ortho-McNeil)	Ethinyl estradiol (35)	Norgestimate (0.25)
Ortho-Novum 1/35 28 (Ortho-McNeil)	Ethinyl estradiol (35)	Norethindrone (1)
Ortho-Novum 1/50 28 (Ortho-McNeil)	Mestranol (50)	Norethindrone (1)
Ovcon 35 21, 28 (Warner-Chilcott)	Ethinyl estradiol (35)	Norethindrone (0.4)
Ovcon 50 28 (Warner-Chilcott)	Ethinyl estradiol (50)	Norethindrone (1)
Ovral 21, 28 (Wyeth-Ayerst)	Ethinyl estradiol (50)	Norgestrel (0.5)
Portia 28 (Barr)	Ethinyl estradiol (30)	Levonorgestrel (0.15)
Sprintec 28 (Barr)	Ethinyl estradiol (35)	Norgestimate (0.25)
Yasmin 28 (Berlex)	Ethinyl estradiol (30)	Drospirenone (3)
Zovia 1/50E 28 (Watson)	Ethinyl estradiol (50)	Ethynodiol diacetate (1)
Zovia 1/35E 28 (Watson)	Ethinyl estradiol (35)	Ethynodiol diacetate (1)

Multiphasics

Drug	Estrogen (mcg)	Progestin (mg)
Cyclessa 28 (Organon)	Ethinyl estradiol (25)	Desogestrel (0.1, 0.125, 0.15)
Enpresse 28 (Barr)	Ethinyl estradiol (30, 40, 30)	Levonorgestrel (0.05, 0.075, 0.125)
Necon 10/11 21, 28 (Watson)	Ethinyl estradiol (35)	Norethindrone (0.5, 1)
Necon 7/7/7 (Watson)	Ethinyl estradiol (35)	Norethindrone (0.5, 0.75, 1)
Nortrel 7/7/7 28 (Barr)	Ethinyl estradiol (35)	Norethindrone (0.5, 0.75, 1)
Ortho Tri-Cyclen 21, 28 (Ortho-McNeil)[b]	Ethinyl estradiol (25)	Norgestimate (0.18, 0.215, 0.25)
Ortho Tri-Cyclen lo 21, 28 (Ortho-McNeil)	Ethinyl estradiol (35, 35)	Norgestimate (0.18, 0.215, 0.25)
Ortho-Novum 10/11 21 (Ortho-McNeil)	Ethinyl estradiol (35, 35)	Norethindrone (0.5, 1.0)
Ortho-Novum 7/7/7 21 (Ortho-McNeil)	Ethinyl estradiol (35, 35)	Norethindrone (0.5, 0.75, 1.0)
Tri-Levlen 28 (Berlex)	Ethinyl estradiol (30, 40, 30)	Levonorgestrel (0.05, 0.075, 0.125)
Tri-Nessa 28 (Watson)	Ethinyl estradiol (35)	Norgestimate (0.18, 0.215, 0.25)
Tri-Norinyl 21, 28 (Watson)	Ethinyl estradiol (35, 35)	Norethindrone (0.5, 1.0, 0.5)
Triphasil 21, 28 (Wyeth)	Ethinyl estradiol (30, 40, 30)	Levonorgestrel (0.05, 0.075, 0.125)
Tri-Sprintec (Barr)	Ethinyl estradiol (35)	Norgestimate (0.18, 0.215, 0.25)
Trivora-28 (Watson)	Ethinyl estradiol (30, 40, 30)	Levonorgestrel (0.05, 0.075, 0.125)
Velivet (Barr)	Ethinyl estradiol (25)	Desogestrel (0.1, 0.125, 0.15)

TABLE 7
(Continued)

Progestin Only

Drug	Estrogen (mcg)	Progestin (mg)
Camila (Barr)	None	Norethindrone (0.35)
Errin (Barr)	None	Norethindrone (0.35)
Jolivette 28 (Watson)	None	Norethindrone (0.35)
Micronor (Ortho-McNeil)	None	Norethindrone (0.35)
Nor-QD (Watson)	None	Norethindrone (0.35)
Nora-BE 28 (Ortho-McNeil)	None	Norethindrone (0.35)
Ovrette (Wyeth-Ayerst)	None	Norgestrel (0.075)

Extended-Cycle Combination

Drug		
Seasonale (Duramed)	Ethinyl estradiol (30)	Levonorgestrel (0.15)

Based in part on data published in the *Medical Letter* Volume 2 (Issue 24) August 2004.

*a*The designations 21 and 28 refer to number of days in regimen available.

*b*Also approved for acne.

TABLE 8
Some Common Oral Potassium Supplements

Brand Name	Salt	Form	mEq Potassium/ Dosing Unit
Glu-K	Gluconate	Tablet	2 mEq/tablet
Kaochlor 10%	KCl	Liquid	20 mEq/15 mL
Kaochlor S-F 10% (sugar-free)	KCl	Liquid	20 mEq/15 mL
Kaochlor Eff	Bicarbonate/ KCl/citrate	Effervescent tablet	20 mEq/tablet
Kaon elixir	Gluconate	Liquid	20 mEq/15 mL
Kaon	Gluconate	Tablet	5 mEq/tablet
Kaon-Cl	KCl	Tablet, SR	6.67 mEq/tablet
Kaon-Cl 20%	KCl	Liquid	40 mEq/15 mL
KayCiel	KCl	Liquid	20 mEq/15 mL
K-Lor	KCl	Powder	15 or 20 mEq/packet
Klorvess	Bicarbonate/ KCl	Liquid	20 mEq/15 mL
Klotrix	KCl	Tablet, SR	10 mEq/tablet
K-Lyte	Bicarbonate/ citrate	Effervescent tablet	25 mEq/tablet
K-Tab	KCl	Tablet, SR	10 mEq/tablet
Micro-K	KCl	Capsule, SR	8 mEq/capsule
Slow-K	KCl	Tablet, SR	8 mEq/tablet
Tri-K	Acetate/bicar- bonate and citrate	Liquid	45 mEq/15 mL
Twin-K	Citrate/gluconate	Liquid	20 mEq/5 mL

SR = sustained release.

TABLE 9
Tetanus Prophylaxis

History of Absorbed Tetanus Toxoid Immunization	Clean, Minor Wounds		All Other Wounds[a]	
	Td[b]	TIG[c]	Td[d]	TIG[c]
Unknown or <3 doses	Yes	No	Yes	Yes
=3 doses	No[e]	No	No[f]	No

[a]Such as, but not limited to, wounds contaminated with dirt, feces, soil, saliva, etc; puncture wounds; avulsions; and wounds resulting from missiles, crushing, burns, and frostbite.

[b]Td = tetanus-diphtheria toxoid (adult type), 0.5 mL IM.
- For children <7 y, DPT (DT, if pertussis vaccine is contraindicated) is preferred to tetanus toxoid alone.
- For persons >7 y, Td is preferred to tetanus toxoid alone.
- DT = diphtheria-tetanus toxoid (pediatric), used for those who cannot receive pertussis.

[c]TIG = tetanus immune globulin, 250 U IM.

[d]If only 3 doses of fluid toxoid have been received, then a fourth dose of toxoid, preferably an adsorbed toxoid, should be given.

[e]Yes, if >10 y since last dose.

[f]Yes, if >5 y since last dose.

Source: Based on guidelines from the Centers for Disease Control and Prevention and reported in *MMWR*.

TABLE 10
Oral Anticoagulant Standards of Practice

Thromboembolic Disorder	INR	Duration
Deep Venous Thrombosis & Pulmonary Embolism		
Treatment single episode		
Transient risk factor	2–3	3 mo
Idiopathic	2–3	6–12 mo
Recurrent systemic embolism	2–3	Indefinite
Prevention of Systemic Embolism		
Atrial fibrillation (AF)[a]	2–3	Indefinite
AF: cardioversion	2–3	3 wk prior; 4 wk post sinus rhythm
Valvular heart disease	2–3	Indefinite
Cardiomyopathy	2–3	Indefinite
Acute Myocardial Infarction		
High risk patients[c]	2–3 + low dose aspirin	3 mo
Prosthetic Valves		
Tissue heart valves	2–3	3 mo
Bileaflet mechanical valves in aortic position	2–3	2–3 mo Indefinite
Other mechanical prosthetic valves[b]	2.5–3.5	Indefinite

[a]With high-risk factors or multiple moderate risk factors.

[b]May add aspirin 81 mg to warfarin in patients with caged ball or caged disk valves or with additional risk factors.

[c]Large anterior MI, significant heart failure, intracardiac thrombus, and/or history of thromboembolic event.

INR = international normalized ratio.

Source: Based on data published in *Chest* 2004 Sep; 126 (Suppl): 1635–6965.

TABLE 11
Serotonin 5-HT₁ Receptor Agonists

Drug	Initial Dose	Repeat Dose	Max. Dose/24h	Supplied
Almotriptan (Axert)	6.25 or 12.5 mg PO	× 1 in 2 h	25 mg	Tabs 6.25, 12.5 mg
Frovatriptan (Frova)	2.5 mg PO	in 2 h	7.5 mg	Tabs 2.5 mg
Naratriptan (Amerge)	1 or 2.5 mg PO[a]	in 4 h	5 mg	Tabs 1, 2.5 mg
Rizatriptan (Maxalt)	5 or 10 mg PO[b]	in 2 h	30 mg	Tabs 5,10 mg Disintegrating tabs 5, 10 mg
Sumatriptan (Imitrex)	25, 50, or 100 mg PO 5–20 mg intranasally 6 mg SQ	in 2 h in 2 h in 1 h	200 mg 40 mg 12 mg	Tabs 25,50 mg Nasal spray 5, 20 mg Inj 12 mg/mL
Zolmitriptan (Zomig)	2.5 or 5 mg PO	in 2 h	10 mg	Tabs 2.5, 5 mg

Precautions/contraindications: [C, M]; ischemic heart disease, coronary artery vasospasm, Prinzmetal's angina, uncontrolled HTN, hemiplegic or basilar migraine, ergots, use of another serotonin agonist within 24 h, use with MAOI. Side effects: dizziness, somnolence, paresthesias, nausea, flushing, dry mouth, coronary vasospasm, chest tightness, HTN, GI upset.

[a]Reduce dose in mild renal and hepatic insufficiency (2.5 mg/d MAX); contraindicated with severe renal (ClCr <15 mL/min) or hepatic impairment.

[b]Initiate therapy at 5 mg PO (15 mg/d max) in patients receiving propranolol.

218

TABLE 12
Antiarrhythmics: Vaughn Williams Classification

Class I: Sodium Channel Blockade

A. **Class Ia:** Lengthens duration of action potential (↑ the refractory period in atrial and ventricular muscle, in SA and AV conduction systems, and Purkinje fibers)
   1. Amiodarone (also class II, III, IV)
   2. Disopyramide (Norpace)
   3. Imipramine (MAO inhibitor)
   4. Procainamide (Pronestyl)
   5. Quinidine
B. **Class Ib:** No effect on action potential
   1. Lidocaine (Xylocaine)
   2. Mexiletine (Mexitil)
   3. Phenytoin (Dilantin)
   4. Tocainide (Tonocard)
C. **Class Ic:** Greater sodium current depression (blocks the fast inward Na^+ current in heart muscle and Purkinje fibers, and slows the rate of ↑ of phase 0 of the action potential)
   1. Flecainide (Tambocor)
   2. Propafenone

Class II: Beta blocker

D. Amiodarone (also class Ia, III, IV)
E. Esmolol (Brevibloc)
F. Sotalol (also class III)

Class III: Prolong refractory period via action potential

G. Amiodarone (also class Ia, II, IV)
H. Sotalol

Class IV: Calcium channel blocker

I. Amiodarone (also class Ia, II, III)
J. Diltiazem (Cardizem)
K. Verapamil (Calan)

TABLE 13
Cytochrome P-450 Isoenzymes and the Drugs They Metabolize, Inhibit, and Induce[a]

CYP1A2

Substrates:	Acetaminophen, caffeine, clozapine, imipramine, theophylline, propranolol
Inhibitors:	Most fluoroquinolone antibiotics, fluvoxamine, cimetidine
Inducer:	Tobacco smoking, charcoal-broiled foods, cruciferous vegetables, omeprazole

CYP2C9

Substrates:	Most NSAIDs (including COX-2), warfarin, phenytoin
Inhibitors:	Fluconazole
Inducer:	Barbiturates, rifampin

CYP2C19

Substrates:	Diazepam, lansoprazole, omeprazole, phenytoin, pantoprazole
Inhibitors:	Omeprazole, isoniazid, ketoconazole
Inducer:	Barbiturates, rifampin

CYP2D6

Substrates:	Most β-blockers, codeine, clomipramine, clozapine, codeine, encainide, flecainide, fluoxetine, haloperidol, hydrocodone, 4-methoxy-amphetamine, metoprolol, mexiletine, oxycodone, paroxetine, propafenone, propoxyphene, risperidone, selegiline (deprenyl), thioridazine, most tricyclic antidepressants, timolol
Inhibitors:	Fluoxetine, haloperidol, paroxetine, quinidine
Inducer:	Unknown

CYP3A

Substrates:	**Anticholinergics:** Darifenacin, oxybutynin, solifenacin, tolterodine
	Benzodiazepines: Alprazolam, midazolam, triazolam
	Ca channel blockers: Diltiazem, felodipine, nimodipine, nifedipine, nisoldipine, verapamil

(continued)

TABLE 13 (continued)
Cytochrome P-450 Isoenzymes and the Drugs They Metabolize, Inhibit, and Induce^a

	Chemotherapy: Cyclophosphamide, erlotinib, ifosfamide, paclitaxel, tamoxifen, vinblastine, vincristine
	HIV protease inhibitors: Amprenavir, atazanavir, indinavir, nelfinavir, ritonavir, saquinavir
	HMG-CoA reductase inhibitors: Atorvastatin, lovastatin, simvastatin
	Immunosuppressive agents: Cyclosporine, tacrolimus
	Macrolide-type antibiotics: Clarithromycin, erythromycin, telithromycin, troleandomycin
	Opioids: Alfentanyl, cocaine, fentanyl, sufentanil
	Steroids: Budesonide, cortisol, 17-β-estradiol, progesterone
	Others: Acetaminophen, amiodarone, carbamazepine, delavirdine, efavirenz, nevirapine, quinidine, repaglinide, sildenafil, tadalafil, trazodone, vardenafil
Inhibitors:	Amiodarone, amprenavir, atazanavir, ciprofloxacin, cisapride, clarithromycin, diltiazem, erythromycin, fluconazole, fluvoxamine, grapefruit juice (in high ingestion), indinavir, itraconazole, ketoconazole, nefazodone, nelfinavir, norfloxacin, ritonavir, telithromycin, troleandomycin, verapamil, voriconazole
Inducer:	Carbamazepine, efavirenz, glucocorticoids, macrolide antibiotics, nevirapine, phenytoin, phenobarbital, rifabutin, rifapentine, rifampin, St. John's wort

^a Increased or decreased (primarily hepatic cytochrome P-450) metabolism of medications may influence the effectiveness of drugs or result in significant drug-drug interactions. Understanding the common cytochrome P-450 isoforms (eg, CYP2C9, CYP209, CYP2C19, CYP3A4) and common drugs that are metabolized by (aka "substrates"), inhibit, or induce activity of the isoform helps minimize significant drug interactions. CYP3A is involved in the metabolism of >50% of drugs metabolized by the liver.

Based on data from Katzung B (ed): *Basic and Clinical Pharmacology*, 9th ed. McGraw-Hill, New York, 2004; *The Medical Letter*, Volume 47, July 4, 2004; http://www.fda.gov/cder/drug/drugreactions (accessed September 16, 2005).

Index

224 Index